Tumour Suppressor Genes, the Cell Cycle and Cancer

CANCER SURVEYS

Advances and Prospects in Clinical, Epidemiological and Laboratory Oncology

Published for the

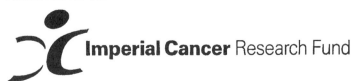

Imperial Cancer Research Fund

Tumour Suppressor Genes, the Cell Cycle and Cancer

Guest Editor
A J Levine

COLD SPRING HARBOR LABORATORY PRESS 1992

CANCER SURVEYS
Tumour Suppressor Genes,
the Cell Cycle and Cancer
Volume 12

Cover and book design by Leon Bolognese & Associates, Inc.

All Cold Spring Harbor Laboratory Press publications may be ordered directly from Cold Spring Harbor
Laboratory Press, 10 Skyline Drive, Plainview, New York 11803-9729. Phone: Continental US & Canada
1-800-843-4388; all other locations (516) 349-1930. FAX: (516) 349-1946.

Contents

Introduction

A J LEVINE

Department of Molecular Biology, Lewis Thomas Laboratory, Princeton University, Princeton, New Jersey 08544-1014

Although the existence of tumour suppressor genes was first postulated more than 20 years ago (Harris *et al*, 1969; Knudson, 1971), it has only been in the past 4–5 years that real insights into their identity and mode of action have emerged. In the interim, the oncogenes have held centre stage in attempts to understand and explain the origins of cancer. The oncogenes, however, have yielded only part of the picture. It is the existence of the tumour suppressor genes that provides a clear understanding of inherited predisposition in cancer, cell or tissue specific cancers, the karyotypic alterations in cancer cells and new concepts in the regulation of the cell cycle. In addition, the surprising interactions between the oncogene products of the DNA tumour viruses and the proteins produced by some tumour suppressor genes have provided remarkable insights into the functions of these gene products. For all of these reasons, it appeared to be a good time to produce an issue of *Cancer Surveys* dedicated to the tumour suppressor genes. The issue covers the GTPase activating proteins (GAP), and neurofibromatosis gene 1 (*NF1*), the Wilms' tumour gene 1 (*WT1*), the familial polyposis and deleted in colon carcinoma (*DCC*) genes, transforming growth factor-β (TGF-β), the retinoblastoma susceptibility gene (*RB*) and *p53*. There is a heavy emphasis in this issue upon *RB* and *p53*, with chapters on their interactions with three different DNA tumour virus groups (SV40, papillomaviruses, adenoviruses) and on *p53* in murine erythroleukaemia and human colon cancer. This has created some redundancy as each chapter unfolds a complementary set of questions asked by different scientists working with different experimental systems. That is the price we have decided to pay to provide for the reader, in one issue, the development of these related concepts by different leaders in this field.

This issue also provides insights into the diverse approaches used to identify tumour suppressor genes and the different mechanisms that negatively regulate cell growth and division. Some chapters explore tumour suppressor genes that are altered in a specific tumour (colon cancer, erythroleukaemia), whereas other chapters focus on a particular tumour suppressor gene itself. There are chapters covering clear examples of a tumour suppressor gene (*RB*) and others reviewing genes and their products that can act like tumour suppressor genes (GAP and TGF-β) but have never been shown to be homozygously altered in cancer cells. At this early stage in the development of this field, this issue defines a tumour suppressor gene broadly.

The concept that one or more gene products could suppress or inhibit the growth of cells in a tumour derives from early experiments in somatic cell genetics (Harris *et al*, 1969). A normal cell in culture fused with a cell able to produce tumours in animals often resulted in a hybrid that grew well in culture but no longer produced tumours in animals. This result could be obtained independently of the aetiology of the tumorigenic cell line (viral, chemically or spontaneously induced tumours) and independently of the cell lineage (epithelial cell, fibroblast or lymphocyte). The hybrid cell lines upon occasion did produce tumours in test animals. In most of these cases, tumour formation was associated with the loss of a specific chromosome derived from the non-tumorigenic parent. These experiments indicated that several different loci were involved in the suppression of tumour growth. In support of this notion was the observation that a somatic cell hybrid made by fusing two different tumorigenic cell lines produced a hybrid that was not tumorigenic in animals, suggesting that genetic complementation could explain this observation and that at least two different genes in different cell lines are involved. These concepts are reviewed by Stanbridge.

These ideas received considerable support from several unlikely sources. In 1971, Knudson, in reviewing the epidemiological evidence for the role of inherited alterations in the origins of the childhood tumour, retinoblastoma, pointed out that 40% of the cases of retinoblastoma occurred in young infants (mean age, 14 months), that the tumours were commonly bilateral and that in many cases, more than one independently derived tumour could be detected in an eye (patients averaged three tumours) (Knudson, 1971). These patients were often found in families with histories of retinoblastoma. The best explanation, Knudson argued, was that the patient had inherited a single mutant allele from one parent and that a mutation in the other (normal) allele (during fetal life or shortly after birth) would result in a tumour. This explained why the distribution of retinoblastomas in carriers followed the Poisson distribution, 60–75% having bilateral tumours, 25–40% having unilateral tumours and 1–10% being unaffected. However, 60% of retinoblastomas did not fit this pattern. In these cases, no family history could be discerned and retinoblastomas occurred at a later age (average, 30 months). These tumours were always unilateral and each patient had only one tumour. These tumours were quite rare (1 in 30 000 people), and they were postulated to arise from two independent mutations, at the same locus, in the same cell. Inherent in this hypothesis, which fits the epidemiological observations, was the concept of a gene and gene product (which came to be named the retinoblastoma susceptibility gene, *RB*) that inhibited tumour growth. The loss of both copies of this gene through mutation resulted in tumour formation. The *RB* gene was mapped to chromosome 13 band 14q and was isolated by DNA cloning at this locus (Friend *et al*, 1987). These DNA clones permitted a test of Knudson's hypothesis, which proved to be correct. The properties of the *RB* gene and product are reviewed by Weinberg.

A second line of support for the concept of tumour suppressor genes arose from numerous observations of the karyotypes of cancer cells. With time, it became clear that tumour cells can reproducibly lose selected chromosomes or specific portions of chromosomes (deletions). During the past 10 years, the use of specific DNA probes detecting restriction site polymorphisms has allowed the quantitation and documentation of these lost DNA species. In human tumours, for example, deletions in chromosomes 11p and 13q are commonly found in breast cancers and deletions of 3p, 13q and 17p in lung cancers and 5q, 17p, 18q and 22q are altered or lost in many colorectal cancers. The Wilms' tumour gene, which maps at 11p13 was identified and isolated from an abnormal chromosome 11 (reviewed by Haber and Housman).

Most recently, the DNA tumour viruses have provided a new means of identifying tumour suppressor gene products and an understanding of their functions. SV40, the papillomaviruses and some adenoviruses encode oncogenes and their products that stimulate cell growth and division. Optimal virus replication occurs in actively growing cells, and the virus encoded oncogene products bind to and act upon the products of two tumour suppressor genes, *RB* and *p53* (see Chapters by Dyson and Harlow; Livingston; and Münger *et al*). Indeed, *p53* (see Chapter by Levine) was discovered by virtue of its interactions with the SV40 large tumour antigen (Lane and Crawford, 1979; Linzer and Levine, 1979), and the early indications that it could act as a tumour suppressor gene came from the study of the *p53* genetic locus in mice with erythroleukaemia (reviewed by Johnson and Benchimol).

One might have predicted that the GTPase activating protein of *ras,* called GAP (see Chapter by Polakis and McCormick) was going to be the product of a tumour suppressor gene. In its absence, the GTP-*ras* state is stable and presumably signalling for growth. Although that does not appear to be the case, the product of the neurofibromatosis gene, *NF1,* which appears as a tumour suppressor gene in cells of neural crest origin, is indeed capable of stimulating GTPase activity with *ras*. Similarly, TGF-β (see Chapter by Massagué *et al*), can negatively regulate cell growth and division but has not turned up as a tumour suppressor gene during genetic analysis. Finally, the study of human colon carcinomas (reviewed by Fearon) has identified at least two candidate tumour suppressor gene products, the gene for inherited predisposition to familial adenoma polyposis coli (*APC*) on chromosome 5 and an extracellular matrix and cellular membrane protein (*DCC*) on chromosome 18.

The experimental studies reviewed in this issue demonstrate the many different approaches that have led to the identification of tumour suppressor genes and the wide variety of mechanisms that the products of these genes employ in negatively regulating cell growth and division. The authors of this issue of *Cancer Surveys* hope that this review of the field will stimulate new directions in research and fresh ideas and concepts that help the understanding of the molecular and genetic basis of cancer.

References

Friend SH, Horowitz JM, Gerber MR *et al* (1987) Deletions of a DNA sequence in retinoblastomas and mesenchymal tumors: organization of the sequence and its encoded protein. *Proceedings of the National Academy of Sciences of the USA* **84** 9059–9063

Harris H, Miller OJ, Klein G, Worst P and Tachebana T (1969) Suppression of malignancy by cell fusion. *Nature* **223** 363–368

Knudson AG Jr (1971) Mutation and cancer: statistical study of retinoblastoma. *Proceedings of the National Academy of Sciences of the USA* **68** 820–823

Lane DP and Crawford LV (1979) T antigen is bound to a host protein in SV40-transformed cells. *Nature* **278** 261–263

Linzer DIH and Levine AJ (1979) Characterization of a 54K dalton cellular SV40 tumor antigen in SV40 transformed cells. *Cell* **17** 43–52

The author is responsible for the accuracy of the references.

Functional Evidence for Human Tumour Suppressor Genes: Chromosome and Molecular Genetic Studies

ERIC J STANBRIDGE[1]

Ludwig Institute for Cancer Research, Melbourne Tumour Biology Branch, Royal Melbourne Hospital, Victoria, 3050, Australia

Introduction
Circumstantial evidence of tumour suppressor loci
Monochromosome transfer studies
    Genetic heterogeneity in Wilms' tumour
    Neuroblastoma: Evidence for a novel tumour suppressor gene on chromosome 17
    Colorectal cancer: Implication of multiple tumour suppressor genes
    Chromosome 11 contains multiple candidate tumour suppressor loci
Functional studies with cloned tumour suppressor genes
The *RB* gene
    Paradox of the *p53* gene
Summary

INTRODUCTION

Approximately a decade ago, the molecular genetic era of human cancer was ushered in with the discovery of "dominantly acting" activated cellular oncogenes (Shih *et al*, 1981). The first activated oncogenes were isolated by transfection of DNA from human cancer cells into mouse NIH3T3 cells, a process that resulted in neoplastic transformation. The activated oncogenes were quickly found to be homologues of retroviral transforming genes (Der *et al*, 1982). This finding, which was predicted on the basis of seminal studies that showed that the avian retroviral *src* oncogene had evolved from the capture of a cellular proto-oncogene (Stehelin *et al*, 1976), led to the further identification of numerous candidate cellular oncogenes.

The discovery that activated oncogenes could be found in 10–30% of human cancers led to theories that activation of single or multiple cooperating cellular oncogenes was in itself sufficient to create a cancerous cell. These theories were all the more attractive when it was found that the expanding list of oncogene functions included growth factors, growth factor receptors, signal transducers, protein kinases and transcriptional factors—all of which, when behaving aberrantly, might lead to uncontrolled cell proliferation.

Permanent address: [1]Department of Microbiology and Molecular Genetics, College of Medicine, University of California, Irvine, California 92717

Cancer Surveys Volume 12: *Tumour Suppressor Genes, the Cell Cycle and Cancer*
© 1992 Imperial Cancer Research Fund. 0-87969-369-X/92. $3.00 + .00

A tacit assumption in many interpretations of these studies was the dominant nature of activated oncogenes. However, earlier studies with somatic cell hybrids had clearly shown that when malignant cells were fused with normal cells, the resulting hybrid cells were non-tumorigenic (Harris *et al*, 1969; Stanbridge, 1976). This phenomenon of tumour suppression indicated that a gene (or genes) from a normal cell might replace a defective function in the cancer cell and render it responsive to normal regulators of cell growth.

The notion of loss of genetic function being a critical event in the genesis of cancer received further support when it was shown with a combination of cytogenetic analyses and molecular studies of restriction fragment length polymorphisms (RFLPs) that specific chromosomal deletions are often associated with certain human malignancies (reviewed in Stanbridge, 1990). The combination of these studies led to the hypothesis that there exists a class of genetic elements, termed tumour suppressor genes, which must be inactivated in some fashion, eg by deletion, point mutation or methylation, before a cell can become malignant (Stanbridge, 1985).

As described in more detail below, the molecular evidence for the existence of tumour suppressor genes is largely circumstantial. The cloning of tumour suppressor genes has proven to be very arduous since, unlike the 3T3 assay, there are very few selective bioassays; therefore, cloning has primarily employed reverse genetic strategies. Although several candidate tumour suppressor genes have been cloned, functional analyses of only two, *p53* and retinoblastoma (*RB*), have been reported.

The initial evidence for tumour suppressor gene function, derived from somatic cell hybrid studies, has been extensively reviewed elsewhere (Sager, 1985; Stanbridge, 1990). In this review, I shall attempt to present the recent and more finely focused evidence derived from monochromosome transfer and cDNA transfection studies.

CIRCUMSTANTIAL EVIDENCE OF TUMOUR SUPPRESSOR LOCI

The critical distinction to be made for tumour suppressor genes is loss of function associated with the emergence of cancerous behaviour of cells—this is in contradistinction to oncogene activation. The earliest indications of such loss of function, although not fully appreciated at the time, were cytogenetic studies documenting non-random chromosome alterations, including deletions, seen in metaphase spreads of various human cancers (Heim and Mitelman, 1989). More intellectually satisfying data were obtained from molecular analyses, utilizing the technique of RFLP analysis (Cavenee *et al*, 1983). It should be noted, however, that the chromosome regions that were analysed with RFLP probes were usually selected on the basis of earlier cytogenetic studies—an excellent example of the complementarity of disparate technologies.

The prototypic example of the identification (and final cloning) of a tumour suppressor gene locus is that of retinoblastoma. This cancer is of considerable scientific interest because, among other notable features, there are both sporadic and familial forms. The tumour arises from cells of the embryonal neural retina and occurs only in young children. In most cases, retinoblastoma arises sporadically with a worldwide incidence of approximately 1:20 000, but in approximately one third of the cases, the tumour is heritable, with the inherited predisposition behaving as a highly penetrant autosomal dominant trait. These properties led Knudson (1971) to postulate his now classical "two-hit" theory, in which he proposed that all types of retinoblastoma involve two separate mutations carried by all retinoblastoma tumour cells. In sporadic retinoblastoma, he argued, both mutations occur somatically in the same retinal precursor cell, whereas in heritable retinoblastoma, one of the mutations is germinal and the second somatic.

Careful karyotypic analysis of retinoblastoma tumour cells had revealed a consistent deletion of the region 13q14 (Yunis and Ramsay, 1978). Cavenee *et al* (1983) used a series of chromosome 13 specific DNA probes that mapped to the long arm of chromosome 13 and were informative, ie heterozygous, with respect to RFLP bands on a Southern blot. Whereas several DNA markers mapping in the 13q14 region were present in a heterozygous state in the normal cells of a patient predisposed to familial retinoblastoma, the same markers were often found in a homozygous state in tumour tissue derived from the same individual (Cavenee *et al*, 1983). This loss of heterozygosity (LOH), or reduction to homozygosity or hemizygosity, involved loss of sequences from the chromosome 13 not carrying the affected *RB* locus, or loss of the entire chromosome 13 in question, with duplication (in the reduction to homozygosity) of the copy containing the defective *RB* allele. Thus, in this particular tumour, the second hit postulated by Knudson involved the other *RB* allele. Sporadic retinoblastomas also arise frequently through the generation of homozygosity at the *RB* locus, the difference being the involvement of two somatic events instead of one germinal and one somatic event in familial cases.

The success of RFLP analysis in identifying the *RB* locus has been followed by a plethora of studies identifying similar losses of genetic material associated with a variety of human cancers. Loss of genetic information is associated with both sporadic cancers and human familial cancer predisposition syndromes. These experimental data have been reviewed elsewhere (Ponder, 1988; Stanbridge, 1990) and will not be covered in detail here. However, several important features arise from these RFLP studies and are implicit in the summary given in Table 1. Almost every classification of solid human tumours is represented, including rare childhood tumours and the more common tumours arising later in adult life. (It should be noted that the data in Table 1 are intended to be representative rather than a comprehensive listing—further examples are reported on a regular basis in cancer journals.) The lack of representation of haematopoietic malignancies may reflect a more extreme focus of scientific investigation into oncogene activation, rather than the absence of a role for tumour suppressor genes in control of these malignant conditions. In certain cancers, only a single tumour suppressor locus has been

TABLE 1. Candidate human tumour suppressor loci[a]

Tumour type	Chromosome region(s) involved	Candidate gene(s) involved
Retinoblastoma	13q14	*RB*
Sporadic Wilms' tumour	11p13, 11p15	*WT1*
Glioblastoma multiforme (astrocytoma)	9p, 10, 17p13	*p53*
Breast carcinoma	1p, 1q, 11p, 13q14, 17p13, 18q	*RB + p53*
Small cell lung cancer	3p, 13q14, 17p13	*PTP, RB + p53*
Non-small cell lung cancer	3p, 9p, 11p, 13q14, 17p13	*PTP, RB + p53*
Bladder carcinoma	9q, 11p, 17p13	*p53*
Colorectal carcinoma	5q21, 17p13, 18q21	*MCC, p53 + DCC*
Renal cell carcinoma	3p, 3q	*PTP*
Neurofibroma	17q	*NF1*
Neuroblastoma	1p, 14q, 17	not known
Melanoma	1, 6q, 7, 10, 19	not known
Myeloid leukaemia	5q	not known
Meningioma	22	not known

[a]These data were derived from a combination of cytogenetic and RFLP analyses. References to these studies are given in the review by Stanbridge (1990)

identified, eg the *RB* locus in retinoblastoma, whereas in others, eg breast, lung and colorectal cancers, multiple loci seem to be involved. The multiple tumour suppressor loci associated with these late onset cancers are certainly consistent with the multistage and "multihit" nature of genetic alterations postulated to be associated with these malignancies (Peto and Easton, 1990). Quite a number of the candidate loci are represented in only a single malignancy, eg the *DCC* gene in colorectal cancer (Fearon *et al*, 1990). This could obviously reflect the fact that "RFLP hunts" are in their infancy, and more widespread involvement in other cancers will be revealed by further investigation; but also it may suggest the existence of certain lineage specific tumour suppressor genes. However, at least two tumour suppressor genes, namely *p53* and *RB*, have been found to be altered (deleted, rearranged or mutated) in many different types of cancer, suggesting aberrations of possible common pathways of growth control in these diverse malignancies (Goodrich and Lee, 1990; Levine *et al*, 1991).

Perhaps the most important feature of the RFLP analyses that is germane to this review is that all of the molecular evidence for tumour suppressor loci is circumstantial and does not constitute functional evidence for the existence of such genes—thereby representing "guilt by association". To provide such evidence, it is necessary to clone candidate tumour suppressor genes and introduce them into cancer cells lacking the relevant functional gene and observe the cells for phenotypic changes, including suppression of growth in vitro and in vivo. Unfortunately, it has proved far more difficult to clone tumour suppressor genes than activated oncogenes because, in most instances, there is no suitable assay other than suppression of tumour growth in vivo (Stanbridge *et al*, 1989). Although a handful of candidate tumour suppressor genes have now been cloned (briefly described below), functional evidence is forthcoming only with *p53* and *RB*, both of which function as potent growth suppressor genes in certain human cancer cells (Huang *et al*, 1988; Baker *et al*, 1990). Thus, for many other candidate genes, other more indirect procedures have been employed. Although somatic cell hybrids provided the first convincing evidence for the genetic basis of tumour suppression, it is clearly a very crude genetic method, since it involves whole genome transfers. The somatic cell fusion approach has been modified in order to facilitate the transfer of single chromosomes (derived from normal cells and presumably carrying wild type tumour suppressor genes) into cancer cells deficient in one or more tumour suppressor functions, via microcell fusion (Saxon *et al*, 1985, 1986).

MONOCHROMOSOME TRANSFER STUDIES

Single chromosome transfer was made possible by the development of the technique of microcell transfer (Fournier and Ruddle, 1977). The key feature of this technique is that the transferred chromosome is retained as a complete structural unit in succeeding generations of recipient cells, unlike the techniques of metaphase chromosome transfer (McBride and Ozer, 1973), where the transferred chromosome is rapidly degraded. The drawback is that chromosome transfer is essentially random. To allow for transfer and selective retention of single specific chromosomes, dominant selectable markers such as the bacterial *gpt* or *neo* genes are integrated into individual human chromosomes via plasmid DNA transfection or retroviral infection (Tunnacliffe *et al*, 1983; Saxon *et al*, 1985). Chromosomes tagged with dominant selectable markers could then be transferred from normal cells into cancer cells previously shown to have deletions in specific chromosome regions. A summary of the published reports of monochromosome transfer studies is given in Table 2. Several features are readily apparent from these findings. In most cases, the expected chromosome containing an intact tumour suppressor gene indeed conveys a tumour suppressing effect, whereas the transfer of irrelevant chromosomes has no such effect. In most, but not all, cases (Shimizu *et al*, 1990), transfer of a single copy of the normal chromosome is sufficient to induce growth inhibition in vitro or tumour suppression in vivo. This strongly suggests a dominant effect of the wild type tumour suppressor allele and supports the evidence that both alleles of a given tumour suppressor gene need to be inactivated in order for a cell to progress to the cancerous state. In at least one example, ie Wilms' tumour, detailed below, it was a region of the chromosome other than the predicted locus that contained tumour suppressor activity. In certain instances, namely endometrial cancers (Yamada *et al*, 1990) and colorectal cancer (Tanaka *et al*, 1991; Goyette MC, Cho K, Fasching C,

TABLE 2. Tumour suppression associated with the transfer of single human chromosomes via microcell fusion

Tumour cell line	Tumour suppressing chromosome[a]		Reference
	expected	observed	
HeLa (cervical carcinoma)	11	11	Saxon et al, 1986
SiHa (cervical carcinoma)	–	11	Oshimura et al, 1990
Retinoblastoma	13	13	Stanbridge, 1989a
Renal cell carcinoma	3	3	Shimizu et al, 1990
Wilms' tumour	11p13	11p15	Dowdy et al, in press
Colorectal carcinoma	5, 17, 18	5, 17, 18	Tanaka et al, 1991;
			Goyette MC et al, unpublished
Endometrial carcinoma	–	1, 6, 9	Yamada et al, 1990
Melanoma	6	6	Trent et al, 1990
Neuroblastoma	1	17	Bader et al, 1991
HT1080 (fibrosarcoma)	1	1, 11	Kugoh et al, 1990

[a]In each study (with the exception of neuroblastoma), transfer of "irrelevant" chromosomes had no effect on cell growth or tumorigenicity

Paraskeva C, Vogelstein B and Stanbridge EJ, unpublished), multiple chromosomes carried a tumour suppressing effect. In the case of neuroblastoma, an unexpected tumour suppressing effect was noted following transfer of an "irrelevant" chromosome, thereby revealing a potential new tumour suppressor gene (Bader et al, 1991). The significance of these observations is now detailed below.

Genetic Heterogeneity in Wilms' Tumour

Wilms' tumour is a paediatric nephroblastoma that occurs in approximately 1/10 000 children and accounts for 85% of all childhood kidney cancer. Wilms' tumour can occur in both hereditary and sporadic forms. The sporadic form accounts for >95% of all Wilms' tumour incidence and generally presents as unilateral foci, whereas the familial form may occur as unilateral or bilateral foci (Knudson and Strong, 1972). Hereditary predisposition to Wilms' tumour has been associated with bilateral aniridia (an autosomal dominant trait characterized by rudimentary development of the iris), urogenital defects and mental retardation. These disorders are collectively referred to as the WAGR syndrome (Miller et al, 1964). In addition, individuals with the Beckwith-Wiedemann syndrome, an autosomal dominant congenital malformation and growth excess disorder, are at increased risk for childhood malignancies including Wilms' tumour, rhabdomyosarcoma and hepatoblastoma (Sotelo-Avila et al, 1980).

Cytogenetic analyses of Wilms' tumours obtained from patients with the WAGR syndrome identified a specific interstitial chromosome deletion, del (11p13), in a minority of cases (Francke et al, 1979).

Molecular mapping, using RFLP analysis, confirmed a loss of hetero-zygosity for DNA probes mapping to the 11p13 region in DNA obtained from Wilms' tumour tissue compared to DNA obtained from normal tissue from the same patient (Koufos *et al*, 1984; Orkin *et al*, 1984). However, it soon became clear that the simple association of LOH of DNA sequences in 11p13 with Wilms' tumour did not fit all situations. Further RFLP studies have identified Wilms' tumours that have no apparent LOH in the 11p13 region. In these cases, LOH was found in 11p15.5, a region considerably distal to 11p13 (Reeve *et al*, 1989). These observations suggest that a subtype of Wilms' tumour may exist that involves inactivation of a tumour suppressor gene that maps to 11p15 rather than 11p13. It should be noted at this juncture that the Beckwith-Wiedemann syndrome maps to 11p15.

Finally, it has been reported that familial forms of Wilms' tumour show no linkage to any region of chromosome 11 (Huff *et al*, 1988). Thus, at least three distinct loci may play a part in the genesis of Wilms' tumour.

The candidate Wilms' tumour suppressor gene that maps to the 11p13 region has recently been cloned (Call *et al*, 1990; Gessler *et al*, 1990) and is now known as the *WT1* gene. The *WT1* gene has a number of properties that make it an attractive candidate for the Wilms' tumour gene. The gene encodes a polypeptide with features that suggest a potential role in transcriptional regulation. There are four zinc finger domains and a region rich in proline and glutamine. The aminoacid sequence of the predicted polypeptide shows sig-nificant homology with two growth regulated mammalian polypeptides, EGR1 and EGR2. A recombinant WT1 protein has been used to show that the zinc finger region binds to an EGR1 consensus sequence (Rauscher *et al*, 1990). A mutation in the zinc finger region, originally identified in a Wilms' tumour patient, abolished its DNA binding activity. It has been suggested that the WT1 protein may act (presumably negatively) at the DNA binding site of a growth factor inducible gene and that loss of DNA binding activity contributes to the tumorigenic process.

Expression of the *WT1* mRNA transcript was found to be restricted to high level expression in fetal kidney and the spleen. There was absent or low level expression in adult kidney tissue. High levels were also expressed in several sporadic Wilms' tumours and haematopoietic cell lines, but no transcripts were detected in cell lines derived from a variety of non-Wilms' solid tumours. On Southern analysis, only a small fraction of Wilms' tumours showed dele-tions, or rearrangements, of the *WT1* gene. However, this obviously does not preclude more subtle alterations, such as point mutations.

The findings that most Wilms' tumours contain an apparently normal *WT1* gene and that levels of *WT1* mRNA expression in the tumours are variable contrast with the frequent deletions and internal rearrangements of the *RB* gene found in retinoblastomas and other neoplasms. However, it could more readily approximate the frequent point mutations found in the *p53* tumour suppressor gene (Nigro *et al*, 1989), although these are most often associated with deletion of the other *p53* allele (Fearon and Vogelstein, 1990).

The classic test of a gene's function is complementation—the introduction of the wild type gene into a cell that has a defective gene to see whether it produces a measurable phenotypic change. In the case of the Wilms' tumour gene, one might expect a tumour suppressor phenotype similar to that seen with the *RB* gene (Huang *et al*, 1988). Unfortunately, to date, no functional tests using cDNA expression vectors have been reported for the *WT1* gene. However, chromosome transfer experiments have clearly indicated that tumour suppression occurs as a result of the introduction of a normal human chromosome 11 into the Wilms' tumour cell line G401 (Weissman *et al*, 1987). Transfer of the complete short arm of chromosome 11 into G401 cells resulted in tumour suppression but did not allow one to determine which region— 11p13, 11p15 or some other location—contained the active tumour suppressor gene. To refine further the microcell technique and to address this question, a radiation reduction method was developed that serves to enrich for deletions and/or rearrangements of discrete regions of a specific chromosome area (Dowdy *et al*, 1990). The procedure involves irradiation of microcells produced from mouse cells that contain a single selectable human chromosome. This human chromosome contains a dominant selectable marker that allows for retention after transfer.

Dowdy and colleagues generated a number of radiation reduced chromosomes using as their starting material a t(X;11p) chromosome containing the entire short arm of 11. Irradiated clones in which the t(X;11) chromosome now contained deletions in the 11p13 region or the 11p15 region were selected. These radiation reduced chromosomes were transferred to G401 cells. The chromosome with the deleted *WT1* gene and a mostly intact 11p15 region retained its tumour suppressing activity, whereas the chromosome with an intact *WT1* gene and a deleted 11p15 region had completely lost its tumour suppressing function (Dowdy *et al*, in press). These results indicate that *WT1* is not a tumour suppressor gene for G401 Wilms' tumour cells and that the 11p14-p15 region contains the tumour suppressor activity. Although these results do not preclude a role for *WT1* in the genesis of Wilms' tumour, they clearly indicate the possibility of genetic heterogeneity with an involvement of 11p14-p15 in certain subtypes of Wilms' tumour (Stanbridge and Dowdy, 1991).

Neuroblastoma: Evidence for a Novel Tumour Suppressor Gene on Chromosome 17

Neuroblastoma is the most common solid tumour of children in the USA, arising from postganglionic sympathetic neurons. Many neuroblastomas have cytogenetic abnormalities in the form of double minutes, homogeneously staining regions or both. Amplification and overexpression of the proto-oncogene N-*myc* are also frequently found in human neuroblastomas and were found to map to the double minutes and homogeneously staining regions (Brodeur, 1990). N-*myc* amplification and overexpression are associated with rapid tumour progression and poor prognosis, but this involvement of N-*myc* may only be important for a subset of particularly aggressive neuroblastomas. The most common alteration in human neuroblastomas, however, is a partial monosomy of chromosome 1p (Brodeur *et al*, 1981). With the development of RFLP analysis, it has been found that the smallest visible region of cytogenetic deletion correlates with the region that shows the most consistent loss of heterozygosity, namely 1p36.1-1pter (Weith *et al*, 1989).

Bader and colleagues (1991) used X;1 translocation chromosomes, as well as chromosomes tagged with the neomycin resistance gene, for microcell transfer into a neuroblastoma cell line containing a 1p deletion and over-expressing N-*myc*. As expected, transfer of a t(X;1q) chromosome had no effect on in vitro growth or in vivo tumour formation. Conversely, the transfer of t(X;1p) or chromosome 11 induced features of differentiation, including neurite outgrowth. Prior experience with somatic cell hybrids has indicated that the biological mechanism of tumour suppression involves the induction of differentiation (Peehl and Stanbridge, 1982). However, although the t(X;1p) chromosome and chromosome 11 induced features of differentiation in vitro, neither transferred chromosome had a tumour suppressing effect. Although the transferred chromosome 11 was retained intact in the cells, no cytogenetically identifiable t(X;1p) chromosome was found in any of the microcell hybrids resulting from this transfer. Thus, it still remains possible that a region of chromosome 1p contains a tumour suppressor gene that perhaps functions as a growth suppressing gene in vitro and precludes selection of proliferating recipient cells. What is obvious, however, is that microcell transfer has clearly demonstrated the dissociation of induction of differentiation from tumour suppression. Conversely, the transfer of chromosome 17 had no effect on growth behaviour in vitro but completely suppressed the tumorigenic phenotype.

A known tumour suppressor gene, *p53*, maps to 17p13, and loss of function of this gene has been implicated in a number of human malignancies, most notably colorectal carcinomas (Baker *et al*, 1989). Preliminary studies involving transfection with wild type *p53* cDNA (Bader S and Stanbridge EJ, unpublished) indicate that this gene is not involved in the observed suppression of neuroblastoma, thereby revealing the presence of a possible new tumour suppressor gene on chromosome 17. The neurofibromatosis gene, *NF1*, which maps to 17q, has recently been cloned and shown to be in a region that contains several potential coding sequences (Cawthon *et al*, 1990). It will be interesting to determine whether any of these are deranged in neuroblastomas.

Finally, the overexpression of the N-*myc* gene is not altered in any of the microcell hybrids (Bader S and Stanbridge EJ, unpublished). This is yet another example of tumour suppression not affecting the expression of an activated oncogene, thereby belying the inference that tumour suppressor genes are anti-oncogenes in the sense of directly controlling the expression of oncogenes.

Colorectal Cancer: Implication of Multiple Tumour Suppressor Genes

Colorectal cancer has become one of the most extensively studied human malignancies. This is due to the availability of tissue at different stages of tumour progression, from normal colonic epithelium to hyperproliferative lesions and from adenomas increasing in dysplasia to carcinomas. Vogelstein *et al* (1988) have screened DNA from tissues at these various stages for genetic alterations indicative of the activation of oncogenes and LOH. In sporadic colorectal tumours, activation of *ras*, predominantly Ki-*ras*, occurs in 40-50% of late stage adenomas and carcinomas examined. In addition, loss of genetic information on chromosome 5q21-22 was observed in 30% of adenomas and in 35% of carcinomas. In contrast, alterations of chromosome 17p12-13 and chromosome 18q21-qter are observed more frequently in carcinomas than in adenomas. However, rather than there being any temporal relationship between these genetic alterations, it is the accumulation of these defects that seems to be important in the progression to the malignant state (see Fearon and Vogelstein, 1990). More than 90% of carcinomas examined have two or more of these genetic alterations, as compared to only 7% of early adenomas.

Candidate tumour suppressor genes mapping to the involved regions of chromosomes 5, 17 and 18 have been identified and at least partially characterized. Linkage analysis has mapped the locus segregating with familial adenomatous polyposis (FAP) to the long arm of chromosome 5, near the region q21-22 (Bodmer *et al*, 1987). Familial adenomatous polyposis is a dominantly inherited disorder characterized by numerous adenomatous polyps in the colon which, if left untreated, develop into carcinomas. Whereas in sporadic carcinomas, alterations associated with chromosome 5 are primarily detected as early as stage II adenomas, in patients with familial cancer, alterations tend to occur later in tumour progression, primarily in carcinomas. A gene termed *MCC* (mutated in colorectal cancer) has recently been cloned from the region of chromosome 5q21 (Kinzler *et al*, 1991). *MCC* encodes an 829 aminoacid protein with a very short region of homology to the G protein coupled m^3 muscarinic acetylcholine receptor. A rearrangement disrupting the coding region of *MCC* has been found in one colorectal tumour, and two additional tumours were discovered to contain somatically acquired point mutations that would have resulted in aminoacid substitutions. Thus, *MCC* may be a tumour suppressor gene, but as yet it is not clear how prevalent *MCC* mutations are in sporadic colorectal tumours, nor has it been determined if *MCC* is involved in FAP.

The previously cloned *p53* gene was found to map to the region of chromosome 17 that is most commonly lost in colorectal cancers. One allele of *p53* was often deleted, and it was found that the remaining allele often contained a point mutation (Baker *et al*, 1989). Thus, *p53* fits the criteria for a tumour suppressor gene, ie inactivation by a combination of allele loss and point mutation. Indeed, when a normal *p53* gene is introduced into colorectal tumour cell lines lacking the wild type alleles, a complete cessation of growth is observed (Baker *et al*, 1990). Mutations of *p53* have been observed in a wide variety of human cancers (Nigro *et al*, 1989).

A gene mapping to the region often deleted on chromosome 18 has been partially cloned (Fearon *et al*, 1990). This candidate tumour suppressor gene is the so-called *DCC* (deleted in colorectal cancer) gene. In addition to deletions, somatic mutations of *DCC* have been observed in a number of colorectal tumours (Vogelstein B, personal communication). This gene is expressed in most tissues, including normal colonic epithelium, but is most abundant in brain tissue. However, its expression is either greatly reduced or absent in many colorectal tumours. The *DCC* gene encodes an mRNA transcript of 10-12 kb. *DCC* shares homology with the neural cell adhesion molecule (N-CAM) and other related cell surface glycoproteins. The *DCC* gene contains four immunoglobulin like domains and a fibronectin type III related domain similar to those present in N-CAMs. Loss of function of such a gene, encoding a cell adhesion molecule, may facilitate the disruption of normal cell-cell contacts and cellular communication.

This compilation of both cytogenetic and molecular data thus provides strong evidence for an accumulation of genetic alterations during progression of colorectal cancer. Accrual of such multiple genetic alterations is also consistent with the late onset of this disease. Since tumour suppressor genes seem to function as negative regulators of cell proliferation, an important question is whether correction of defects in any one of the candidate tumour suppressor genes (ie *MCC*, *DCC* or *p53*) is sufficient to suppress tumorigenicity or whether correction of some combination, or all, of the defects is required. The most direct answer to these questions would be to introduce the relevant wild type gene into a cancer cell that is mutant or deleted for that particular gene; however, this has been demonstrated only in *p53* cDNA transfection studies.

Monochromosome transfer studies have provided compelling evidence that correction of any single defect is sufficient to control negatively the tumorigenic behaviour of colorectal cancer cells. One group of investigators has found that transfer of chromosome 5 or 18 had a significant growth inhibiting effect in vitro, abolished anchorage independent growth and completely suppressed tumorigenicity (Tanaka *et al*, 1991). Goyette and colleagues (Goyette MC, Cho K, Fasching C, Paraskeva C, Vogelstein B and Stanbridge EJ, unpublished) found a gradient of potency of tumour suppression with each individual chromosome transfer. The introduction of chromosome 17 into the colorectal cancer cell line SW480 resulted in complete suppression of growth in vitro. This potent in vitro growth inhibitory effect is the same as that seen when SW480 cells are transfected with wild type *p53* cDNA (Baker *et al*, 1990). Transfer of chromosome 5 had marginal effects on in vitro population doubling times but completely suppressed tumorigenicity. Chromosome 18 transfer had no effect upon in vitro growth and a variable tumour suppressing effect; some clones formed no tumours, and others formed tumours that progressed in size significantly more slowly than parental SW480 tumours.

These findings indicate that although multiple defects in tumour suppressor genes seem to be required for progression to the malignant state in colorectal cancer, correction of only a single defect is necessary to revert the cells to a non-tumorigenic phenotype.

Chromosome 11 Contains Multiple Candidate Tumour Suppressor Loci

A combination of chromosome transfer and molecular genetic evidence suggests that multiple tumour suppressor loci map to chromosome 11. The first compelling functional evidence for tumour suppressor genes via mono-chromosome transfer demonstrated a candidate gene on chromosome 11 that is capable of suppressing the tumorigenic phenotype of the cervical cancer cell line, HeLa (Saxon *et al*, 1986). The region containing this candidate gene has been more finely mapped to 11q13 (Srivatsan E, personal communication). Introduction of chromosome 11 into another cervical carcinoma cell line, SiHa, also suppressed tumorigenicity (Oshimura *et al*, 1990). Transfer of chromosome 11 was also found to suppress the tumorigenic behaviour of a Wilms' tumour (Weissman *et al*, 1987), a rhabdomyosarcoma (Oshimura *et al*, 1990) and a fibrosarcoma (Kugoh *et al*, 1990). In the case of the Wilms' tumour cell line G401, the tumour suppressor function mapped to 11p14-p15 (Dowdy *et al*, 1991), whereas another candidate Wilms' tumour gene, *WT1*, maps to 11p13 (Call *et al*, 1990). Thus, there is ample evidence that multiple tumour suppressor genes reside on chromosome 11. Transfer of chromosome 11 does not suppress all tumour cell lines (Oshimura *et al*, 1990) and therefore does not reflect a "general" tumour suppressor property.

FUNCTIONAL STUDIES WITH CLONED TUMOUR SUPPRESSOR GENES

As mentioned earlier, the cloning of tumour suppressor genes has proved to be an arduous task that often involves labour intensive reverse genetic strategies. Despite these formidable barriers, several candidate tumour suppressor genes have recently been cloned and are listed in Table 3. However, functional evidence for their tumour suppressing properties is available only for *p53* and *RB* genes. The structures and functions of these two genes are reviewed extensively elsewhere in this issue, and I shall review only certain salient features of *RB* and *p53* that are important in our thinking of tumour suppressor gene function.

The *RB* Gene

The retinoblastoma (*RB*) gene was first cloned by Friend *et al* (1986). It is a large gene, containing 27 exons dispersed within approximately 200 kb of genomic DNA (Hong *et al*, 1989). The 4.7 kb mRNA transcript encodes a 110 kDa protein, which has functionally important posttranslational phosphory-

TABLE 3. Cloned candidate tumour suppressor genes

Tumour suppressor gene	Chromosome location	Possible function	Reference
RB	13q14	transcription factor	Chellappen *et al*, 1991
p53	17p13	transcription factor	Raycroft *et al*, 1990
WT1	11p13	transcription factor	Rauscher *et al*, 1990
NF1	17q11	GAP related	Xu *et al*, 1990
DCC	18q21	cell adhesion-communication	Fearon *et al*, 1990
MCC	5q21	G protein activation	Kinzler *et al*, 1991
PTP	3p21	protein-tyrosine phosphatase	Laforgia *et al*, 1991

lated states (Lee *et al*, 1987a). Rather surprisingly, the gene was found to be expressed in virtually all tissues. However, in malignant retinoblastoma cells, there is either no RB protein expressed or, if there is, it is a truncated or mutant form of the protein. Several intriguing properties of the RB protein have been revealed. It was quickly found to be localized in the nucleus and appears to be associated with DNA, although no specific DNA binding sequences have been identified (Lee *et al*, 1987a). However, it has recently been reported that the underphosphorylated form of the RB protein interacts with the transcription factor E2F (Chellappan *et al*, 1991). The phosphorylation state of the RB protein varies through the cell cycle, with maximum phosphorylation occurring in S phase and reduced phosphorylation occurring after M phase (Buchkovich *et al*, 1989; DeCaprio *et al*, 1989). It was also noted that end stage differentiation of cells in culture was accompanied by reduced phosphorylation (Mihara *et al*, 1989) and that senescent human diploid fibroblasts also contained predominantly underphosphorylated forms of the RB protein (Stein *et al*, 1990). These observations suggest that RB acts in a cell cycle specific fashion and that the oscillation of phosphorylation-dephosphorylation states may be a principal mechanism in controlling the cycling of cells. A particularly intriguing property of the RB protein is its propensity to form tight complexes with the protein products of transforming genes of DNA tumour viruses, including SV40 large T antigen (DeCaprio *et al*, 1988), adenovirus E1A protein (Whyte *et al*, 1988) and the E7 protein of human papillomavirus (Dyson *et al*, 1989). This property of complexing with DNA tumour virus transformation related proteins is also shared by the p53 protein (discussed below). The importance of these associations is underscored by the fact that non-functional mutants of the retinoblastoma protein are characterized by defects in phosphorylation, inability to complex with the E1A oncoprotein and failure to become tightly associated with nuclear structures (Templeton *et al*, 1991). Also, the large T antigens of many non-transforming mutants of SV40 fail to complex with wild type RB protein.

Mutations and/or deletions of the *RB* gene were first identified in retino-blastomas but have been documented in an increasing variety of human malignancies including osteosarcomas (Fung *et al*, 1987; Lee *et al*, 1987b), prostate carcinoma (Bookstein *et al*, 1990), small cell lung carcinomas (Harbour *et al*, 1988; Yokota *et al*, 1988), bladder carcinomas (Horowitz *et al*, 1989) and breast carcinomas (Varley *et al*, 1989). Correction of such defects has been accomplished by introducing a wild type *RB* cDNA in a retroviral vector into retinoblastoma, osteosarcoma and prostate carcinoma cells (Huang *et al*, 1988; Bookstein *et al*, 1990). In each case, a potent growth suppressing effect was noted in vitro and, if sufficient cells could be cultured, tumorigenicity assays indicated a strong tumour suppressing effect. Introduction of the wild type *RB* cDNA into cells containing wild type *RB* genes had no effect on cell proliferation or tumorigenicity.

The *RB* gene therefore represents the prototypic tumour suppressor gene. The tight complexing of RB (and p53) protein with various viral oncoproteins has stimulated renewed interest in how DNA tumour viruses transform cells. It is clearly tempting to conclude that the oncoproteins subvert normal cell cycle control in some way by complexing with RB and p53 proteins, neutralizing their cell cycle regulatory function in some way, thereby leading to the uncontrolled proliferation characteristic of cancer cells. A significant problem with this straightforward and rather simple hypothesis is that transformation of human diploid fibroblasts and epithelial cells by these viruses or their transforming genes is a rare event (Stanbridge, 1989b). For example, infection of fibroblasts with SV40 leads to 100% of cells positive for nuclear T antigen, but the cells eventually cease dividing—a possible manifestation of cellular senescence—and only rare populations of dividing cells are recovered. These cells are immortal, but non-tumorigenic. Thus, factors in addition to the complexing of SV40 large T with RB and p53 may have critical roles in the process of neoplastic transformation.

Paradox of the *p53* Gene

The chequered history of the *p53* gene—originally thought to be an oncogene and now identified as a tumour suppressor gene—has been extensively reviewed elsewhere (Levine, 1990; Levine *et al*, 1991). The *p53* gene has been implicated in many inherited and sporadic forms of human cancers (see Table 1). Loss of function of both alleles—one through a deletion, the other through a point mutation—is most commonly encountered in these malignancies. Loss of function at both alleles is consistent with the recessive nature of this and other tumour suppressor genes, eg retinoblastoma. The point mutations seen are often missense and can occur at many different positions in the 393 codons of the human *p53* gene, although there are certain "hot spots" (Levine *et al*, 1991). A recent exciting finding was the report that germline *p53* mutations are found in the rare autosomal dominant Li-Fraumeni syndrome, which is characterized by diverse tumours at multiple sites in the body (Malkin *et al*, 1990).

The *p53* gene product seems to act, like RB protein, as a negative regulator of cell growth. It is located in the nucleus and has DNA binding properties. Recently, a 33 base pair DNA sequence has been identified that binds specifically to wild type human p53 protein in vitro (Kern *et al*, 1991). Like RB, the p53 protein complexes with several viral oncoproteins, including SV40 large T antigen, the adenovirus E1B protein and the E6 protein of human papillomaviruses (Sarnow *et al*, 1982; Werness *et al*, 1990). The E6 protein binds to and promotes the proteolytic breakdown of p53 (Scheffner *et al*, 1990), the first direct proof that an oncoprotein may inactivate p53 function. Also, all *p53* mutants studied fail to bind SV40 large T antigen, thereby indicating that p53 interacts with a cellular homologue of T antigen that may be critical for cell cycle control (Levine *et al*, 1991).

Correction of p53 defects has been accomplished by transfecting various cancer cells containing mutant alleles with a wild type *p53* cDNA or by chromosome 17 transfer, also containing a wild type copy of the *p53* gene. In all cases, transfer of the wild type gene resulted in a potent growth suppressing effect in vitro. Studies with vectors containing inducible promoters suggest that the cells are growth arrested in the G_1 phase of the cell cycle following mitosis (Mercer *et al*, 1990).

Cancer cells that contain mutant alleles of *p53* and are growth suppressed following introduction of wild type p53 include colorectal carcinoma (Baker *et al*, 1990; Goyette MC, Cho K, Fasching C, Paraskeva C, Vogelstein B and Stanbridge EJ, unpublished), glioblastoma (Mercer *et al*, 1990), breast carcinoma (Casey *et al*, in press) and lung carcinoma (Cajot JF, Harris C and Stanbridge EJ, unpublished). It has also been reported that Saos-2 osteosarcoma cells, which contain no endogenous *p53*, have prolonged doubling times following introduction of wild type *p53* cDNA and are suppressed for tumorigenicity (Chen *et al*, 1990). Mutant *p53* induced the cells to grow faster than parental Saos-2 cells in culture and to form more aggressive tumours. This apparent gain in function following mutation of *p53* has been observed in rodent cells (Martinez *et al*, 1991; Michalovitz *et al*, 1991). However, if both wild type and mutant *p53* cDNAs are expressed in Saos-2 cells, the wild type suppressing effect is dominant (Chen *et al*, 1990). Another perplexing feature is that although there is a dramatic growth inhibiting effect following introduction of wild type *p53* into colorectal carcinoma cells containing mutant alleles of *p53*, the same vector has no effect on growth of cells that contain only wild type alleles (Baker *et al*, 1990). It should also be noted that in the natural case of cells containing one mutant and one wild type allele of *p53*, as seen in Li-Fraumeni syndrome, the growth properties of cultured fibroblasts are similar to those derived from normal donors, including cellular senescence. Thus, although it seems fairly clear that *p53* behaves as a tumour suppressor gene, there are many puzzling aspects to its role in controlling cell cycle events. The notion that mutation of *p53* results in a gain of function remains unresolved and may differ between mice and humans. One possible complicating factor in this scenario is that different mutants of *p53* differ in their ability to cooperate with *ras* in rodent cell transforming assays (Michalovitz *et al*, 1991).

SUMMARY

There is now ample genetic and some functional evidence for the existence of tumour suppressor genes. Although much of the functional evidence has been derived from somatic cell hybrid and chromosome transfer studies, it is critical that cloned candidate tumour suppressor genes be used in such functional assays. Our experience with *RB* and *p53* indicates that much will be learned about the control of the cell cycle from studies of tumour suppressor genes. However, the handful of candidate genes cloned to date also indicates a variety of cellular localizations and cellular functions. Thus, just as oncogenes seem to act to promote growth at many levels of metabolic control, it would seem that tumour suppressor genes act in complementary ways to control cell proliferation. The molecular genetic study of cancer has truly entered an exciting phase.

Acknowledgements

I wish to thank Tony Burgess and Ashley Dunn for their warm hospitality at the Ludwig Institute, where this review was written. Special thanks are due to Miss Colleen Backus for expert secretarial assistance. The author's studies were supported by grants from the National Cancer Institute and the Council for Tobacco Research, USA.

References

Bader SA, Fasching C, Brodeur GM and Stanbridge EJ (1991) Dissociation of suppression of tumourigenicity and differentiation in vitro effected by transfer of single human chromosomes into human neuroblastoma cells. *Cell Growth and Differentiation* **2** 245–255

Baker SJ, Fearon ER, Nigro JM *et al* (1989) Chromosome 17 deletions and p53 gene mutations in colorectal carcinomas. *Science* **244** 217–221

Baker SJ, Markowitz S, Fearon ER, Willson JKV and Vogelstein B (1990) Suppression of human colorectal carcinoma cell growth by wild-type p53. *Science* **249** 912–915

Bodmer WF, Bailey CJ, Bodmer J *et al* (1987) Localization of the gene for familial adenomatous polyposis on chromosome 5. *Nature* **328** 614–616

Bookstein R, Shew J-Y, Chen P-L, Scully P and Lee W-H (1990) Suppression of tumorigenicity of human prostate carcinoma cells by replacing a mutated RB gene. *Science* **247** 712–715

Brodeur GM (1990) Neuroblastoma: clinical significance of genetic abnormalities. *Cancer Surveys* **9** 673–688

Brodeur GM, Green AA, Hayes FA, Williams KJ, Williams DL and Tsiatis AA (1981) Cytogenetic features of human neuroblastomas and cell lines. *Cancer Research* **41** 4678–4686

Buchkovich K, Duffy LA and Harlow E (1989) The retinoblastoma protein is phosphorylated during specific phases of the cell cycle. *Cell* **58** 1097–1105

Call KM, Glaser TM, Ito CY *et al* (1990) Description and characterisation of a zinc finger polypeptide gene at the human chromosome 11 Wilms' tumor locus. *Cell* **60** 509–520

Casey G, Lo-Hsueh M, Vogelstein B and Stanbridge EJ Growth suppression of human breast cancer cells by the introduction of a wild type p53 gene. *Oncogene* (in press)

Cavenee WK, Dryja TP, Phillips RA *et al* (1983) Expression of recessive alleles by chromosomal mechanisms in retinoblastoma. *Nature* **305** 779–784

Cawthon RM, Weiss R, Xu G *et al* (1990) A major segment of the neurofibromatosis type 1 gene: cDNA sequence, genomic structure, and point mutations. *Cell* **62** 193–201

Chellappan SP, Hiebert S, Mudryj M, Horowitz JM and Nevins JR (1991) The E2F transcription factor is a cellular target for the RB protein. *Cell* **65** 1053–1062

Chen P-L, Chen Y, Bookstein R and Lee W-H (1990) Genetic mechanisms of tumor suppression by the human p53 gene. *Science* **250** 1576–1580

DeCaprio JA, Ludlow JW, Figge J *et al* (1988) SV40 large tumor antigen forms a specific complex with the product of the retinoblastoma susceptibility gene. *Cell* **54** 275–283

DeCaprio JA, Ludlow JW, Lynch D *et al* (1989) The product of retinoblastoma susceptibility gene has properties of a cell cycle regulatory element. *Cell* **58** 1085–1095

Der CJ, Krontiris TG and Cooper GM (1982) Transforming genes of human bladder and lung carcinoma cell lines are homologous to the ras genes of Harvey and Kirsten sarcoma viruses. *Proceedings of the National Academy of Sciences of the USA* **79** 3637–3640

Dowdy SF, Scanlon DJ, Fasching CL, Casey G and Stanbridge EJ (1990) Irradiation microcell-mediated chromosome transfer (XMMCT): the generation of specific chromosomal arm deletions. *Genes, Chromosomes and Cancer* **2** 318–327

Dowdy SF, Fasching C, Araujo D *et al* Suppression of tumorigenicity in Wilms' tumor by the p14:p15 region of chromosome 11. *Science* (in press)

Dyson N, Howley PM, Munger K and Harlow E (1989) The human papilloma virus-16 E7 oncoprotein is able to bind to the retinoblastoma gene product. *Science* **243** 934–937

Fearon E and Vogelstein B (1990) A genetic model for colorectal tumorigenesis. *Cell* **61** 759–767

Fearon ER, Cho KR, Nigro JM *et al* (1990) Identification of a chromosome 18q gene that is altered in colorectal cancers. *Science* **247** 49–56

Fournier REK and Ruddle FH (1977) Microcell-mediated transfer of murine chromosomes into mouse, Chinese hamster, and human somatic cells. *Proceedings of the National Academy of Sciences of the USA* **4** 319–323

Francke U, Holmes LB, Atkins L and Riccardi VM (1979) Aniridia-Wilms' tumor association: evidence for specific deletion of 11p13. *Cytogenetics and Cell Genetics* **24** 185–192

Friend SH, Horowitz JM, Gerber MR *et al* (1986) Deletions of a DNA sequence in retinoblastomas and mesenchymal tumours: organisation of the sequence and its encoded protein. *Proceedings of the National Academy of Sciences of the USA* **84** 9059–9063

Fung YKT, Murphree AL, T'Ang A, Qian J, Hinrichs SH and Benedict WF (1987) Structural evidence for the authenticity of the human retinoblastoma gene. *Science* **236** 1657–1661

Gessler M, Poustka A, Cavenee W, Neve RL, Orkin SH and Bruns GAP (1990) Homozygous deletion in Wilms' tumour of a zinc-finger gene identified by chromosome jumping. *Nature* **343** 774–778

Goodrich D and Lee WH (1990) The molecular genetics of retinoblastoma. *Cancer Surveys* **9** 529–554

Harbour JW, Lai W-H, Whang-Peng J, Gazar AF, Minna JD and Kaye FJ (1988) Abnormalities in structure and expression of the human retinoblastoma gene in SCLC. *Science* **241** 353–357

Harris H, Miller OJ, Klein G, Worst P and Tachibana T (1969) Suppression of malignancy by cell fusion. *Nature* **223** 363–368

Heim S and Mitelman F (1989) Primary chromosome abnormalities in human neoplasia. *Advances in Cancer Research* **52** 2–44

Hong FD, Huang H-JS, To H *et al* (1989) Structure of the human retinoblastoma gene. *Pro-*

ceedings of the National Academy of Sciences of the USA **86** 5502–5506

Horowitz JM, Yandell DW, Park SH *et al* (1989) Point mutational inactivation of the retinoblastoma antioncogene. *Science* **243** 937–940

Huang H-JS, Yee J-K, Shew J-Y *et al* (1988) Suppression of the neoplastic phenotype by re-placement of the retinoblastoma gene product in human cancer cells. *Science* **242** 1563–1566

Huff V, Compton DA, Chao LY, Strong LC, Geiser CF and Saunders GF (1988) Lack of linkage of familial Wilms' tumour to chromosomal band 11p13. *Nature* **336** 377–378

Kern SE, Kinzler KW, Bruskin A *et al* (1991) Identification of p53 as a sequence-specific DNA-binding protein. *Science* **252** 1708–1711

Kinzler KW, Nilbert MC, Vogelstein B *et al* (1991) Identification of a gene located at chromosome 5q21 that is mutated in colorectal cancers. *Science* **251** 1366–1370

Koufos A, Hansen MF, Lampkin BC *et al* (1984) Loss of alleles at loci on human chromosome 11 during genesis of Wilms' tumour. *Nature* **309** 170–172

Knudson AG (1971) Mutation and cancer: statistical study of retinoblastoma. *Proceedings of the National Academy of Sciences of the USA* **68** 820–823

Knudson AG and Strong LC (1972) Mutation and cancer: a model for Wilms' tumor of the kid-ney. *Journal of the National Cancer Institute* **48** 313–324

Kugoh HM, Hashiba H, Shimizu M and Oshimura M (1990) Suggestive evidence for functional-ly distinct, tumor suppressor genes on chromosomes 1 and 11 for a human fibrosarcoma cell line, HT1080. *Oncogene* **5** 1637–1644

Laforgia S, Morse B, Levy J *et al* (1991) Receptor protein-tyrosine phosphatase γ is a candidate tumor suppressor gene of human chromosome region 3p21. *Proceedings of the National Academy of Sciences of the USA* **88** 5036–5040

Lee W-H, Shew J-Y, Hong F *et al* (1987a) The retinoblastoma susceptibility gene product is a nuclear phosphoprotein associated with DNA binding activity. *Nature* **329** 642–645

Lee W-H, Bookstein R, Hong F, Young L-J, Shew J-Y and Lee EY-HP (1987b) Human retinoblastoma susceptibility gene: cloning, identification, and sequence. *Science* **235** 1394–1399

Levine AJ (1990) Tumor suppressor genes. *Bioessays* **12** 60–66

Levine AJ, Momand J and Finlay CA (1991) The p53 tumour suppressor gene. *Nature* **351** 453–456

McBride OW and Ozer HL (1973) Transfer of genetic information by purified metaphase chromosomes. *Proceedings of the National Academy of Sciences of the USA* **70** 1258–1262

Malkin D, Li FP, Strong LC *et al* (1990) Germ line p53 mutations in a familial syndrome of breast cancer, sarcomas, and other neoplasms. *Science* **250** 1233–1238

Martinez J, Georgoff I, Martinez J and Levine AJ (1991) Cellular localization and cell cycle regulation by a temperature-sensitive p53 protein. *Genes and Development* **5** 151–159

Mercer WE, Shields MT, Amin M *et al* (1990) Negative growth regulation in a glioblastoma tumor cell line that conditionally expresses wild type p53. *Proceedings of the National Acad-emy of Sciences of the USA* **87** 6166–6170

Michalovitz D, Halevy O and Oren M (1991) p53 mutations: gains or losses? *Journal of Cellular Biochemistry* **45** 22–29

Mihara K, Cao X-R, Yen A *et al* (1989) Cell cycle-dependent regulation of phosphorylation of the human retinoblastoma gene product. *Science* **246** 1300–1303

Miller RW, Fraumeni JF and Manning MD (1964) Association of Wilms' tumour with aniridia, hemihypertrophy and other congenital abnormalities. *New England Journal of Medicine* **207** 922–927

Nigro JM, Baker SJ, Preisinger AC *et al* (1989) Mutations in the p53 gene occur in diverse tumour types. *Nature* **342** 705–708

Orkin SH, Goldman DS and Sallan SE (1984) Development of homozygosity for chromosome 11p markers in Wilms' tumour. *Nature* **309** 172–174

Oshimura M, Kugoh H, Koi M *et al* (1990) Transfer of a normal human chromosome 11 suppresses tumorigenicity of some but not all tumor cell lines. *Journal of Cellular Biochemistry* **42** 135–142

Peehl DM and Stanbridge EJ (1982) The role of differentiation in the control of tumorigenic expression in human cell hybrids. *International Journal of Cancer* **30** 113–120

Peto J and Easton D (1990) The contribution of inherited predisposition to cancer incidence. *Cancer Surveys* **9** 395–416

Ponder B (1988) Gene losses in human tumours. *Nature* **335** 400–402

Rauscher FJ, Morris JF, Tournay OE, Cook DM and Curran T (1990) Binding of the Wilms' tumor locus zinc finger protein to the EGR-1 consensus sequence. *Science* **250** 1259–1262

Raycroft L, Wu H and Lozano G (1990) Transcriptional activation by wild type but not transforming mutants of the p53 anti-oncogene. *Science* **249** 1049–1051

Reeve AE, Sih SA, Raizis AM and Feinberg AP (1989) Loss of heterozygosity at a second locus on chromosome 11 in sporadic Wilms' tumor cells. *Molecular and Cellular Biology* **9** 1799–1803

Sager R (1985) Genetic suppression of tumor formation. *Advances in Cancer Research* **44** 43–68

Sarnow P, Ho YS, Williams J and Levine AJ (1982) Adenovirus E1b-58kd tumor antigen and SV40 large tumor antigen are physically associated with the same 54 kd cellular protein in transformed cells. *Cell* **28** 387–394

Saxon PJ, Srivatsan ES, Leipzig GV, Sameshima JH and Stanbridge EJ (1985) Selective transfer of individual human chromosomes to recipient cells. *Molecular and Cellular Biology* **5** 140–146

Saxon PJ, Srivatsan ES and Stanbridge EJ (1986) Introduction of human chromosome 11 via microcell transfer controls tumorigenic expression of HeLa cells. *EMBO Journal* **15** 3461–3466

Scheffner M, Werness BA, Huibregtse JM, Levine AJ and Howley PM (1990) The E6 oncoprotein encoded by human papillomavirus types 16 and 18 promotes the degradation of p53. *Cell* **63** 1129–1136

Shih C, Padhy LC, Murray M and Weinberg RA (1981) Transforming genes of carcinomas and neuroblastomas introduced into mouse fibroblasts. *Nature* **290** 261–264

Shimizu M, Yokoto J, Mori N *et al* (1990) Introduction of normal chromosome 3p modulates the tumorigenicity of a human renal cell carcinoma cell line YCR. *Oncogene* **5** 185–194

Sotelo-Avila C, Gonzalez-Crussi F and Fowler JW (1980) Complete and incomplete forms of Beckwith-Wiedemann syndrome: their oncogenic potential. *Journal of Pediatrics* **96** 47–50

Stanbridge EJ (1976) Suppression of malignancy in human cells. *Nature* **260** 17–20

Stanbridge EJ (1985) A case for human tumor suppressor genes. *Bioessays* **3** 252–255

Stanbridge EJ (1989a) *The Genetic Basis of Tumor Suppression*, CIBA Symposium No 142, pp 149–159, John Wiley and Sons, New York

Stanbridge EJ (1989b) An argument for using human cells in the study of the molecular genetic basis of human cancer, In: Chadwick K, Seymour C and Barnhart B (eds). *Cell Transformation and Radiation-Induced Cancer*, pp 1–10, Adam Hilger, New York

Stanbridge EJ (1990) Human tumor suppressor genes. *Annual Review of Genetics* **24** 615–658

Stanbridge EJ and Dowdy SF (1991) Genetic heterogeneity in Wilms' tumor, In: Brandt ML (ed). *Hereditary Tumors,* vol 83, pp 141–151, Serono Symposia Publications, Italy

Stanbridge EJ, Dowdy SF, Latham KM, Muller MM and Gross MM (1989) Strategies for cloning human tumor suppressor genes, In: Cavenee W, Hastie N and Stanbridge EJ (eds). *Current Communications in Molecular Biology: Recessive Oncogenes and Tumor Suppression*, pp 189–196, Cold Spring Harbor Laboratory Press, Cold Spring Harbor, New York

Stehelin D, Varmus HE, Bishop JM and Vogt PK (1976) DNA related to transforming gene(s) of avian sarcoma viruses is present in normal avian DNA. *Nature* **260** 170–173

Stein GH, Beeson M and Gordon L (1990) Failure to phosphorylate the retinoblastoma gene product in senescent human fibroblasts. *Science* **249** 666–669

Tanaka K, Oshimura M, Kikuchi R, Seki M, Hayashi T and Miyaki M (1991) Suppression of tumorigenicity in human colon carcinoma cells by introduction of normal chromosome 5 or 18. *Nature* **349** 340–342

Templeton DJ, Park SH, Lanier L and Weinberg RA (1991) Nonfunctional mutants of the retinoblastoma protein are characterized by defects in phosphorylation, viral oncoprotein association, and nuclear tethering. *Proceedings of the National Academy of Sciences of the USA* **88** 3033–3037

Trent JM, Stanbridge EJ, McBride HL *et al* (1990) Tumorigenicity in human melanoma cell lines controlled by introduction of human chromosome 6. *Science* **247** 568–571

Tunnacliffe A, Parker M, Povey S *et al* (1983) Integration of Eco-gpt and SV40 early-region sequences into human chromosome 17: a dominant selection system in whole-cell and microcell human-mouse hybrids. *EMBO Journal* **2** 1577–1584

Varley JM, Armour J, Swallow JE *et al* (1989) The retinoblastoma gene is frequently altered leading to loss of expression in primary breast tumours. *Oncogene* **4** 725–729

Vogelstein B, Fearon ER, Hamilton SR *et al* (1988) Genetic alterations during colorectal-tumor development. *New England Journal of Medicine* **319** 525–532

Weissman BE, Saxon PJ, Pasquale SR, Jones GR, Geiser AG and Stanbridge EJ (1987) Introduction of a normal human chromosome 11 into a Wilms' tumor cell line controls its tumorigenic expression. *Science* **236** 175–180

Weith A, Martinsson T, Cziepluch C, Bruderlein S, Amler LC and Berthold F (1989) Neuroblastoma consensus deletion maps to 1p36 1-2. *Genes, Chromosomes and Cancer* **1** 159–166

Werness BA, Levine AJ and Howley PM (1990) Association of human papillomavirus types 16 and 18 E6 proteins with p53. *Science* **248** 76–79

Whyte P, Buchkovich KJ, Horowitz JM *et al* (1988) Association between an oncogene and an anti-oncogene: the adenovirus E1A proteins bind to the retinoblastoma gene product. *Nature* **334** 124–129

Xu G, Lin B, Tanaka D *et al* (1990) The catalytic domain of the neurofibromatosis type 1 gene product stimulates ras GTPase and complements ira mutants of S. cerevisiae. *Cell* **63** 835–841

Yamada H, Wake N, Fujimoto S, Barrett JC and Oshimura M (1990) Multiple chromosomes carrying tumor suppressor activity for a uterine endometrial carcinoma cell line identified by microcell-mediated chromosome transfer. *Oncogene* **5** 1141–1147

Yokota J, Akiyama T, Fung Y-KT *et al* (1988) Altered expression of the retinoblastoma (RB) gene in small-cell carcinoma of the lung. *Oncogene* **3** 471–475

Yunis JJ and Ramsay N (1978) Retinoblastoma and subband deletion of chromosome 13. *American Journal of Diseases of Children* **132** 161–163

The author is responsible for the accuracy of the references.

Interactions between p21^{ras} Proteins and Their GTPase Activating Proteins

P POLAKIS • F MCCORMICK

Cetus Corporation, 1400 53rd Street, Emeryville, California 94608

INTRODUCTION: PROPERTIES OF p21^{ras} PROTEINS AND THE DISCOVERY OF GTPase ACTIVATING PROTEIN (GAP)

p21^{ras} proteins are members of a large family of GTPases that share many structural properties and are involved in a variety of different biological functions (Bourne *et al*, 1990). The family includes proteins involved in membrane trafficking (the rab/YPT group) and in organization of the cytoskeleton (the rho group). p21^{ras} proteins themselves have been implicated in a variety of biological events: they are capable of transforming certain types of mammalian cells (eg fibroblasts, epithelial cells) and of causing differentiation or growth arrest in others (pheochromocytomas, Schwann cells). Mutant forms of p21^{ras} proteins have a causal role in the development of more than 30% of all human cancers (Bos, 1989). Recently, p21^{ras} proteins have been shown to interact with the product of the gene that causes neurofibromatosis type 1 (NF1: Ballester *et al*, 1990; Martin *et al*, 1990; Xu *et al*, 1990a). In *Saccharomyces cerevisiae*, they regulate adenylyl cyclase (see recent reviews in Gibbs and Marshall, 1989; Broach and Deschenes, 1990); in *Schizosaccharomyces pombe*, they are necessary for the mating response (Fukui *et al*, 1986; Nadin-Davis *et al*, 1986). In *Drosophila melanogaster*, they are involved in development of the eye (Bishop and Corces, 1988); in *Caenorhabditis elegans*, they are involved in development of the vulva (Beitel *et al*, 1990). In none of these cases is it clear how they elicit the appropriate response. This lack of understanding persists despite detailed structural analysis of a number of p21^{ras} proteins and a wealth

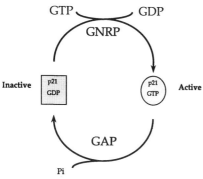

Fig. 1. Relation between the GTPase activating protein (GAP) and a guanine nucleotide releasing protein (GNRP) in regulating the activity of p21ras in vivo

of biochemical and biological information derived from study of p21ras mutants.

One critical aspect of p21ras function is clear, however: their activity is determined by guanine nucleotides. p21ras proteins cycle between active GTP bound forms and inactive GDP bound forms (Fig. 1). Interconversion of these forms depends on regulatory proteins that mediate exchange of GDP for GTP (guanine nucleotide releasing proteins, GNRPs) and hydrolysis of bound GTP to GDP (GTPase activating proteins, GAPs; Bourne *et al,* 1991).

The existence of such factors was suggested by analyzing properties of purified, recombinant p21ras proteins produced in *Escherichia coli:* we observed that the biochemical properties of the oncogenic aspartate-12 mutant of p21ras did not differ substantially from its wild type counterpart (Trahey *et al,* 1987). Therefore, the dramatic differences in biological activities of these isolated proteins could not be explained in terms of their measured biochemical properties. These findings led us to look for differences between these proteins in vivo rather than in vitro. Estimation of GTPase activities of normal and mutant p21ras proteins in *Xenopus* oocytes revealed the presence of a protein (GAP) that greatly stimulated normal p21ras GTPase activity but failed to affect oncogenic mutants (Trahey and McCormick, 1987). The ability of GAPs to downregulate oncogenic p21ras proteins but not oncogenic mutants accounted for their different biological potencies.

In this chapter, we discuss four topical aspects of GAP: firstly, the possibility that binding of GAP to p21ras is coupled to a signalling event, so that GAP itself could be thought to be part of the ras effector complex. Secondly, we summarize interactions between GAP and tyrosine phosphoproteins and suggest that GAP may provide a functional connection between signalling pathways involving p21ras proteins and tyrosine kinases. We then review recent evidence that the product of the gene responsible for NF1 is a second GAP for p21ras, and finally, we discuss the role of GAPs in the inhibition of ras function by the *ras* relative, Ki-*rev1/rap1.*

GAPs AS *ras* EFFECTORS

Shortly after the discovery of GAP activity in extracts from mammalian cells, the site on p21^{ras} with which GAP interacts was mapped (Adari *et al,* 1988; Calés *et al,* 1988). To our surprise, GAP seemed to bind to a site previously defined as the "effector binding site". Mutations in this region (aminoacids 32–42) had been shown to destroy the ability of v-Ha-*ras* to transform cells, without affecting guanine nucleotide binding or membrane localization (Sigal *et al,* 1986; Willumsen *et al,* 1986). These mutations therefore appeared to define a new domain, essential for ras effector function. Interaction with GAP at this critical site suggested that binding to GAP might be necessary for ras function, as well being necessary for its downregulation. According to this model, in normal cells, p21^{ras} interacts with GAP and sends a signal. This signal is terminated by subsequent hydrolysis of GTP to GDP, mediated by the effector itself, so that signalling and downregulation are intimately coupled together. In ras transformed cells, mutant p21^{ras} proteins bind GAP, send a signal, but signal transmission is not terminated.

A necessary prediction of this model was that oncogenic p21^{ras} mutants should indeed bind to GAP, and this was shown to be the case (Vogel *et al,* 1988). Oncogenic mutants do not escape from regulation by failing to bind GAP: in some cases, oncogenic mutants actually bind GAP much more tightly than their wild type counterparts. These observations are consistent with the hypothesis that GAP is part of an effector complex, but they do not prove that GAP is an effector of ras action: other cellular proteins may bind to p21^{ras} at a site that overlaps the GAP binding site, but, in binding, these other proteins fail to stimulate GTPase activity.

More direct support for the effector hypothesis came from analysis of a cell free system, in which a heterotrimeric G protein (referred to as Gk, or Gi-3) couples to a muscarinic receptor and activates a K channel (Yatani *et al,* 1990). In this system, application of agonist (carbachol) to the external face of the cell membrane results in GTP dependent channel opening. When agonist is removed, channel opening stops, with a $t_{1/2}$ of inactivation thought to be determined by the GTPase activity of the G protein. Evidence that this GTPase acts more slowly in vitro than in vivo prompted us to test whether GAP accelerated Gk-GTPase activity; this was not the case. However, addition of picomolar concentrations of recombinant GAP to the inside surface of the membrane had a totally unexpected effect: it caused uncoupling of the muscarinic receptor from Gk. Furthermore, this effect was ras dependent. We then found that addition of recombinant p21^{ras} proteins had the same effect as addition of GAP: they uncoupled the receptor, in this case in a GAP dependent manner. Oncogenic mutants of p21^{ras} were more effective than wild type p21^{ras}. Channel opening seemed to require interaction of p21^{ras} with GAP, suggesting a biochemical activity associated with the p21^{ras}/GAP complex. The biochemical basis of these effects is not yet understood. Perhaps GAP is an enzyme that generates second messengers in a p21^{ras} dependent fashion, and these second messengers may cause uncoupling of the muscarinic receptor from Gk. In any event, the demonstration of a function of the p21^{ras}/GAP complex clearly implies that GAP has activities additional to GTPase stimulation and supports its proposed role as a p21^{ras} effector. The real importance of these observations must await further understanding of the biochemical mechanism underlying receptor uncoupling. Genetic and biochemical analysis of RAS function in yeast argues strongly that the known GTPase activating proteins (IRA1 and IRA2) in this organism are not effectors for p21^{ras} action (Tanaka *et al*, 1989, 1990b, 1991). Disruption of these genes leads to upregulation of RAS function, apparently by constitutive activation of adenylyl cyclase. Thus, the ira1 phenotype resembles that of constitutively activated RAS. Expression of mammalian GAPs in ira1 mutants restores normal RAS function (Ballester *et al*, 1989; Tanaka *et al*, 1990a). It therefore appears that cyclase activation and RAS regulation by IRA proteins are separate and distinct events. Some caveats need to be considered, however. Firstly, the possibility that the adenyl cyclase complex has GAP activity has not been formally ruled out. Secondly, IRA proteins may have functions additional to their roles as RAS regulators. For instance, they could be RAS effectors that control pathways that have yet to be identified.

If GAP is indeed necessary for ras action in mammalian cells, it is clear that it does not act alone. This was shown by Zhang *et al* (1990b), who overexpressed GAP cDNAs in cells transformed by normal c-Ha-*ras* and observed reversion of the transformed phenotype in response to increased GAP expression. No reversion was seen when GAP was overexpressed in cells transformed by v-Ha-*ras*. These experiments confirm the role of GAPs as downregulators of normal ras, but show no signs of a signalling function. Therefore, we must conclude that if GAP has an effector function, it is not limiting with respect to this function. According to this interpretation, when GAP is overexpressed, other components of the signalling complex become limiting, so that GAP becomes uncoupled from its signalling activity and merely downregulates p21^{ras}. Another interpretation is raised by the discovery that cells have another type of GAP, encoded by the *NF1* gene (discussed below). GAP and NF1 protein may both be effectors, each coupled to distinct signalling pathways (Fig. 2). Overexpression of GAP would reduce the level of p21^{ras}·GTP, and so inhibit signalling via the NF1 pathway.

TYROSINE KINASES AND THEIR CONNECTION WITH p21^{ras} GAP SIGNALLING

Tyrosine kinases regulate many of the events associated with both the promotion and arrest of cell growth and division. Some of these kinases, such as the cell surface growth factor receptors, are responsible for initiating the mitogenic programme. The induction of cellular proliferation by p21^{ras} suggests that it may share common downstream elements with these tyrosine

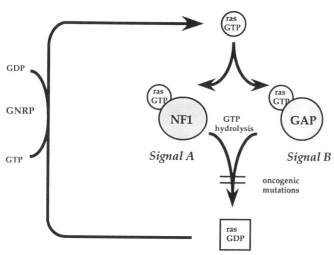

Fig. 2. Representation of the interactions of p21^ras with GAP and NF1 protein. The guanine nucleotide releasing protein (GNRP) promotes the formation GTP bound p21^ras which can then either bind GAP or NF1 protein, resulting in the production of distinct signals. Binding also results in the hydrolysis of GTP bound to wild type p21^ras but not to oncogenic p21^ras mutants

kinases in mitogenic signalling. In fact, there are several strong arguments in favour of a role for p21^ras in mediating signals initiated by tyrosine kinases. Among these are the findings that epidermal growth factor (EGF) and platelet derived growth factor (PDGF) induced proliferation of fibroblasts, insulin induced maturation of *Xenopus* oocytes and nerve growth factor (NGF) induced differentiation of PC-12 cells are all blocked by the microinjection of neutralizing antibodies to p21^ras (Mulcahy *et al*, 1985; Hagag *et al*, 1986; Korn *et al*, 1987). It has also been shown that p21^ras accumulates in the active GTP bound state in fibroblasts stimulated with PDGF, EGF or after their transformation by the v-*src* or *abl* oncogenes (Gibbs *et al*, 1990; Satoh *et al*, 1990a,b). Additionally, a dominant interfering mutant of p21^ras, K17N, prevented EGF induced DNA synthesis when overexpressed in fibroblasts (Cai *et al*, 1990). In all of these examples, p21^ras seems to be downstream from tyrosine kinases in mitogenic signalling pathways.

GAP and Receptor Tyrosine Kinases

In view of the strong implications for p21^ras in growth factor receptor signalling, it was encouraging to discover that GAP, a key regulator of p21^ras, associates with and is phosphorylated by activated tyrosine kinase receptors (Molloy *et al*, 1989; Anderson *et al*, 1990; Kaplan *et al*, 1990; Kazlauskas *et al*, 1990; Margolis *et al*, 1990). Furthermore, GAP association with the activated PDGF receptor correlates with receptor activity: a mutant receptor that fails to associate with GAP also fails to induce mitogenesis, even though the receptor phosphorylates itself and other substrates, including phospholipase C-gamma (Kaplan *et al*, 1990). This finding suggests that the association of GAP is essential for fulfilling the requirements of a complete mitogenic signal from the PDGF receptor.

Support for the essential role of GAP in PDGF receptor signalling comes from analysis of the function of this receptor in fibroblasts transformed by *ras* oncogenes. In these cells, PDGF fails to stimulate phospholipases C and A2 activity (Benjamin *et al*, 1987), even though the receptor undergoes normal PDGF dependent autophosphorylation and phospholipase C-gamma binding. However, GAP does not bind to activated receptors in these cells (Kaplan *et al*, 1990). This result could be because of modifications (eg phosphorylation) to GAP, the receptor or both. The effect could be less direct: ras transformation may stimulate GAP to associate with other cellular phosphoproteins (eg p190 and p62, as discussed below) in a manner that precludes its simultaneous association with the PDGF receptor. Alternatively, *ras* transformation may promote association of other proteins with the receptor that directly compete with GAP for binding. This effect could represent a feedback mechanism normally used by the receptor after signal transduction through p21^{ras}. In *ras* transformed cells, persistent signalling through p21^{ras} may result in persistent feedback, resulting in permanent abolition of GAP binding to the receptor.

The functional consequences of PDGF induced tyrosine phosphorylation on GAP are not clear. Speculation that phosphorylation reduces GAP activity towards p21^{ras} is appealing because it accounts for an accumulation of p21^{ras} in the GTP bound state. However, estimates of the stoichiometry of tyrosine phosphorylation seem to be too low to account for a substantial modulation of total cellular GAP activity. Even in the membrane fraction from PDGF stimulated cells, where the ratio of tyrosine phosphorylated GAP is highly enriched, only about 15–20% of the GAP molecules are phosphorylated (Molloy *et al*, 1989). If tyrosine phosphorylation completely inhibited GAP, a 15–20% loss of total GAP activity would be unlikely to lead to a substantial increase of p21^{ras} in the GTP bound state. We have also purified tyrosine phosphorylated GAP with an anti-phosphotyrosine affinity support and found that its specific activity was not detectably different from that of non-phosphorylated GAP (Clark R, McCormick F, unpublished). This is not to preclude the potential importance of tyrosine-phosphorylation on some aspect of GAP function, but its effect on GAP activity towards p21^{ras} seems to be marginal.

What then is the relevance of GAP binding to the activated PDGF receptor? Localization of GAP to the membrane through association with the receptor may serve to facilitate interaction with p21^{ras}. Experiments in our laboratory indicate that GAP, which is physically associated with the PDGF receptor, can still interact functionally with p21^{ras}. Purified recombinant GAP was incubated with plasma membranes containing the activated receptor. GAP associated with the membranes and was still able to stimulate the GTPase activity of added p21^{ras}. Membranes containing receptors that were not autophosphorylated also bound GAP, albeit less than activated receptors, but no recoverable GAP activity was found in these membranes. However, activity was recovered when the membranes were solubilized with detergent. These results suggest that the ability of GAP to localize to the plasma membrane in an active state is enhanced by the presence of autophosphorylated PDGF receptors. Thus, the PDGF receptor may permit GAP to approach the membrane bound p21^{ras} while remaining functionally active. By contrast, in the absence of activated receptors, GAP can only localize to the membrane as a reversibly inactivated species.

The finding that GAP can simultaneously associate with the PDGF receptor and interact with p21^{ras} is consistent with the structural regions of GAP proposed to be involved in these two processes. Mutational analysis of GAP indicates that the binding sites for p21^{ras} and the PDGF receptor are located in distinct parts of the GAP molecule. The association of GAP with the receptor has been demonstrated with several in vitro reconstitution systems. We have found that purified GAP specifically recognizes the autophosphorylated PDGF receptor immobilized on nitrocellulose after its transfer from an SDS-polyacrylamide gel. This system showed that GAP binds to the receptor directly and not through a protein intermediate. We have found with this same system that the aminoterminal region of GAP, containing the *src* homology (SH) domains, is necessary for binding to the immobilized receptor (Fig. 3). Moreover, immune complexes of TrpE fusion proteins containing the GAP-SH2 domain also bind PDGF receptors when exposed to lysates from cells pretreated with PDGF (Anderson *et al*, 1990). By contrast, the carboxyterminal 40 kDa fragment of GAP, which is sufficient for the stimulation of p21^{ras} GTPase activity (Marshall *et al*, 1989), fails to associate with the PDGF receptor (Fig. 3). Since GAP is capable of independent interactions with the PDGF receptor and with p21^{ras}, the two processes may function in a coordinated manner. Four potential outcomes of such an interaction are represented in Fig. 4. As noted above, the receptor may facilitate an interaction between GAP and p21^{ras} at the plasma membrane. In the simplest interpretation (Fig. 4a), this would result in a downregulation of p21^{ras}. This prediction is contrary to the observed increase of p21^{ras} in the GTP bound state after receptor stimulation (Gibbs *et al*, 1990; Satoh *et al*, 1990b). Alternatively, GAP may be a signalling molecule itself that requires interaction with both the receptor and p21^{ras} for signal output (Fig. 4b).

Association of GAP with the PDGF receptor may be necessary for receptor function: correct or efficient interaction may be p21^{ras} dependent (Fig. 4c). However, this possibility is difficult to reconcile with the observation that GAP fails to interact with the receptor in cells transformed by *ras* oncogenes. Finally, GAP may modulate activities of other proteins that bind to the PDGF receptor (phospholipase C-gamma, raf1, p60^{src} and phosphatidyl inositol 3'-kinase; reviewed by Ullrich and Schlessinger, 1990). If so, GAP's effects may be ras dependent (Fig. 4d).

In three of these scenarios (b, c and d), GAP is assumed to have positive effects on PDGF signalling, and these effects all require interaction of GAP with p21^{ras}. Because binding of GAP to p21^{ras} is known to be GTP dependent (Vogel *et al*, 1988), conditions that contribute to the accumulation of p21^{ras} in

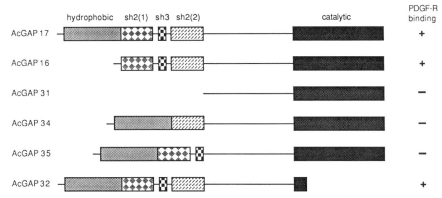

Fig. 3. The *src* homology domains of GAP bind to the PDGF receptor. The various regions of GAP, indicated above, were deleted, and the mutant proteins were tested for binding to the PDGF receptor. sh2 and sh3 indicate *src* homology domains. "Catalytic" refers to the region of GAP that independently stimulates the GTPase activity of p21^{ras}. The hydrophobic domain is of unknown function

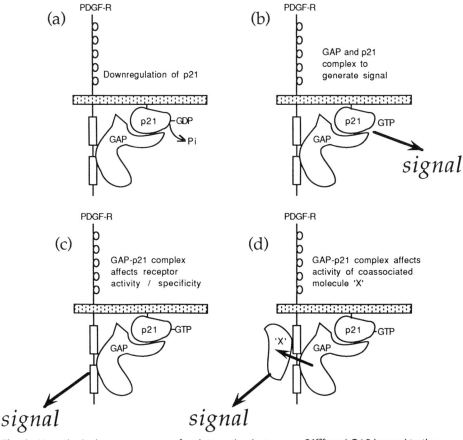

Fig. 4. Hypothetical consequences of an interaction between p21^{ras} and GAP bound to the PDGF receptor

the GTP bound state might also stimulate GAP-PDGF-receptor interactions. Recently, insulin treatment of fibroblasts has been shown to promote a rapid and dramatic accumulation of p21^{ras} in the GTP bound state (Boudewijn *et al*, 1991). This finding may explain the synergy between insulin and other growth factors in stimulating DNA synthesis (Rozengurt, 1986).

GAP and Non-receptor Tyrosine Kinases

In addition to the involvement of GAP with receptor tyrosine kinases, GAP might also provide a vital link in the mitogenic signalling of the so-called cytoplasmic tyrosine kinases. In fibroblasts transformed by *src*, *fps* and *abl* oncogenes, a substantial proportion of GAP is found in a stable complex with a phosphorylated 190 kDa polypeptide (Ellis *et al*, 1990). This complex is also rapidly formed in cells stimulated with EGF (Moran *et al*, 1991). On the basis of co-immunoprecipitation of p190 with GAP, we have estimated that 25–50% of the GAP in cells transformed by v-*src* is associated with this protein (Wong G and McCormick F, unpublished data). The p190 in the GAP immunocomplex contains a low level phosphorylated tyrosine and considerably higher levels of phosphoserine (Moran *et al*, 1991). Athough it is not clear whether phosphorylation of p190 is essential for GAP binding, treatment of the GAP-p190 immunocomplex with phosphatase promotes its dissociation (Moran *et al*, 1991).

The observation that transformation of fibroblasts with p60^{v-src}, or their stimulation with EGF, caused an accumulation of p21^{ras} in the GTP bound state suggested that overall GAP activity in these cells may be inhibited. Since these same conditions also promoted the formation of the GAP-p190 complex, it was conceivable that p190 inhibited GAP activity. A comparison of the specific activities of monomeric and p190 complexed GAP, resolved from lysates of cells transformed by v-*src*, revealed that p190-GAP was approximately fourfold lower (Moran *et al*, 1991). Binding of up to half the cellular GAP by p190 may be sufficient to promote the modest increase in GTP bound p21^{ras} observed in cells transformed by *src* (Satoh *et al*, 1990a). By contrast, p190 may not simply serve to inhibit GAP. The GAP-p190 complex may constitute a downstream effector for mediating p21^{ras} signals or p190 may also have a catalytic function of its own that is activated through a GAP-p21^{ras} interaction. This would require the simultaneous binding of GAP to p190 and p21^{ras}. This has already been demonstrated by showing that p190-GAP has some activity towards p21^{ras} (Moran *et al*, 1991). Moreover, we have found that the SH2 regions of GAP are sufficient for binding p190 (Martin G *et al*, unpublished), indicating that, as with the PDGF receptor, the "catalytic" region of GAP is not involved in this association.

In addition to binding p190, GAP also binds tightly to a 62 kDa protein that is highly phosphorylated on tyrosine in cells transformed by cytoplasmic tyrosine kinases (Ellis *et al*, 1990). p62 is one of the major substrates for protein tyrosine kinases in these cells. Furthermore, phosphorylation of p62 by a number of mutant tyrosine kinases correlated with the ability of these mutants to cause cellular transformation. For instance, v-*fps* mutants that lack functional SH2 domains were defective in both transformation and p62 phosphorylation, even though these mutants retained tyrosine kinase activity and normally phosphorylated a number of other cellular substrates (Koch *et al*, 1989) In a second study, non-transforming variants of BCR/*abl*, produced by mutating BCR sequences, failed to phosphorylate p62 even though these mutants were competent in both autophosphorylation and phosphorylation of other substrates (Muller *et al*, 1991). On the basis of their chromatographic behaviour, it is probable that GAP-p190 and GAP-p62 complexes are exclusive (Moran *et al*, 1991). This hypothesis can also be surmised from binding studies showing that, as with p190 and the PDGF receptor, it is the GAP-SH2 regions that are critical for its association with p62 (Martin G *et al*, unpublished). The functional outcome of GAP binding to p62 has not yet been defined. There does not seem to be an affect on GAP activity towards p21^{ras}, but there is some evidence indicating that p62 may localize GAP to a membrane compartment (Moran *et al*, 1991).

GAP AND *NF1*

The gene responsible for von Recklinghausen's neurofibromatosis (*NF1*) has recently been cloned (Cawthon *et al*, 1990; Viskochil *et al*, 1990; Wallace *et al*, 1990; Zhang *et al*, 1990a). *NF1* is characterized by abnormal proliferation of cells of neural crest origin. In its mildest form, this is manifest as "cafe-au-lait" spots: these are thought to be caused by abnormal growth of melanocytes. More severe forms consist of disfiguring neurofibromas, composed primarily, but not exclusively, of Schwann cells. *NF1* affects about 1 in 3500 people worldwide, and about half of these cases are the result of transmission of a defective *NF1* allele from an affected parent. In these cases, the disease seems to be inherited as an autosomal dominant trait. In the rest of the cases, spontaneous mutations occur in the *NF1* allele.

Molecular cloning of the *NF1* gene revealed a region of sequence similarity with GAP and yeast IRA proteins (the GAP related domain, NF1-GRD; Xu *et al*, 1990b). When expressed in *E coli*, yeast or insect cells, NF1-GRD is capable of stimulating p21^{ras} GTPase activity (Ballester *et al*, 1990; Martin *et al*, 1990; Xu *et al*, 1990a). Furthermore, NF1-GRD binds to p21^{ras} more tightly than does GAP: leucine-61 Ha-*ras* for instance binds to NF1-GRD with a K_d of about 5 nmol (Bollag and McCormick, 1991). This binding can be inhibited by relatively low concentrations of lipids, such as phosphatidyl-5,4-bisphosphate (PIP2) and phosphatidic acid (PA), whereas GAP is insensitive to these compounds at comparable concentrations. NF1 protein and GAP seem to be expressed ubiquitously. We have detected both NF1 and GAP activity in most cells and tissues by applying assay conditions that discriminate between the two activities (Bollag and McCormick, 1991).

These results raise several questions: firstly, which protein is responsible for regulating p21^{ras} activity, or do they both contribute to this function? For instance, after activation of T cells, ras p21 accumulates rapidly in the GTP bound state; this seems to be due to inhibition of GTPase activity rather than increase in nucleotide exchange. Is the change in GTPase activity due to inhibition of NF1 protein or GAP, or both? Clearly, if both were equally active in resting cells, inhibiting one activity would only change total GTPase activity by a factor of two: this is insufficient to allow significant accumulation of p21·GTP (McCormick *et al*, 1988). We must therefore conclude either that one form of GTPase activating protein (GAP or NF1 protein) is the major negative regulator of ras GTPase and is the target of inactivation during T cell activation or that both types of GAP are inhibited. Secondly, in cells containing oncogenic ras proteins, would NF1 protein or GAP be the primary target of interaction of these mutant proteins? The answer would seem to be NF1 protein, assuming that levels of NF1 protein are comparable to GAP. This is simply because ras proteins bind to NF1 protein much more tightly than to GAP, by a factor of more than 20 in most cases. If GAPs are also effectors, then it would seem that NF1 protein is a stronger candidate than GAP itself as a signalling molecule. Figure 2 shows a model in which both GAP and NF1 protein regulate p21^{ras} GTPase activity. In this model, p21·GTP may return to its inactive state via either pathway, the relative contribution of each pathway being determined by the activity of GAP and NF1 protein in cells, as well as by the concentration of ras p21·GTP. At high concentrations of p21^{ras}, the GAP pathway may be dominant, since GAP has a higher K_m than NF1 protein (Martin *et al*, 1990). In this model, we assume that interaction of ras p21 with GAP and NF1 protein generates two distinct signal outputs and that these signals are interdependent. For instance, inhibition of NF1, for example, by phospholipids, would increase signalling via the GAP pathway. Alternatively, overexpression of GAP would reduce the level of ras p21·GTP and thus prevent signalling via NF1. This could be the basis of the suppression of cellular transformation by GAP overexpression discussed above. Thirdly, what is the significance of NF1 protein's interaction with p21^{ras} in the context of neurofibromatosis? A simple model might be that a mutant *NF1* allele would fail to downregulate p21^{ras} and thus allow abnormal proliferation of cells through increased p21^{ras} signalling. However, mutations that have been identified so far in *NF1* alleles fall outside the GAP related domain and may not alter NF1/p21^{ras} interaction. In addition, activated *ras* proteins cause growth arrest in Schwann cells in vitro rather than abnormal proliferation. Finally, Schwann cells from NF1 patients may contain a normal *NF1* allele, as well as GAP itself, and may therefore have sufficient capacity to downregulate p21^{ras} in the absence of a defective *NF1* allele. All of these possibilities are under investigation. For example, although there is no genetic evidence for inactivation of the second *NF1* allele in neurofibromas (ie no evidence of reduction to homozygosity), this possibility cannot be excluded until this allele has been completely sequenced. Another model for *NF1* activation assumes that *NF1* is involved in signalling from p21^{ras}. Since ras p21·GTP is cytostatic in Schwann cells (Ridley *et al*, 1988), the signal would presumably be a negative regulator of proliferation. In this model, the signal output is defective or unregulated as a result of mutation, allowing for abnormal proliferation. The striking resemblance of NF1 protein to the yeast IRA proteins offers hope that studying the latter proteins with the power of yeast genetics may soon reveal new aspects of their function. Further insights into NF1 action will lead to a new level of understanding of *ras* genes themselves.

p21^{rap1}, rap1GAP, AND THEIR RELATIONSHIP TO p21^{ras} FUNCTION

Over 30 small GTPases with varying degrees of homology with p21^{ras} have been described (see recent reviews in Downward, 1990; Sanders, 1990). Many of these proteins have been characterized biochemically and all of these seem to possess relatively low intrinsic rates of GTP hydrolysis. These findings suggest that each will require a GTPase activating protein to convert active to inactive forms. However, the ability of rasGAP to stimulate GTP hydrolysis seems to be confined to the immediate *ras* family that includes the Ha-, Ki-, N- and R-*ras* gene products. NF1 protein probably has a similar specificity, although its ability to interact with R-*ras* has not yet been tested. GAP has been shown to bind to the p21^{rap1} without affecting its GTPase activity (Frech *et al*, 1990; Hata *et al*, 1990). p21^{rap1} protein is 53% identical to p21^{ras} (Pizon *et al*, 1988) and has an identical effector binding region. In the GTP bound state, p21^{rap1} binds to GAP with an affinity 10- to 100-fold higher than that of p21^{ras} (Frech *et al*, 1990; Hata *et al*, 1990). These results may explain why transfection of *ras* transformed fibroblasts with cDNA encoding p21^{rap1} results in suppression of the transformed phenotype (Kitayama *et al*, 1989): p21^{rap1} may act by competing with p21^{ras} for GAP, or perhaps NF1, binding. In a separate system, p21^{rap1} blocked *ras* induced germinal vesicle breakdown of *Xenopus* oocytes (Campa *et al*, 1991). Again, we can explain these observations by assuming that binding of GAP and/or NF1 is necessary for p21^{ras} and that p21^{rap1} acts as a competitive inhibitor of this interaction. It should be noted that proteins other than GAP and NF1 may interact at the "effector" binding domain of p21^{ras} and that these may be the true effectors of ras action: it is reasonable to assume that p21^{rap1} would also compete with p21^{ras} for binding to these proteins.

The suppressor activity of p21^{rap1} in the *ras* transformed cell is likely to be dependent on its binding GTP, as does its interaction with GAP. A mutation at position 12, known to reduce GTPase activity in p21^{ras}, results in a rap1 protein with increased suppressor activity (Kitayama *et al*, 1990). It is difficult to explain how this mutation could enhance the level of the GTP-bound form of p21^{rap1} since wild type p21^{rap1} already exhibits a strikingly low intrinsic GTP hydrolytic rate: in the order of 0.004/min (Frech *et al*, 1990). In view of this slow rate, and that the cell contains excess GTP over GDP, one would pre-

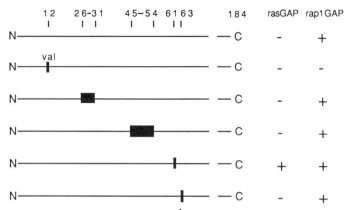

Fig. 5. Mutational analysis of p21^{rap1}. Mutants were generated containing either a G12V substitution or substitutions corresponding to aminoacids in the analogous position of p21^{ras} as indicated by the blocked areas. The purified mutant proteins were tested for stimulation of GTPase activity by rasGAP and rap1GAP

dict that wild type p21^{rap1} would exist predominantly in the GTP bound state in the cell. However, as is the case with p21^{ras,} there exists a GTPase activating protein that specifically stimulates the GTPase activity of p21^{rap1} (rap1GAP). Consistent with the enhanced suppressor activity of p21$^{rap1-val12}$, we have found that this mutant does not respond to stimulation by purified rap1GAP (Haubruck *et al*, 1991). By resisting stimulation by rap1GAP, p21$^{rap1-val12}$ would be maintained in the GTP-bound state and serve as a more effective antagonist of p21^{ras} function.

We have recently isolated rap1GAP, and cloned a cDNA expressing it (Rubinfeld *et al*, 1991). Surprisingly, the primary structure deduced from the cDNA shows no similarity to p21^{ras} GAP, suggesting that the two proteins may stimulate GTPase activity by completely different mechanisms. This was also suggested from our analysis of p21^{rap1} mutants containing the corresponding p21^{ras} residues in regions where the two proteins are divergent. Some of these mutants are shown schematically in Fig. 5. Substitution of p21^{ras} residues aminoterminal to position 60 had no affect on p21^{rap1} sensitivity to rap1GAP and it remained insensitive to rasGAP. This result showed that the aminoterminal regions of the proteins were interchangeable for GAP activation. Based on the crystal structure, the region of p21^{ras} between residues 59 and 65, referred to as loop four, was proposed to interact with p21^{ras} GAP (Krengel *et al*, 1990). Substituting p21^{rap1} residue 63 for the corresponding p21^{ras} residue did not substantially affect sensitivity to p21^{ras} GAP. However, substitution at position 61 resulted in a rap1 protein that was sensitive to both p21^{ras} GAP and rap1GAP. By contrast, mutations at position 61 in p21^{ras} are known to be transforming and render the protein insensitive to p21^{ras} GAP. Moreover, p21^{ras}, which contains glutamine at position 61, is not responsive to rap1GAP. These results show that the position 61 residue in p21^{ras} is critical for its sensitivity to p21^{ras} GAP and in fact can confer p21^{ras} GAP sensitivity to

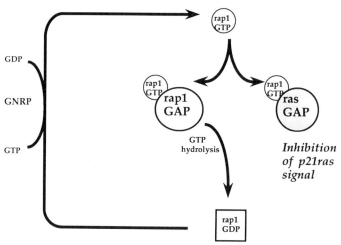

Fig. 6. Representation of the proposed inhibition of p21^{ras} signalling by p21^{rap1}. A specific guanine nucleotide releasing protein (GNRP) promotes the formation of p21^{rap1} GTP, which is either downregulated by rap1GAP or competes with p21^{ras} for binding to rasGAP

p21^{rap1}. However, position 61 in p21^{rap1} does not seem to be critical for its sensitivity to rap1GAP

If we assume that the role of rap1GAP is to convert p21^{rap1} GTP to p21^{rap1} GDP, then rap1GAP might indirectly enhance the activity of p21^{ras}. This hypothesis is based on the proposition that the ras transformation suppressor activity of p21^{rap1} is GTP dependent. A scheme outlining the possible interplay between p21^{ras}, p21^{rap1} and their GAPs is shown in Fig. 6. In this scenario, an interaction between p21^{ras} and p21^{ras} GAP would lead to a productive signal for growth as discussed in the first section of this chapter. However, competitive binding of p21^{rap1} to p21^{ras} GAP would preclude a productive interaction with p21^{ras}. rap1GAP would function by inactivating the competitor and facilitating p21^{ras}-rasGAP interaction. In the event that p21^{ras} GAP or NF1 protein are not downstream effectors t for p21^{ras}, a similar scenario involving competition of p21^{ras} and p21^{rap1} for the true effector would also apply.

Based on the scheme presented in Fig. 6, high levels of rap1GAP expression would be expected to contribute cell growth and division. We have examined the relative levels of rap1GAP in various cells and tissues using a polyclonal antibody raised against purified recombinant rap1GAP. The protein does not seem to be ubiquitously expressed and is present in highest amounts in developing tissues and certain cancer cell lines (Rubinfeld *et al*, 1991). Most intriguing is the high level of rap1GAP in undifferentiated HL60 cells. After their induced differentiation to a granulocytic cell, the immunoreactivity is strikingly reduced. We have also observed this decrease following differentiation of human erythroleukaemia cells. rap1GAP is also present in human fetal tissues at much higher levels than in the corresponding adult tissues. Notably, a Wilms' kidney tumour cell line, SK-NEP-1, contained substantial levels of immunoreactivity, but a second Wilms' tumor cell, G-401, as well as the human kidney 293 cell, did not contain detectable levels. These observations suggest that in certain cell types, rap1GAP may play a part in regulating cell proliferation, possibly by indirectly regulating p21^{ras}.

SUMMARY

Two proteins that regulate p21^{ras} GTPase activity have been identified. These proteins interact with a region of ras p21 that is necessary for p21^{ras} function and may themselves be components of signalling complexes. The first of these proteins to be identified, GAP, contains domains that interact with receptor tyrosine kinases and other tyrosine phosphoproteins, providing a direct link between signalling pathways involving these proteins and p21^{ras}. The second, the product of the *NF1* gene, is less well characterized but seems to connect p21^{ras} to other signalling pathways which are perturbed in the NF1 disease. The ability of p21^{ras} to interact with GAP may be compromised by competitive binding to the product of the Ki-*rev1* gene, p21^{rap1}. This competition for binding to GAP, or other proteins that interact with the effector site of ras p21, may explain the ability of Ki-*rev1* to suppress cellular transformation by *ras* oncogenes.

References

Adari H, Lowy DR, Willumsen BM, Der CJ and McCormick F (1988) Guanosine triphosphatase activating protein (GAP) interacts with the p21ras effector binding domain. *Science* **240** 518–521

Anderson D, Koch CA, Grey L, Ellis C, Moran MF and Pawson T (1990) Binding of SH2 domains of phospholipase C gamma 1 GAP, and Src to activated growth factor receptors. *Science* **250** 979–982

Ballester R, Michaeli T, Ferguson K, Xu HP, McCormick F and Wigler M (1989) Genetic analysis of mammalian GAP expressed in yeast. *Cell* **59** 681–686

Ballester R, Marchuk D, Boguski M *et al* (1990) The NF1 locus encodes a protein functionally related to mammalian GAP and yeast IRA proteins. *Cell* **63** 851–859

Beitel GJ, Clark SG and Horvitz HR (1990) *Caenorhabditis elegans ras* gene *let*-60 acts as a switch in the pathway of vulval induction. *Nature* **348** 503–509

Benjamin CW, Tarpley WG and Gorman RR (1987) Loss of platelet-derived growth factor-stimulated phospholipase activity in NIH-3T3 cells expressing the EJ-ras oncogene. *Proceedings of the National Academy of Sciences of the USA* **84** 546550

Bishop JG and Corces VG (1988) Expression of an activated *ras* gene causes developmental abnormalities in transgenic *Drosophila melanogaster*. *Genes and Development* **2** 567–577

Bollag G and McCormick F (1991) Differential regulation of ras GAP and neurofibromatosis gene product activities. *Nature* **351** 576–579

Bos JL (1989) ras oncogenes in human cancer: a review. *Cancer Research* **49** 4682–4689

Boudewijn MTB, Medema RH, Maassen JA *et al* (1991) p21Hras mediates insulin-induced gene expression in fibroblast cell lines. *EMBO Journal* (in press)

Bourne HR, Sanders DA and McCormick F (1990) The GTPase superfamily: a conserved switch for diverse cell functions. *Nature* **348** 125–132

Bourne HR, Sanders DA and McCormick F (1991) The GTPase superfamily: conserved structure and molecular mechanism. *Nature* **349** 117–127

Broach JR and Deschenes RJ (1990) The function of RAS genes in *Saccharomyces cerevisiae.* *Advances in Cancer Research* **54** 79–139

Cai H, Szeberényi J and Cooper GM (1990) Effect of a dominant inhibitory Ha-ras mutation on mitogenic signal transduction in NIH 3T3 cells. *Molecular and Cellular Biology* **10** 5314–5323

Calés C, Hancock JF, Marshall CJ and Hall A (1988) The cytoplasmic protein GAP is implicated as the target for regulation by the ras gene product. *Nature* **332** 548–551

Campa MJ, Chang K-G, Molina y Vedia L, Reep BR and Lapetina EG (1991) Inhibition of ras-induced germinal vesicle breakdown in Xenopus oocytes by rap-1B. *Biochemical and Biophysical Research Commununications* **174** 1–5

Cawthon RM, Weiss R, Xu GF *et al* (1990) A major segment of the neurofibromatosis type 1 gene: cDNA sequence, genomic structure, and point mutations. *Cell* **62** 193–201

Downward J (1990) The ras superfamily of small GTP-binding proteins. *Trends in Biochemical Sciences* **15** 469–472

Ellis C, Moran M, McCormick F and Pawson T (1990) Phosphorylation of GAP and GAP-associated proteins by transforming and mitogenic tyrosine kinases. *Nature* **343** 377–381

Frech M, John J, Pizon V *et al* (1990) Inhibition of GTPase activating protein stimulation of Ras-p21 GTPase by the Krev-1 gene product. *Science* **249** 169–171

Fukui Y, Kozasa T, Kaziro Y, Takeda T and Yamamoto M (1986) Role of a *ras* homolog in the life cycle of *Schizosaccharomyce pombe*. *Cell* **44** 329–336

Gibbs JB and Marshall MS (1989) The ras oncogene—an important regulatory element in lower eucaryotic organisms. *Microbioliological Reviews* **53** 171–185

Gibbs JB, Marshall MS, Scolnick EM, Dixon RA and Vogel US (1990) Modulation of guanine nucleotides bound to Ras in NIH3T3 cells by oncogenes, growth factors, and the GTPase activating protein (GAP). *Journal of Biological Chemistry* **265** 20437–20442

Hagag N, Halegoua S and Viola M (1986) Inhibition of growth factor-induced differentiation of PC12 cells by microinjection of antibody to ras p21. *Nature* **319** 680–682

Hata Y, Kikuchi A, Sasaki T, Schaber MD, Gibbs JB and Takai Y (1990) Inhibition of the ras p21 GTPase-activating protein-stimulated GTPase activity of c-Ha-ras p21 by smg p21 having the same putative effector domain as ras p21s. *Journal of Biological Chemistry* **265** 7104–7107

Haubruck H, Polakis P, McCabe P *et al* (1991) Mutational analysis of rap1/Krev protein; sensitivity to GTPase activating proteins and suppression of the yeast cdc24 budding defect. *Journal of Cellular Biochemistry* **138 (Supplement 15B)**

Kaplan DR, Morrison DK, Wong G, McCormick F and Williams LT (1990) PDGF beta-receptor stimulates tyrosine phosphorylation of GAP and association of GAP with a signaling complex. *Cell* **61** 125–133

Kazlauskas A, Ellis C, Pawson T and Cooper JA (1990) Binding of GAP to activated PDGF receptors. *Science* **247** 1578–1581

Kitayama H, Sugimoto Y, Matsuzaki T, Ikawa Y and Noda M (1989) A ras-related gene with transformation suppressor activity. *Cell* **56** 77–84

Kitayama H, Matsuzaki T, Ikawa Y and Noda M (1990) Genetic analysis of the Kirsten-*ras*-revertant 1 gene: potentiation of its tumor suppressor activity by specific point mutations. *Proceedings of the National Academy of Sciences of the USA* **87** 4284–4288

Koch CA, Moran M, Sadowski I and Pawson T (1989) The common src homology region 2 domain of cytoplasmic signaling proteins is a positive effector of v-fps tyrosine kinase function. *Molecular and Cellular Biology* **9** 4131–4140

Korn LJ, Siebel CW, McCormick F and Roth RA (1987) *Ras* p21 as a potential mediator of insulin action in *Xenopus* oocytes. *Science* **236** 840–843

Krengel U, Schlichting L, Scherer A *et al* (1990) Three-dimensional structures of H-ras p21 mutants: molecular basis for their inability to function as signal switch molecules. *Cell* **62** 539–548

Margolis B, Li N, Koch A, Mohammadi M *et al*(1990) The tyrosine phosphorylated carboxy-terminus of the EGF receptor is a binding site for GAP and PLC-gamma. *EMBO Journal* 9 4375–4380

Marshall MS, Hill WS, Ng AS *et al* (1989) A C-terminal domain of GAP is sufficient to stimulate ras p21 GTPase activity. *EMBO Journal* 8 1105–1110

Martin GA, Viskochil D, Bollag G *et al* (1990) The GAP-related domain of the neurofibromatosis type 1 gene product interacts with ras p21. *Cell* 63 843–849

McCormick F, Adari H, Trahey M *et al* (1988) Interaction of ras p21 proteins with GTPase activating protein. *Cold Spring Harbour Symposia on Quantitative Biology* 2 849–854

Molloy CJ, Bottaro DP, Fleming TP, Marshall MS, Gibbs JB and Aaronson SA (1989) PDGF induction of tyrosine phosphorylation of GTPase activating protein. *Nature* 342 711–714

Moran MF, Polakis P, McCormick F, Pawson T and Ellis C (1991) Protein-tyrosine kinases regulate the phosphorylation, protein interactions, subcellular distribution, and activity of p21ras GTPase activating protein. *Molecular and Cellular Biology* 11 1804–1812

Mulcahy LS, Smith MR and Stacey DW (1985) Requirement for *ras* proto-oncogene function during serum stimulated growth of NIH-3T3 cells. *Nature* 313 241–243

Muller AJ, Young JC, Pendergast A *et al* (1991) BCR first exon seqeunces specifically activate the BCR/ABL tyrosine kinase oncogene of Philadelphia chromosome-positive human leukemias. *Molecular and Cellular Biology* 11 1785–1792

Nadin-Davis SA, Nasim A and Beach D (1986) Involvement of *ras* in sexual differentiation but not in growth control in fission yeast *Schizosaccharomyce pombe*. *EMBO Journal* 5 2963–2972

Pizon V, Chardin P, Lerosey I, Olofsson B and Tavitian A (1988) Human cDNAs rap1 and rap2 homologous to the *Drosophila* gene Dras3 encode proteins closely related to *ras* in the "effector" region. *Oncogene* 3 201–204

Ridley AJ, Paterson HF, Noble M and Land H (1988) ras-mediated cell cycle arrest is altered by nuclear oncogenes to induce Schwann cell transformation. *EMBO Journal* 7 1635–1645

Rozengurt E (1986) Early signals in the mitogenic response. *Science* 234 161–166

Rubinfeld B, Munemitsu S, Clark R *et al* (1991) Molecular cloning of a GTPase activating protein specific for the Krev-1 protein p21rap1. *Cell* 65 1033–1042

Sanders DA (1990) A guide to low molecular weight GTPases. *Cell Growth & Differentiation* 1 251–258

Satoh T, Endo M, Nakafuku M, Akiyama T, Yamamoto T and Kaziro Y (1990a) Accumulation of p21ras·GTP in response to stimulation with epidermal growth factor and oncogene products with tyrosine kinase activity. *Proceedings of the National Academy of Sciences of the USA* 87 7926–7929

Satoh T, Endo M, Nakafuku M, Nakamura S and Kaziro Y (1990b) Platelet-derived growth factor stimulates formation of active p21ras GTP complex in Swiss mouse 3T3 cells. *Proceedings of the National Academy of Sciences of the USA* 87 5993–5997

Sigal IS, Gibbs JB, D'Alonzo JS and Scolnick EM (1986) Identification of effector residues and a neutralizing epitope of Ha-ras-encoded p21. *Proceedings of the National Academy of Sciences of the USA* 83 4725–4729

Tanaka K, Matsumoto K and Toh-e A (1989) IRA1, an inhibitory regulator of the RAS-cyclic AMP pathway in Saccharomyces cerevisiae. *Molecular and Cellular Biology* 9 757–68

Tanaka K, Nakafuku M, Satoh T *et al* (1990a) S cerevisiae genes IRA1 and IRA2 encode proteins that may be functionally equivalent to mammalian ras GTPase activating protein. *Cell* 60 803–807

Tanaka K, Nakafuku M, Tamanoi F, Kaziro Y, Matsumoto K and Toh-e A (1990b) IRA2, a second gene of Saccharomyces cerevisiae that encodes a protein with a domain homologous to mammalian ras GTPase-activating protein. *Molecular and Cellular Biology* 10 4303–4313

Tanaka K, Lin BK, Wood DR and Tamanoi F (1991) IRA2, an upstream negative regulator of RAS in yeast, is a RAS GTPase-activating protein. *Proceedings of the National Academy of Sciences of the USA* 88 468–472

Trahey M and McCormick F (1987) A cytoplasmic protein stimulates normal N-ras p21 GTPase, but does not affect oncogenic mutants. *Science* **238** 542–545

Trahey M, Milley RJ, Cole GE *et al* (1987) Biochemical and biological properties of the human N-ras p21 protein. *Molecular and Cellular Biology* **7** 541–544

Ullrich A and Schlessinger J (1990) Signal transduction by receptors with tyrosine kinase activity. *Cell* **61** 203–212

Viskochil D, Buchberg AM, Xu G *et al* (1990) Deletions and a translocation interrupt a cloned gene at the neurofibromatosis type 1 locus. *Cell* **62** 187–192

Vogel US, Dixon RA, Schaber MD *et al* (1988) Cloning of bovine GAP and its interaction with oncogenic ras p21. *Nature* **335** 90–93

Wallace MR, Marchuk DA, Andersen LB *et al* (1990) Type 1 neurofibromatosis gene: identification of a large transcript disrupted in three NF1 patients. *Science* **249** 181–186

Willumsen BM, Papageorge AG, Kung HF *et al* (1986) Mutational analysis of a *ras* catalytic domain. *Molecular and Cellular Biology* **6** 2646–2654

Xu GF, Lin B, Tanaka K *et al* (1990a) The catalytic domain of the neurofibromatosis type 1 gene product stimulates ras GTPase and complements ira mutants of S cerevisiae. *Cell* **63** 835–841

Xu GF, O'Connell P, Viskochil D *et al* (1990b) The neurofibromatosis type 1 gene encodes a protein related to GAP. *Cell* **62** 599–608

Yatani A, Okabe K, Polakis P, Halenbeck R, McCormick F and Brown AM (1990) ras p21 and GAP inhibit coupling of muscarinic receptors to atrial K+ channels. *Cell* **61** 769–776

Zhang K, DeClue JE, Vass WC, Papageorge AG, McCormick F and Lowy DR (1990a) Suppression of c-ras transformation by GTPase-activating protein. *Nature* **346** 754–756

The authors are responsible for the accuracy of the references.

The Retinoblastoma Gene and Gene Product

ROBERT A WEINBERG

Whitehead Institute for Biomedical Research, Cambridge, Massachusetts 02142

Introduction
Isolation of the *RB* gene
Involvement of the *RB* gene in tumours
Biology of pRB function
pRB and viral oncoproteins
A model of pRB action
Summary

INTRODUCTION

Study of the rare eye tumour retinoblastoma would seem to offer insights confined to a unique, highly specialized mechanism of tumour pathogenesis. But results of the past 5 years have shown otherwise: the *RB* gene, which is centrally involved in the formation of retinoblastomas, has proven to be at the centre of a growth controlling machinery that is critical to many cell types throughout the body, and its inactivation underlies the creation of a variety of common tumours. Further, aspects of *RB* gene function have implications for a number of areas of cancer biology, including the pathogenetic mechanisms exploited by DNA tumour viruses.

Historically, the genetics of familial susceptibility to retinoblastoma led the way towards defining a paradigm that is now applied to a rapidly increasing cohort of tumour suppressor genes, many of which are described in this issue. The peculiarities of retinoblastoma greatly facilitated these pioneering studies. The tumour is of early onset, occurring from birth up to the age of 6 or 7 years, and its diagnosis is usually straightforward and unambiguous—individual foci of incipient tumours can be visualized and counted through the ophthalmoscope without resort to invasive surgery. The usually rare tumour (1 in 20 000 live births) can occur in familial clusters, where its incidence would suggest the involvement of a discrete Mendelian allele having strong but not total penetrance.

These familial cases were first observed a century ago, when cure of childhood retinoblastoma made possible the survival into adulthood of genetically afflicted individuals who could then pass heritable disease susceptibility on to offspring (DeGouvea, 1886; Dunphy, 1964). Such familial cases of retino-blastoma presented as multifocal tumours involving both eyes. In this respect, they contrasted with another form of retinoblastoma, known as the "sporadic" form of the disease, in which a single tumour focus involves one or the other eye and there is no suggestion of a familial disease history. Children with this form of retinoblastoma do not pass on the disease susceptibility trait to their offspring.

Confronting these two forms of the disease, Alfred Knudson postulated in 1971 that both forms of the disease require two genetic alterations in order for tumour formation to begin (Knudson, 1971). In the sporadic form of the disease, he argued, two genetic lesions, both occurring as somatic mutations, are sustained in the genome of a single retinal precursor cell, which then proceeds to spawn a tumour focus. Upon studying the kinetics and multiplicity of tumours in familial cases, he proposed that one of the two required mutations was already present in the genome of the conceptus and thus carried in the genomes of all cells of the target organ, the retina. In these cases, only a single somatic mutation needed to occur in order for one or another retinal cell to reach the doubly mutated configuration that triggered outgrowth of a tumour focus.

In fact, the term "familial retinoblastoma" is not the most appropriate description for these cases. To be sure, it includes the cases involving children who have inherited a mutant allele from a similarly afflicted parent. But more often than not, the mutant allele present in the fertilized egg has arisen de novo during gametogenesis in a genetically normal parent, usually the father (Dryja et al, 1989; Toguchida et al, 1989; Zhu et al, 1989). Accordingly, "familial" retinoblastoma includes those cases in which recent germinal mutations result in a child carrying a "constitutional" mutation in his or her genome.

Knudson's early work shed no light on either the genes affected in this process or the nature of the mutations that precipitate disease. Clues to this came later, initially through cytological studies that revealed the deletion of chromosomal material surrounding and including the q14 band of chromosome 13 in some retinoblastomas (Yunis and Ramsey, 1978). Such interstitial deletions suggested the involvement of a gene mapping to this chromosomal region, loss of which was critical to tumorigenesis. These deletions could be observed in only a small proportion of tumours, yet one could surmise that more subtle mutations affecting this gene might be present in the remaining tumours but escape detection because they resulted in only sub-microscopic alteration of the chromosome.

The 13q14 gene was termed *RB*. The hypothesis that this gene represented the first of Knudson's postulated targets provided no clear indication of the nature of the second target. One educated guess identified the second, surviving *RB* gene copy present on the homologous chromosome as the second target gene. According to such speculation, Knudson's two mutational events represented the successive elimination of the two copies of *RB*.

This particular model was vindicated in 1983 when it was shown that the chromosomal region associated with the *RB* gene often undergoes a conversion to homozygosity in tumour cells (Benedict *et al*, 1983; Cavenee *et al*, 1983; Godbout *et al*, 1983; Sparkes *et al*, 1983; Dryja *et al*, 1984; Gilbert, 1986). This reduction to homozygosity, or the equivalent loss of heterozygosity, was proposed as a means of eliminating the surviving wild type *RB* allele following mutational inactivation of the first one. If the 13q14 chromosomal region carrying the wild type allele were discarded and replaced with a duplicated copy of the homologous region bearing the mutant allele, the cell would lose both functional *RB* genes. As an alternative, independent somatic mutations of the surviving wild type allele could intervene to inactivate the second *RB* gene copy, but this particular sequence of events occurs with much lower probability per cell generation.

Most important is the final consequence of these accumulated germinal and somatic mutational events—the total elimination of *RB* gene function. Such an endpoint made it apparent that the *RB* gene acts in normal cells to limit or suppress growth; its loss would seem to deprive a cell of the ability to brake or shut down its own proliferation. Because children who are constitutionally hemizygous for *RB* are essentially normal developmentally, it is clear that the single copy of the wild type gene present in virtually all of their cells suffices to program normal cell growth. In this sense, the mutant, inactive *RB* allele present in their cells is recessive in its effects on the proliferation of individual cells, although its presence in the conceptus virtually assures (with 90% penetrance) that the organism as a whole will sustain one or more retinal tumours. Such a high rate of tumorigenesis in heterozygous children derives from the large size of the retinal target cell population and the probability per cell division that one or another of these cells will lose its single intact *RB* gene copy. To summarize, a mutant, null *RB* allele functions recessively at the cellular level but acts dominantly at the level of the whole organism.

ISOLATION OF THE *RB* GENE

The *RB* gene was isolated by molecular cloning in 1986 (Friend *et al*, 1986) and shown to encompass 200 kb of human chromosome 13 (Hong *et al*, 1989; McGee *et al*, 1989). The initial identification depended on detection of deletions involving large segments of this gene that were present in a small group of tumour DNAs and could be visualized by means of Southern blotting analysis. However, it soon became apparent that the majority of inactive, tumour associated *RB* alleles had lost function through subtle alterations, specifically point mutations. A number of these have been catalogued to date (Fung *et al*, 1987; Lee *et al*, 1987a; Dunn *et al*, 1988; Canning *et al*, 1989; Dunn *et al*, 1989; Horowitz *et al*, 1989; Yandell *et al*, 1989; Gallie *et al*, 1990; Kaye *et al*, 1990). Many affect splice donor or acceptor sequences and wreak havoc because of the attendant deletion of entire exons from the processed *RB* mRNA. In addition, several mutations in the reading frame creating missense and nonsense mutations have been documented. These various point mutations, which create the great majority of tumour associated *RB* alleles, are apparently as effective in knocking out gene function as the initially detected gross deletions. Loss of a segment from the transcriptional promoter of the *RB* gene also serves to inactivate this gene (Huang *et al*, 1988).

Although this catalogue of tumour associated mutations would seem to provide compelling genetic proof that the cloned DNA sequence indeed represents the long sought *RB* gene, an even more convincing demonstration might come from functional testing of the cloned gene. For example, since retinoblastoma cells and other tumour cell types (see below) appear to owe their growth deregulation to loss of *RB* gene function, reintroduction of an intact *RB* allele into these cells should lead to restoration of more normal growth control. The resulting reversion of these cells to a more normal phenotype would represent a striking proof that the introduced sequence is indeed identical with the *RB* gene. Moreover, it would open the door to a new form of anti-tumour treatment in which malignant cell growth could be controlled if not reversed by gene therapy.

These experiments have proved highly successful in the hands of some. Thus, use of retrovirus transducing vectors has made it possible to introduce cDNA copies of the wild type *RB* gene into large numbers of retinoblastoma, sarcoma and prostate carcinoma cells. The cells respond with some inhibition of growth in vitro and a profound loss of tumorigenicity in vivo (Huang *et al*, 1988; Bookstein *et al*, 1990a). Yet others have found that cloned *RB* gene copies are strongly growth suppressive for both Rb$^+$ and Rb$^-$ cell lines in vitro and that this suppression is so profound that cell growth can in practice not be tested in vivo (Fung Y-K T, personal communication; Weinberg RA, unpublished). Perhaps a well regulated cloned *RB* gene rather than one driven by a strong constitutive transcriptional promoter will yield cells that have lost tumorigenicity without loss of in vitro growth potential. These discrepancies in experimental results will likely be sorted out in coming years. In any event, it is apparent that these initial successes at reversion represent strong support for the candidacy of the cloned gene as the essential regulator of cell growth that is lost during retinoblastoma pathogenesis.

The mutations of the *RB* gene found in tumour cell genomes affect the ability of the cell to synthesize an intact *RB* gene product, termed here pRB and now known to be a 105–110 kDa nuclear phosphoprotein (Friend *et al*, 1987; Lee *et al*, 1987b). This protein is encoded by an mRNA that is synthesized through the joining of 27 exons present in the primary transcript of the 200 kb gene. The encoded aminoacid sequence gives few clues to function. There have been suggestions of leucine zipper and zinc finger domains, but it remains unclear whether these various sequences have such roles in the active protein (Lee *et al*, 1987b; Bernards *et al*, 1989). The nuclear localization of pRB suggests a role in replication or transcriptional control, but, as discussed below, little beyond this is apparent from data available until now. The presence of a DNA binding domain, which is usually not altered by mutations, may signal the ability of pRB to interact physiologically with DNA, perhaps even on a sequence specific basis (Wang *et al*, 1990).

INVOLVEMENT OF THE *RB* GENE IN TUMOURS

The use of *RB* DNA probes and anti-pRB antibodies has made it possible to survey *RB* gene expression in a variety of organisms and tissues (Bernards *et al*, 1989). The gene would seem to be present in all chordates. Its widespread if not ubiquitous expression in a variety of tissues would suggest an essential role in growth regulation in virtually all cell types. This is hard to reconcile with the much smaller catalogue of tissue types in which *RB* inactivation seems to contribute to tumorigenesis.

The list of tumour types that do indeed carry inactive *RB* alleles extends far beyond the initially characterized retinoblastomas but still represents only a small sampling of the cell types in the body. Initial use of DNA probes showed that sarcomas, notably osteosarcomas, figure prominently (Friend *et al*, 1987; Weichselbaum *et al*, 1988; Reissmann *et al*, 1989; Shew *et al*, 1989). This was no surprise, since children cured of retinoblastomas early in life but carrying constitutional *RB* mutations have long been known to have greatly increased risk for these connective tissue tumours in their later years (DerKinderen *et al*, 1988).

More surprising was the discovery, made through use of DNA and antibody probes, that *RB* alleles are lost in some prostate carcinomas, perhaps a third of bladder and mammary carcinomas and virtually all small cell lung cancers. These epithelial tumours are not known to threaten children carrying constitutional *RB* mutations. The involvement of *RB* in these common cancers must occur almost exclusively as a consequence of somatic mutations (Harbour *et al*, 1988; Lee *et al*, 1988; T'Ang *et al*, 1988; Yokota *et al*, 1988; Bookstein *et al*, 1989, 1990b; Varley *et al*, 1989; Horowitz *et al*, 1990).

Presently available data provide no means for rationalizing the peculiar set of target tissues that are affected by germline and somatic *RB* mutations. These various target cell types are not allied through common developmental or evolutionary origins, and attempts at explanation invariably fall back on vague models which argue that *RB* gene loss is rate limiting in tumour pathogenesis in certain cell types but not in others. Thus, some cell types may be protected from transformation by multiple, redundant mechanisms that succeed in maintaining a normal growth program even in the face of *RB* inactivation. Yet another model would state that *RB* inactivation is lethal to certain cell types; as a consequence, tissues composed of these cells never originate *RB*-nullizygous tumours.

RB specific DNA probes have proven to be useful tools in human genetic diagnosis. Thus, the presence of mutant *RB* alleles can be traced through certain families and ascertained even in fetal tissues through amniocentesis or chorionic villus sampling. Regrettably, these genetic diagnoses have proven to be most laborious, since each family studied carries a novel mutant allele, often created by a point mutation that is detectable only after painstaking survey of the 27 *RB* exons and flanking splice regulating sequences (Cavenee *et al*, 1986; Yandell *et al*, 1989).

BIOLOGY OF pRB FUNCTION

For the cell biologist, the interest attached to the *RB* gene centres on its encoded protein and the mechanisms through which it normally regulates cell proliferation. At the level of cell physiology, one might propose that pRB acts as a transducer of extracellular signals into the cell nucleus. These extracellular signals may normally serve to induce a cell to stop proliferating so that it will conform to the developmental and physiologic requirements of the surrounding tissue. When these afferent anti-mitogenic signals reach the nucleus, pRB may act to process and transduce them, releasing efferent signals that ultimately cause a shutdown of cell growth. By this logic, a cell that has lost pRB function will continue to receive afferent growth inhibitory signals but will lose the ability to respond to them appropriately, leading in turn to the inappropriate proliferation of cancer.

Such broad biological models require detailed verification at the molecular level. Here, the clues are tantalizing but still few in number. One apparently important clue has been provided by the observation that the state of phosphorylation of pRB is modulated in concert with passage of the cell through its growth cycle. Thus, pRB is seen as a relatively underphosphorylated molecule when it is prepared from cells in the G_1 phase of the cell cycle. A hyperphosphorylated form of pRB, which migrates more slowly on gel electrophoresis, is seen in S, G_2 and M phase cells (Buchkovich *et al*, 1989; DeCaprio *et al*, 1989; Ludlow *et al*, 1990).

This behaviour is compatible with the phosphorylation of pRB occurring during the G_1/S transition, perhaps at the hands of a cdc2 like, cyclin regulated kinase. There are more than half a dozen sites of pRB phosphorylation, all involving serine (or threonine) residues, and the primary sequence of pRB contains a number of sites that could represent substrates for cdc2 kinase (Templeton *et al*, 1991). The G_1/S phosphorylation of pRB may then alter its functioning, perhaps placing it in a state where it permits progression of the cell through further steps in its growth cycle.

This programmed modulation of pRB phosphorylation is correlated with the behaviour of pRB on cell fractionation. The phosphorylated form of pRB seen in S, G_2 and M cells is found in the cytoplasmic supernate on cell lysis in low ionic strength buffer, whereas the underphosphorylated form(s) of pRB in G_1 cells is bound tightly to some unidentified nuclear structure (Mittnacht and Weinberg, 1991; Templeton *et al*, 1991). This suggests that the observed phosphorylation regulates association of pRB with some nuclear partner protein and that binding to this partner serves to tether pRB tightly to the nuclear structure.

The importance of this particular interaction is underscored by analysis of mutant pRB proteins present in a variety of tumour cell lines. All have lost their ability to become tightly tethered to this nuclear anchor (Mittnacht and Weinberg, 1991; Templeton *et al*, 1991). The simplest, although hardly exclusive, interpretation of this finding is that the association of pRB with its nuclear anchor is critical to its growth suppressing powers and that tumour cells gain growth advantage when this binding is disrupted through alterations of pRB structure. Moreover, since tight RB binding to this anchor is lost on G_1/S phosphorylation, this might suggest that the phosphorylated form of pRB is inactive in suppressing growth.

But this "nuclear anchor" may represent only the tip of a much more complex iceberg. One domain of pRB has been synthesized in large amounts by recombinant technology and used as an affinity reagent to identify and isolate cellular proteins that specifically bind to pRB. As many as ten distinct polypeptide species have been found that bind to this pRB fragment but fail to bind to mutant versions (Huang *et al*, 1991; Kaelin *et al*, 1991). This suggests that pRB mediated growth regulation may in fact involve direct interactions with a large, diverse constituency of partner proteins, only one of which is the previously mentioned anchoring protein.

pRB AND VIRAL ONCOPROTEINS

An independent line of work in an ostensibly unrelated research area has converged unexpectedly and dramatically with these studies of pRB function. This research documents the ability of DNA tumour virus oncoproteins to form complexes with pRB in virus transformed cells and is described in detail in three other chapters in this issue. In short, the E1A oncoprotein of human adenovirus type 5, the large T oncoprotein (LT) of simian virus 40 (SV40) and the E7 oncoproteins of human papillomavirus types 16 and 18 are each able to bind directly to the pRB present in virus transformed cells (DeCaprio *et al*, 1988; Dyson *et al*, 1989, 1990; Whyte *et al*, 1988, 1989).

This direct confrontation between viral growth promoting proteins and the cell's growth constraining pRB, first uncovered in 1988, suggests a simple model of how these oncoproteins are able to induce cellular transformation. By binding to pRB, each of these may compromise or inactivate pRB function. In doing so, these oncoproteins may liberate the cell from the growth constraints imposed by pRB.

This most attractive model remains only a speculation. A proof that pRB activity is indeed neutralized following association with viral oncoproteins will come only after pRB function is elucidated through in vivo and in vitro assays. Further, any attempts at understanding the functional consequences of oncoprotein:pRB association are complicated by the fact that each of these oncoproteins also seeks out other alternative cellular targets. For example, adenovirus E1A protein seeks out and forms complexes with at least six other cellular proteins in addition to pRB (Yee and Branton, 1985; Harlow *et al*, 1986). Consequently, it becomes arbitrary to attribute any specific biological change elicited by wild type E1A to alteration of pRB rather than to another of these cellular targets. Mutant forms of E1A, engineered through directed mutagenesis, has been found to lose selectively the affinity for some of these cell proteins and to show a concomitant loss in one or another biological function (Egan et al, 1988; Jelsma et al, 1989; Whyte et al, 1989; Howe et al, 1990; Stein RW et al, 1990). These results provide good clues to the biological roles of some of these targets and to the consequences of their alteration by E1A.

The ability of the viral oncoproteins to associate with pRB has provided a powerful experimental tool for studying pRB function. pRB domains that are involved in oncoprotein binding have been defined through direct mutagenesis of RB cDNA clones (Hu et al, 1990; Kaelin et al, 1990). The residues of pRB involved in E1A, LT and E7 binding are clustered in large part in two distinct polypeptide domains that presumably lie in close juxtaposition in the native pRB. The oncoprotein binding site that they form would seem to fit in a lock and key fashion with a complementary domain that is shared in common by the three viral proteins. Indeed, the regions of the viral proteins involved in pRB binding contain certain residues in common and are presumed to present a similar steric conformation to their pRB partner on binding (Figge et al, 1988).

A number of mutant pRB proteins derived from a variety of human tumours have been shown to have lost their ability to complex with E1A or SV40 LT (Shew et al, 1990). This includes mutant pRB forms that differ from wild type structure by only a single aminoacid replacement (Kaye et al, 1990; Templeton et al, 1991). This is a striking and puzzling finding because neither E1A nor LT is present in the cells that serve as precursors to these tumours. As such, it is hardly apparent how loss of the ability of pRB to bind these viral proteins could confer growth advantage on an evolving tumour cell clone.

One solution to this puzzle is provided by a model which states that these viral oncoproteins mimic the structure of a cellular protein(s), binding to which is critical to the growth suppressing powers of pRB. Mutations occurring in tumour cells may alter the binding pocket of pRB and affect simultaneously its association with both the viral oncoproteins and the similarly structured cell protein(s). Having lost the ability to bind to this cellular protein(s), pRB would lose its ability to shut down cell growth. By extension, the ability of the viral oncoproteins to bind pRB may preempt its association with the endogenous E1A-like partner protein.

The importance of this pRB oncoprotein binding pocket is underscored by some of the results presented earlier. It would seem that the nuclear tethering of pRB is mediated in large part through this pRB domain, since single aminoacid substitutions in this region cause pRB to be released into the cytoplasmic fraction on cell lysis (Mittnacht and Weinberg, 1991; Templeton et al, 1991). Moreover, it was this domain of pRB which, as a recombinant product, served as the affinity reagent for binding multiple cellular proteins in the previously mentioned experiments; conversely, mutant forms of this domain failed to attract these cellular binding partners (Huang et al, 1991; Kaelin et al,

1991). Taken together, these various lines of evidence indicate that the integrity of this domain is essential for binding of pRB to various viral oncoproteins as well as to multiple cellular proteins.

One other set of observations further refines our understanding of pRB function. Observations with SV40 LT showed that this viral protein binds exclusively to the underphosphorylated form of pRB, ie that form present in G_1 cells (Ludlow *et al*, 1989). The adenovirus E1A and human papillomavirus E7 oncoproteins show a similar preference (Templeton DJ, Hinds P and Weinberg RA, unpublished; Howley P, personal communication). These various data suggest that the viral oncogene proteins can accomplish their task— deregulation of cellular growth control—by focusing their attention exclusively on the underphosphorylated form of pRB. This implies that the underphosphorylated G_1 form of pRB is active in growth control, whereas the hyperphosphorylated S, G_2, M form may be physiologically inert.

In consonance with this are observations of pRB phosphorylation in growing and quiescent cells (Chen *et al*, 1989; Furukawa *et al*, 1990). For example, the pRB of resting lymphocytes, which is underphosphorylated, undergoes extensive phosphorylation upon stimulation with a phytohaemagglutinin. Conversely, the largely phosphorylated pRB present in rapidly growing HL60 promyelocytic leukaemia cells loses its phosphate groups when these cells are induced to enter a non-mitotic, endstage differentiation pathway. Yet another line of research reports the dephosphorylation of pRB when cells enter into senescence (Stein GH *et al*, 1990). Since phosphorylation of pRB is correlated with active growth, this would suggest, as before, that the underphosphorylated form is used by cells to constrain growth.

An apparently contradictory finding comes from observations showing that the mutant pRB forms found in various human tumours are invariably underphosphorylated or unphosphorylated. This would seem paradoxical, in that it is precisely this underphosphorylated form of pRB that is postulated to be active in normal cells in growth suppression, and yet these tumour cells have been liberated from pRB's growth suppressing effects. The proposed resolution of this paradox is simple: as a consequence of structural alterations, pRB simultaneously loses all growth suppressing powers and its ability to become phosphorylated. Consequently, any subsequent phosphorylation becomes moot, since the protein is in any case functionally inert. Why mutant pRB forms cannot undergo G_1/S phosphorylation remains unclear. One possible model is that pRB must be part of a multiprotein complex in order to be an effective substrate for phosphorylation and that the mutant pRB has lost its ability to participate in complex formation (Hamel *et al*, 1990).

A MODEL OF pRB ACTION

A synthesis of all this allows one to construct a tentative model of pRB action in the normal cell. Upon emergence from mitosis, a cell will dephosphorylate its complement of pRB molecules. This dephosphorylation itself will not cause pRB to suppress growth; rather, it will only make pRB available to suppress growth should the cell require it to do so. Having emerged from M, the cell may exit the cell cycle into quiescence (G_0) or proceed to the G_1 phase and exploit pRB either to maintain the quiescence of G_0 (if the former) or to block growth at some stage in its progression through or exit from G_1 (if the latter).

In the G_0 state, a centrally acting controller, which determines whether or not the cell should remain quiescent, may exploit pRB to enforce and maintain this quiescence. Alternatively, in G_1 the cell may monitor whether external conditions (eg available growth factors) permit progression to the end of G_1 and entrance into S. In the absence of such permissive conditions, the cell may engage underphosphorylated pRB to shut down progression through the cycle, either at an intermediate stopping point in G_1 or at the G_1/S transition. Should external conditions be conducive to passage all the way through G_1, then the cell will activate a kinase (perhaps a cdc2 kinase) and use it to phosphorylate pRB. As a direct consequence of phosphorylation, pRB will be taken out of action until much later, when the cell has passed through S and G_2 and finally emerges from mitosis.

How does pRB shut down growth in response to signals from the cell's central controller? It would seem to require its oncoprotein binding domain to perform this function, as suggested by the loss of growth suppressing ability following alterations of this domain in the mutant pRB forms present in human tumours. By binding to cellular partners having oncoprotein like structure, pRB succeeds in shutting down growth. Within the normal cell, phosphorylated pRB loses its ability to bind such cellular partner proteins and by this logic, its ability to suppress growth.

What do we know about these cellular partners? One manifestation of their existence may be the cell cycle dependent binding of pRB to the nuclear structure, which is strong in G_1 and weak in S, G_2 and M (Mittnacht and Weinberg, 1991). Thus, one candidate for a cellular partner is the nuclear protein that seems to anchor pRB to the nuclear structure. Within the intact cell, the binding of viral oncoproteins to this pRB domain would preempt its ability to interact physically with this nuclear anchor as well as other partner proteins, thereby precluding its ability to shut down growth. To summarize, there are three conditions that would seem to compromise pRB's ability to bind partner proteins and shut down growth: G_1/S phosphorylation, mutation in the oncoprotein binding domain and oncoprotein binding.

Two recent reports provide possible clues about events further downstream in this regulatory cascade. In one, pRB expressed by an introduced plasmid is reported to repress use of a c-*fos* transcriptional promoter (Robbins *et al*, 1990). A second report implicates pRB as an intermediate in the downregulation of the c-*myc* gene, which is observed when keratinocytes are exposed to the growth inhibitory factor TGF-β (Pietenpol *et al*, 1990). Transforming growth factor-β mediated shutoff of *myc* occurs within 1 hour after exposure to this factor, and studies of the *myc* transcriptional promoter ascribe TGF-β responsiveness to a specific sequence element. In the presence of the SV40 LT, E1A or E7 oncoproteins, *myc* becomes refractory to the transcriptional shutdown normally elicited by TGF-β. The suggestion is that when pRB is sequestered by one or another of these viral oncoproteins, then a vital link in the TGF-β *myc* signalling pathway is removed, resulting in turn in the inability of TGF-β to evoke a c-*myc* shutoff.

These observations may suggest how pRB can act as a modulatable suppressor of centrally important, growth promoting proto-oncogenes such as c-*fos* and c-*myc*. In the absence of pRB, proto-oncogene expression becomes derepressed, perhaps mimicking the deregulation seen when these proto-oncogenes are converted into oncogenes through *cis* acting mutations. Another explanation for proto-oncogene suppression could be that *myc* shutoff is due to the actions of other cellular proteins which, like pRB, are known to be complexed by E1A and SV40 LT.

A more biological line of thinking also provides some support for models that depict pRB as a negative regulator of proto-oncogenes such as *myc*. The three viral oncoproteins that bind to pRB (E1A, LT and E7) are each known to mimic a *myc* oncogene in "oncogene collaboration" tests (ie each on its own is able, like a *myc* oncogene, to collaborate with a *ras* oncogene in the transformation of embryo cells [Land *et al*, 1983; Ruley *et al*, 1983; Phelps *et al*, 1988; Vousden and Jat, 1989]). This might suggest that by inactivating pRB, a putative *trans* acting negative regulator of *myc,* these oncoproteins are able to elicit constitutively expressed *myc* genes, thus mimicking the *cis* acting lesions that create *myc* oncogene alleles.

For the future, at least three interconnected lines of work hold promise for elucidating the signalling pathways in which pRB participates: study of its DNA interactions, characterization of its cellular binding partners and unravelling the connections between pRB and the cdc2 cell cycle clock. With this information in hand, the biochemical mechanisms of pRB will come into clear view, and then we will understand with some precision how loss of pRB leads to malignancy.

SUMMARY

Retinoblastoma, an uncommon childhood cancer of the eye, sometimes occurs in families but is often sporadic. Cytological analysis suggested that the retinoblastoma gene resided on chromosome 13 band q14. Subsequent isolation of the *RB* gene from this locus allowed a more detailed analysis, showing that both copies of *RB* are mutated or lost in retinoblastoma, a finding that has been extended to a surprising number of other malignancies. In familial retinoblastoma, one copy of *RB* is mutant in the conceptus, consistent with the familial predisposition to the disease and indicating that a single wild type copy is sufficient for normal development. These studies provided the first good evidence that loss of a gene function correlated with tumorigenesis and led to the concept of "tumour suppressor genes", which have an important negative influence on the regulation of cell growth. Examinations of the biological properties of the gene product are consistent with this proposed role in cell proliferation. Further insight into the potential molecular mechanisms concerned has come from observations showing an association of some viral oncoproteins with the *RB* gene product. Thus, there is strong evidence that the RB protein has a key role in the integrated network of signals that control the cell cycle.

References

Benedict WF, Murphree AL, Banerjee A, Spina CA, Sparkes MC and Sparkes RS (1983) Patient with 13 chromosome deletion: evidence that the retinoblastoma gene is a recessive cancer gene. *Science* **219** 973–975

Bernards R, Schackleford GM, Gerber MR *et al* (1989) Structure and expression of the murine retinoblastoma gene and characterization of its encoded protein. *Proceedings of the National Academy of Sciences of the USA* **86** 6474–6478

Bookstein R, Lee EY-HP, Peccei A and Lee W-H (1989) Human retinoblastoma gene: long-range mapping and analysis of its deletion in a breast cancer cell line. *Molecular and Cellular Biology* **9** 1628–1634

Bookstein R, Shew JY, Chen P-L, Scully P and Lee W-H (1990a) Suppression of tumorigenicity of human prostate carcinoma cells by replacing a mutated Rb gene. *Science* **247** 712–715

Bookstein R, Rio P, Madreperla SA *et al* (1990b) Promoter deletion and loss of retinoblastoma gene expression in human prostate carcinoma. *Proceedings of the National Academy of Sciences of the USA* **87** 7762–7766

Buchkovich K, Duffy LA and Harlow E (1989) The retinoblastoma protein is phosphorylated during specific phases of the cell cycle. *Cell* **58** 1097–1105

Canning S and Dryja TP (1989) Short, direct repeats at the breakpoints of deletions of the retinoblastoma gene. *Proceedings of the National Academy of Sciences of the USA* **86** 5044–5048

Cavenee WK, Dryja TP, Phillips RA *et al* (1983) Expression of recessive alleles by chromosomal mechanisms in retinoblastoma. *Nature* **305** 779–784

Cavenee WK, Murphree AL, Shull MM *et al* (1986) Prediction of familial predisposition to retinoblastoma. *The New England Journal of Medicine* **314** 1201–1207

Chen P-L, Scully P, Shew J-Y, Wang JYJ and Lee W-H (1989) Phosphorylation of the retinoblastoma gene product is modulated during the cell cycle and cellular differentiation. *Cell* **58** 1193–1198

DeCaprio JA, Ludlow JW, Figge J *et al* (1988) SV40 large tumor antigen forms a specific complex with the product of the retinoblastoma susceptibility gene. *Cell* **54** 275–283

DeCaprio JA, Ludlow JW, Lynch D *et al* (1989) The product of the retinoblastoma susceptibility gene has properties of a cell cycle regulatory element. *Cell* **58** 1085–1095

DeGouvea H (1886) *Bull Soc de MedSurg Rio de Janeiro* (August 25th issue)

DerKinderen DJ, Koten JW, Nagelkerke NJD, Tan KE Beemer FA and Den Otter W (1988) Non-ocular cancer in patients with hereditary retinoblastoma and their relatives. *International Journal of Cancer* **41** 499–504

Dryja TP, Mukai S, Petersen R, Rapaport JM, Walton D and Yandell DW (1989) Parental origin of mutations of the retinoblastoma gene. *Nature* **339** 556–558

Dryja TP, Webster MD, White R *et al* (1984) Homozygosity of chromosome 13 in retinoblastoma. *New England Journal of Medicine* **310** 550–553

Dunn JM, Phillips RA, Becker AJ and Gallie BL (1988) Identification of germline and somatic mutations affecting the retinoblastoma gene. *Science* **241** 1797–1800

Dunn JM, Phillips RA, Zhu X, Becker A and Gallie B (1989) Mutations in the Rb1 gene and their effects on transcription. *Molecular and Cellular Biology* **9** 4596–4604

Dunphy EB (1964) The story of retinoblastoma. *American Journal of Ophthalmology* **58** 539–552

Dyson N, Bernards R, Friend SH *et al* (1990) Large T antigens of many polyomaviruses are able to form complexes with the retinoblastoma protein. *Journal of Virology* **64** 1353–1356

Dyson N, Howley PM, Münger K and Harlow E (1989) The human papilloma virus-16 E7 oncoprotein is able to bind to the retinoblastoma gene product. *Science* **243** 934–937

Egan C, Jelsma TN, Howe JA, Bayley ST, Ferguson B and Branton PE (1988) Mapping of cellular protein-binding sites on the products of early-region 1A of human adenovirus type 5 *Molecular and Cellular Biology* **8** 3955–3959

Figge J, Webster T, Smith TF and Paucha E (1988) Prediction of similar transforming regions in simia virus 40 large T, adenovirus E1A and *myc* oncoproteins. *Journal of Virology* **62** 1814–1818

Friend SH, Bernards R, Rogelj S *et al* (1986) A human DNA segment with properties of the gene that predisposes to retinoblastoma and osteosarcoma. *Nature* **323** 643–646

Friend SH, Horowitz JM, Gerber MR *et al* (1987) Deletions of DNA sequence in both retinoblastomas and mesenchymal tumors: organization of the sequence and its encoded protein. *Proceedings of the National Academy of Sciences of the USA* **24** 9059–9063

Fung Y-K T, Murphree AL, T'Ang A, Qian J, Hinriches SH and Benedict WF (1987) Structural evidence for the authenticity of the human retinoblastoma gene. *Science* **236** 1657–1661

Furukawa Y, DeCaprio J A, Freedman A *et al* (1990) Expression and state of phosphorylation of the retinoblastoma susceptibility gene product in cycling and noncycling human hematopoietic cells. *Proceedings of the National Academy of Sciences of the USA* **87** 2770–2774

Gallie BL, Dunn JM, Hamel PA and Phillips RA (1990) Point mutations in retinoblastoma. *New England Journal of Medicine* **322** 1397–1398

Gilbert F (1986) Retinoblastoma and cancer genetics. *New England Journal of Medicine* **314** 1248–1249

Godbout R, Dryja TP, Squire J, Gallie B and Phillips RA (1983) Somatic inactivation of genes on chromosome 13 is a common event in retinoblastoma. *Nature* **304** 451–453

Hamel PA, Cohen BL, Sorce LM, Gallie BM and Phillips RA (1990) Hyperphosphorylation of the retinoblastoma gene product is determined by domains outside the simian virus 40 large T-antigen-binding regions. *Molecular and Cellular Biology* **10** 6586–6595

Harbour JW, Lai S-L, Whang-Peng J, Gazdar AF, Minna JD and Kaye FJ (1988) Abnormalities in structure and expression of the human retinoblastoma gene in SCLC. *Science* **241** 353–357

Harlow E, Whyte P, Franza BR Jr and Schley C (1986) Association of adenovirus early-region 1A proteins with cellular polypeptides. *Molecular and Cellular Biology* **6** 1579–1589

Hong FD, Huang H-S, To H *et al* (1989) Structure of the human retinoblastoma gene. *Proceedings of the National Academy of Sciences of the USA* **86** 5502–5506

Horowitz JM, Yandell DW, Park S-H *et al* (1989) Point mutational inactivation of the retinoblastoma antioncogene. *Science* **243** 937–940

Horowitz JM, Park S-H, Bogenmann E *et al* (1990) Frequent inactivation of the retinoblastoma antioncogene is restricted to a subset of human tumors. *Proceedings of the National Academy of Sciences of the USA* **87** 2775–2779

Howe JA, Mymryk JS, Egan C, Branton PE and Bayley ST (1990) Retinoblastoma growth suppressor and a 300kDa protein appear to regulate cellular DNA synthesis. *Proceedings of the National Academy of Sciences of the USA* **87** 5883–5887

Hu Q, Dyson N and Harlow E (1990) Regions of the retinoblastoma protein needed for binding to adenovirus E1A or SV40 large T antigen are common sites for mutations. *EMBO Journal* **9** 1147–1155

Huang H-J S, Yee J-K, Shew J-Y *et al* (1988) Suppression of the neoplastic phenotype by replacement of the Rb gene in human cancer cells. *Science* **242** 1563–1566

Huang S, Lee W-H and Lee Y-H (1991) A cellular protein that competes with SV40 T antigen for binding to the retinoblastoma gene product. *Nature* **350** 160–162

Jelsma JN, Howe JA, Mymryk JS, Evelegh CM, Cunniff and Bayley ST (1989) Sequences in E1A proteins of human adenovirus 5 required for cell transformation, repression of a transcriptional enhancer, and induction of proliferating cell nuclear antigen. *Virology* **170** 120–130

Kaelin, WG Jr, Ewen ME and Livingston DM (1990) Definition of the minimal simian virus 40 large T antigen- and adenovirus E1A-binding domain in the retinoblastoma gene product. *Molecular and Cellular Biology* **10** 3761–3769

Kaelin WG Jr, Pallas DC, DeCaprio JA, Kaye FJ and Livingston DM (1991) Identification of cellular proteins that can interact specifically with the T/E1A-binding region of the retinoblastoma gene product. *Cell* **64** 521–532

Kaye FJ, Kratzke RA, Gerster JL and Horowitz JM (1990) A single amino acid substitution results in a retinoblastoma protein defective in phosphorylation and oncoprotein binding. *Proceedings of the National Academy of Sciences of the USA* **87** 6922–6926

Knudson AG Jr (1971) Mutation and cancer: statistical study of retinoblastomas. *Proceedings of the National Academy of Sciences of the USA* **68** 820–823

Land H, Parada LF and Weinberg RA (1983) Tumorigenic conversion of primary embryo fibroblasts requires at least two cooperating oncogenes. *Nature* **304** 596–602

Lee EY-HP, To H, Shew J-Y, Bookstein R, Scully P and Lee W-H (1988) Inactivation of the retinoblastoma susceptibility gene in human breast cancer. *Science* **241** 218–221

Lee W-H, Bookstein R, Hong F *et al* (1987a) Human retinoblastoma susceptibility gene: cloning, identification, and sequence. *Science* **235** 1394–1399

Lee W-H, Shew JY, Hong FD *et al* (1987b) The retinoblastoma susceptibility gene encodes a nuclear phosphoprotein associated with DNA binding activity. *Nature* **329** 642–645

Ludlow JW, DeCaprio JA, Huang C-M, Lee W-H, Paucha E and Livingston DM (1989) SV40 large T antigen binds preferentially to an underphosphorylated member of the retinoblastoma susceptibility gene product family. *Cell* **56** 57–65

Ludlow JW, Shon J, Pipas JM, Livingston DM and DeCaprio A (1990) The retinoblastoma susceptibility gene product undergoes cell cycle-dependent dephosphorylation and binding to and release from SV40 large T. *Cell* **60** 387–396

McGee TL, Yandell DW and Dryja TP (1989) Structure and partial genomic sequence of the human retinoblastoma susceptibility gene product. *Gene* **80** 119–128

Mittnacht S and Weinberg RA (1991) G1/S phosphorylation of the retinoblastoma protein is associated with an altered affinity for the nuclear compartment. *Cell* **65** 381–393

Phelps WC, Yee CL, Münger K and Howley PM (1988) The human papillomavirus type 16E7 gene encodes transactivation and transformation functions similar to those of adenovirus E1A. *Cell* **53** 539–547

Pietenpol JA, Stein RW, Moran E *et al* (1990) TGF-β1 inhibition of c-myc transcription and growth in keratinocytes is abrogated by viral transforming proteins with pRb binding domains. *Cell* **61** 777–785

Reissmann PT, Simon MA, Lee W and Slamon DJ (1989) Studies of the retinoblastoma gene in human sarcomas. *Oncogene* **4** 839–843

Robbins PD, Horowitz JM and Mulligan RC (1990) Negative regulation of human c-fos expression by the retinoblastoma gene product. *Nature* **346** 668–670

Ruley HE (1983) Adenovirus early region 1A enables viral and cellular transforming genes to transform primary cells in culture. *Nature* **304** 602–606

Shew J-Y, Ling N, Yang X, Fodstad O and Lee W-H (1989) Antibodies detecting abnormalities of the retinoblastoma susceptibility gene product (pp110^{Rb}) in osteosarcomas and synovial sarcomas. *Oncogene Research* **1** 205–214

Shew J-Y, Chen P-L, Bookstein R, Lee Y-H P and Lee W-H (1990) Deletion of splice donor site ablates expression of the following exon and produces a unphosphorylated Rb protein unable to bind SV40 T antigen. *Cell Growth and Differentiation* **1** 17–25

Sparkes RS, Murphree AL, Lingua RW *et al* (1983) Gene for hereditary retinoblastoma assigned to human chromosome 13 by linkage to esterase D. *Science* **219** 971–973

Stein GH, Beeson M and Gordon L (1990) Failure to phosphorylate the retinoblastoma gene product in senescent human fibroblasts. *Science* **249** 666–668

Stein RW, Corrigan M, Yaciuk P, Whelan J and Moran E (1990) Analysis of E1A-mediated growth regulation functions: binding of the 300-kilodalton cellular product correlates with E1A enhancer repression function and DNA synthesis-inducing activity. *Journal of Virology* **64** 4421–4427

T'Ang A, Varley JM, Chakraborty S, Murphree AL and Fung Y-KT (1988) Structural rearrangement of the retinoblastoma gene in human breast carcinoma. *Science* **242** 263–266

Templeton DJ, Park S-H, Lanier L and Weinberg RA (1991) Nonfunctional mutants of the retinoblastoma protein are characterized by defects in phosphorylation, viral oncoprotein association, and nuclear tethering. *Proceedings of the National Academy of Sciences of the USA* **88** 3033–3037

Toguchida J, Ishizaki K, Sasaki MS *et al* (1989) Preferential mutation of paternally derived RB gene as the initial event in sporadic osteosarcoma. *Nature* **338** 156–158

Varley JM, Armour J, Swallow JE *et al* (1989) The retinoblastoma gene is frequently altered leading to loss of expression in primary breast tumors. *Oncogene* **4** 725–729

Vousden KH and Jat PS (1989) Functional similarity between HPV16 E7, SV40 large T and adenovirus E1A proteins. *Oncogene* **4** 153–158

Wang NP, Chen P-L, Huang S, Donoso LA, Lee W-H and Lee EY-HP (1990) DNA-binding activity of retinoblastoma protein is intrinsic to its carboxyl-terminal region. *Cell Growth and Differentiation* **1/5** 233–239

Weichselbaum RR, Beckett M and Diamond A (1988) Some retinoblastomas, osteosarcomas, and soft tissue sarcomas may share a common etiology. *Proceedings of the National Academy of Sciences of the USA* **85** 2106–2109

Whyte P, Buchkovich K, Horowitz JM *et al* (1988) Association between an oncogene and an anti-oncogene: the adenovirus E1A proteins bind to the retinoblastoma gene product. *Nature* **334** 124–129

Whyte P, Williamson NM and Harlow E (1989) Cellular targets for transformation by the adenovirus E1A proteins. *Cell* **56** 67–75

Yandell DW, Campbell TA, Dayton SH *et al* (1989) Oncogenic point mutations in the human retinoblastoma gene: their application to genetic counseling. *New England Journal of Medicine* **321** 1689–1695

Yee S-P and Branton PE (1985) Detection of cellular proteins associated with human adenovirus type 5 early region E1A polypeptides. *Journal of Virology* **147** 142–153

Yokota J, Akiyama T, Fung Y-KT *et al* (1988) Altered expression of the retinoblastoma (Rb) gene in small-cell carcinoma of the lung. *Oncogene* **3** 471–475

Yunis JJ and Ramsey N (1978) Retinoblastoma and sub-band deletion of chromosome 13. *American Journal of Diseases of Children* **132** 161–163

Zhu X, Dunn JM, Phillips RA, Godbout AD, Paton KA and Gallie BL (1989) Preferential germline mutation of the paternal allele in retinoblastoma. *Nature* **340** 312–313

The author is responsible for the accuracy of the references.

The *p53* Tumour Suppressor Gene and Product

A J LEVINE

Department of Molecular Biology, Lewis Thomas Laboratory, Princeton University, Princeton, New Jersey 08544-1014

Historical perspectives
The genotypes of *p53* mutations in tumours
Inherited forms of *p53* mutations
Somatic *p53* mutations in tumours
The phenotypes of wild type and mutant *p53* genes
Mutant *p53* alleles
Wild type *p53* alleles
Properties of the p53 mutant and wild type proteins
The wild type *p53* gene
The wild type and mutant p53 proteins
Functions of the *p53* gene and protein
Conclusions

HISTORICAL PERSPECTIVES

Simian virus 40 (SV40) is able to infect and transform cells in culture (Tooze, 1973), and these cells have an enhanced ability to replicate in culture and produce tumours in isogenic animals. The virus encoded oncogene product that confers this enhanced growth potential upon these transformed cells is called the large T or tumour antigen (Tooze, 1973). When SV40 transformed cells are injected into an isogenic animal, they produce a tumour. The host animal recognizes the viral large T antigen, expressed in the tumour cells, as foreign and produces antibodies that react with this protein. Antibodies of this type have been used to bind to and identify the SV40 large T antigen in transformed cells. When this is done, the SV40 large T antigen may be immunoprecipitated from soluble protein extracts of transformed cells, and a second protein of 53 000 daltons (p53) is frequently detected in these immunoprecipitates. When serial dilutions of the antibody taken from animals bearing SV40 induced tumours are made, the ratio of the SV40 large T antigen to p53 is constant at all dilutions. These findings suggest that antibody directed against one protein, large T antigen, coimmunoprecipitated a second protein by virtue of its being associated or complexed with the T antigen (Lane and Crawford, 1979). It is unlikely that antibodies directed against both proteins would have identical titres or identical levels upon serial dilution. On the basis of these data, it was concluded that the SV40 large T antigen in transformed cells complexed or associated with a second protein of 53 000 daltons (Lane and Crawford, 1979). In a different series of experiments (Linzer and Levine, 1979), antisera from animals bearing SV40 induced tumours were shown by immunoprecipitation to detect a 53 000 dalton protein in embryonal carcinoma cells as well as SV40 transformed cells. These 53 kDa proteins, either associated with T antigen in SV40 transformed cells or in the absence of T antigen in embryonal carcinoma cells, were identical according to their partial peptide maps (Linzer and Levine, 1979). Thus, antisera from tumour bearing animals contained antibodies directed against p53 epitopes as well as T antigen epitopes. Furthermore, monoclonal antibodies directed against SV40 T antigen did not cross react with p53 from embryonal carcinoma cells but co-immunoprecipitated p53 in SV40 transformed cells, thus demonstrating the SV40 T antigen–p53 complex (Linzer and Levine, 1979). In a third series of experiments, murine cells transformed with a chemical carcinogen, methylcholanthrene (MethA cells), were used to immunize isogenic animals. These animals produced antibodies directed against a 53 kDa protein (DeLeo *et al*, 1979). Subsequent experiments proved this was the same protein detected in association with large T antigen and in embryonal carcinoma cells.

On the basis of these early observations, it was concluded that p53 was a cellular encoded protein that interacted and complexed with the SV40 large T antigen and was present in relatively abundant levels in transformed tumorigenic cells in culture. Because animals bearing tumours frequently produced antibodies directed against p53, it was classified as a tumour antigen. In fact, about 10% of humans with cancer tested produced antibodies directed against this p53 protein (Crawford *et al*, 1982).

It was next demonstrated that the SV40 large T antigen could regulate the levels of p53 in a cell. A temperature sensitive mutant of SV40 large T antigen in transformed cells grown at 32°C bound to p53, and these cells expressed high levels of p53. When grown at 39°C, these cells no longer contained functional SV40 large T antigen and were no longer transformed; nor did they bind T antigen to p53, and they expressed much reduced levels of p53 (Linzer *et al*, 1979). Furthermore, it could be shown that a wide variety of transformed cells in culture or tumours in animals expressed much higher levels of p53 than their normal cell or tissue counterparts, regardless of the transforming agent (Benchimol *et al*, 1982; Thomas *et al*, 1983). Tumours caused by viruses or chemicals, spontaneous tumours and transformed cells all produced or contained cells that expressed high levels of p53 protein. The major mechanism of regulation of p53 levels in normal and transformed cells was posttranslational, modulating the half-life or stability of the p53 protein (Oren *et al*, 1981; Reich *et al*, 1983). Normal cells had low levels of p53 with a half-life of about 20 minutes, whereas transformed cells often had much higher levels of p53 with half lives of hours (Reich *et al*, 1983).

The complementary DNA (cDNA) and genomic clones of the *p53* gene were isolated and characterized (Oren *et al*, 1983; Bienz *et al*, 1984; Pennica *et al*, 1984; Harlow *et al*, 1985; Arai *et al*, 1986). Some *p53* cDNA clones could immortalize cells in culture (Jenkins *et al*, 1984), and the same clones when co-transfected into rat embryo fibroblasts along with the activated *ras* oncogene contributed to transformation of these cells in culture (Eliyahu *et al*, 1984; Parada *et al*, 1984). On the basis of these observations, *p53* was classified as an oncogene, but it was then demonstrated that only mutant *p53* cDNA or genomic clones could immortalize cells in culture or cooperate with the *ras* oncogene to transform these cells. The wild type form of the *p53* gene did not transform cells (Eliyahu *et al*, 1988; Hinds *et al*, 1989). In fact, the wild type *p53* gene or cDNAs could inhibit or block the transformation of cells by other oncogenes (Finlay *et al*, 1989). Whereas the mutant forms of *p53* behaved as oncogenes, the wild type *p53* acted as a transformation or tumour suppressor gene, blocking the oncogenic process. In several murine (Mowat *et al*, 1985) and human (Baker *et al*, 1989; Nigro *et al*, 1989) tumours, both alleles of the *p53* gene were found to be mutant. One allele commonly contained a missense mutation, whereas the other allele was lost, via deletion or gene conversion, reducing the tumour cell to homozygosity at the *p53* locus (Levine *et al*, 1991). This is a property of a tumour suppressor gene. Indeed, returning a wild type *p53* allele back into a tumorigenic cell containing no *p53* (a deletion mutant) suppressed the tumorigenic potential of these cells (Chen *et al*, 1990). Because of these finding, the wild type *p53* gene was classified as a tumour suppressor gene.

During the past 13 years, *p53* has thus evolved from a tumour antigen to an oncogene to a tumour suppressor gene. Indeed, it has elements of all three activities. Tumour suppressor gene products are commonly thought of as negative regulators of cell growth. When the wild type p53 protein is overexpressed in cells in culture, it blocks cell division in the G_1 phase of the cell cycle (Michalovitz *et al*, 1990; Martinez *et al*, 1991). A temperature sensitive *p53* allele expressed in a p53 plus *ras* transformed cell line behaves as a wild type protein at 32°C and as a mutant protein at 39°C (Michalovitz *et al*, 1990). These cells replicate at 39°C but are blocked for cell division at 32°C, and the block appears to be in the late G_1 phase of the cell cycle. Thus, p53 appears to be a negative regulator of cell division acting at a specific stage of the cell cycle (late G_1) to prevent progression into S phase (DNA synthesis). At present, there are two hypotheses to explain the functioning of p53 during the late G_1 phase of the cell cycle. Some evidence points to a role of p53 as a transcription factor or a protein regulating transcription factors in the cell (Fields and Jang, 1990; Raycroft *et al*, 1990). In this case, p53 could directly or indirectly regulate several genes or products essential for entry into the S phase of the cell cycle. Alternatively, there is some evidence indicating a role for p53 in DNA replication or initiation of DNA replication. p53 could regulate the assembly or function of DNA replication complexes in the cell (Lane and Benchimol, 1990). These two ideas are not mutually exclusive.

This chapter reviews the genotypes and phenotypes of mutant p53 proteins and contrast them with the activities of the wild type p53 protein. The properties of mutant or wild type p53 proteins are elucidated, and their possible functions are reviewed and discussed. *p53* mutations now constitute the single most common genetic alteration (somatic mutation) in human cancers. About 75–80% of colon cancers and 50% of lung and breast cancers contain *p53* mutations. For this reason, it is an important subject for study, and it is critical that we learn more about the structure and function of the *p53* gene and its protein.

THE GENOTYPES OF *p53* MUTATIONS IN TUMOURS

Inherited Forms of *p53* Mutations

Some individuals with the Li-Fraumeni syndrome come from families with inherited *p53* mutations (Li, 1988; Malkin *et al*, 1990; Srivastava *et al*, 1990). In Li-Fraumeni families, several closely related individuals acquire cancer at a young age (25–35 years) and are also at risk for the development of multiple independent cancers over their lifetime. The cancers are varied, but certain tissue types tend to be more commonly affected (eg osteogenic sarcoma) than in the population at large. Thus, there is a tissue bias but not a strict specificity in this inherited predisposition for cancer at a young age. Inherited *p53* mutations are transmitted in the heterozygous state and are all missense mutations producing a faulty or altered protein (Malkin *et al*, 1990). Mutations occur in several different codons but are not randomly distributed in the gene. Presumably, with one allele of *p53* in the mutant form, the time it would take for a second mutation or a reduction to homozygosity at the *p53* locus and additional mutations in oncogenes or other tumour suppressor genes is reduced, and cancer appears at a younger age and independently at more than one site. The presence of a missense mutant allele of *p53*, at least at these limited codons in the *p53* gene, does not disrupt development of the organism.

The introduction of a missense mutant *p53* gene into transgenic mice produces a similar phenotype. In families of mice expressing a mutant *p53* gene (one missense mutation and two wild type copies), cancer develops at a higher than normal frequency (about 20% of the family) 6–9 months after birth (Lavigueur *et al*, 1989). Again, the time interval suggests the need for additional, time dependent events such as mutations before a cancer develops. The fact that these mice start life with two wild type alleles (as opposed to Li-Fraumeni patients with one wild type allele) yet develop cancer at a young age may suggest a role for gene conversion (from wild type to mutant) or a promoting function of the missense mutant protein. It could enhance the rate of other mutations or promote a cancer in another way.

Because many human (Levine *et al*, 1991) and some murine (Mowat *et al*, 1985) tumours select against both wild type *p53* alleles and contain only mutant *p53* gene products, a mouse with both *p53* genes deleted (a knockout of *p53*) would be an interesting animal. If *p53* function is not required for the development of the mouse or if the *p53* gene product is redundant in development, such a mouse with no p53 ought to develop tumours at a young age. The production of mice without *p53* is in progress in several laboratories.

Somatic *p53* Mutations in Tumours

The first indication that *p53* mutations eliminating p53 function in both alleles occur in tumours came from studies of murine erythroleukaemia induced by Friend virus infection (Mowat *et al*, 1985; Rovinski *et al*, 1987; Munroe *et al*, 1988). In these erythroleukaemic cells, both *p53* alleles may suffer deletions, insertions or rearrangements, suggesting a loss of function being selected for in the tumour (Lane and Benchimol, 1990). In some cases, one *p53* allele has a missense mutation that produces an altered protein and the other allele is lost or inactivated and produces no gene product. These observations first led Benchimol and his colleagues to postulate that *p53* could act as a tumour suppressor gene in these tumours.

In a wide variety of human tumours, one *p53* allele contains a missense mutation producing a faulty protein and the second allele is reduced to homozygosity, either by gene conversion or by deletion. This was first shown to be the case in colon carcinomas (Baker *et al*, 1989; Nigro *et al*, 1989) by Vogelstein and his colleagues, but this pattern is common for tumours from a variety of tissues. Mutations of *p53* have been demonstrated in human tumours of the anus (Crook *et al*, 1991), bone (Miller *et al*, 1990; Mulligan *et al*, 1990), bladder (Sidransky *et al*, 1991), brain (Nigro *et al*, 1989), breast (Prosser, *et al*, 1990; Davidoff *et al*, 1991; Varley *et al*, 1991), colon (Baker *et al*, 1990), oesophagus (Hollstein *et al*, 1990, 1991), stomach (Tamura *et al*, 1991), liver (Bressac *et al*, 1991; Hsu *et al*, 1991), lung (both small cell and non-small cell carcinomas) (Takahashi *et al*, 1989; Chiba *et al*, 1990; Iggo *et al*, 1990; Hensel *et al*, 1991), lymphoid system (Ahuja *et al*, 1989; Gaidano *et al*, 1991), ovary (Marks *et al*, 1991) and prostate (Isaacs *et al*, 1991). About 75% of the time, these tumour cells contain missense mutations, suggesting a selection for a faulty protein which then may play a part in promoting cell growth or division. The human *p53* gene contains 393 codons, and the position of these missense mutations in the gene is not random. A graphic representation of the altered codon of 148 missense mutations found in human tumours is plotted in Fig. 1. All of these mutations cluster between codons 118 and 309 (out of 393 codons). Furthermore, most of these mutations occur in the most highly conserved regions of aminoacid sequences when p53 proteins from different species are compared (Soussi *et al*, 1987). The aminoacid residues between codons 117 and 142, 171 and 181, 236 and 258 and 270 and 286 show sequence conservation of 90–100% between *Xenopus* and human p53 proteins (Soussi *et al*, 1987; Levine and Momand, 1990). This sequence conservation suggests a functional role or significance, and the clustering of missense mutations in this region of the gene reinforces the importance of these residues in protein function. The non-random nature of these mutations in this gene is in-all tumors

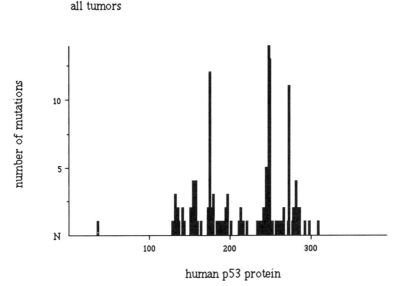

Fig. 1. Distribution of *p53* missense mutations found in human tumours of all origins. The frequency of a mutation in the gene is plotted as a function of its location or codon in the *p53* gene. These data are compiled from the publications referenced in the text

dicated by the presence of hot spots or codons frequently found in a mutant form (Fig. 1). These residues at aminoacids 175 (17/148), 248 and 249 (25/148), 273 (9/148) and 282 (8/148) account for 40% of the total missense mutations observed to date in primary human tumours. These hot spot mutations are dependent on the tissue of origin of the cancer. For example, the codon 175 mutant allele is found commonly in colorectal carcinomas (8/25), Burkitt's lymphoma (3/10) and have been found at least once in breast carcinoma, glioblastoma and oesophageal carcinoma (Nigro *et al*, 1989; Baker *et al*, 1990; Prosser *et al*, 1990; Gaidano *et al*, 1991; Hollstein *et al*, 1991). This mutation is not found in lung or hepatocellular carcinomas. By contrast, codon 249 mutations were common (almost 50%) in hepatocellular carcinomas from Qidong, China, and from South Africa but were not observed in colon, lung or breast carcinomas (Bressac *et al*, 1991; Hsu *et al*, 1991). There are two possible explanations for this striking and unusual tissue specific distribution of hot spot mutations in human cancers (Fig. 2). This may reflect the exposure of different body cell surfaces, such as the lung, colon or liver, to diverse environmental mutagens or carcinogens. These different mutagens, such as aflatoxin B_1 in the liver or benzo(*a*)pyrene (from smoking) in the lung, could induce different mutations at different (preferred sites of action) codons in this gene. If this were the case, the distribution of these mutations in the *p53* gene is an example of an Ames test for environmental mutagens and their specificity that is being carried out in the human population. In support of this idea is the observation that the type of mutations found in the lung are both transversions and transitions. By contrast, colon mutations in the *p53* gene are always transitions,

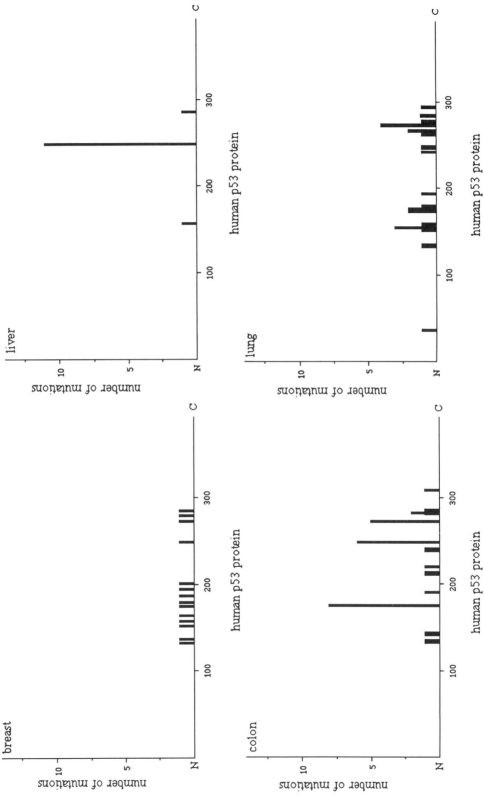

Fig. 2. Distribution of *p53* missense mutations detected in specific human tumours. The location of a missense mutation in the *p53* gene and the frequency of these mutations are examined for breast, colon, liver and lung tumours. These data are compiled from publications referenced in the text

in some cases resulting from changes at CpG dinucleotides (G:C to A:T changes). It is known that methylated C residues in CpG dinucleotides have a mutation rate higher than that of the non-methylated residues. It would be useful to examine methylation patterns in different normal tissue types at specific codons in the $p53$ gene (Hollstein $et\ al$, 1991).

An alternative to tissue specific mutagenesis at the $p53$ locus is the possibility that different $p53$ mutations are selected for their enhanced growth potential in a tissue specific fashion. In this case, codon 175 mutations may produce a faulty protein that efficiently stimulates growth of colon epithelial cells but not liver cells. Conversely, the 249 codon mutant would produce a protein that interacts well with proteins that promote cell division in liver cells. Thus, mutations might arise more randomly across the $p53$ gene, perhaps at all codons, but selection results in only some subset of mutants being observed in the final cancer cells analysed in these studies (Figs. 1 and 2). Mutational tissue specificity and selection for cell division are not mutually exclusive explanations of these data. Both processes may be acting here.

In colon cancers, the presence of a mutant $p53$ allele strongly selects for the loss of the remaining (wild type) $p53$ allele. In colorectal carcinomas that express just one $p53$ allele (those cells that have undergone a reduction to homozygosity at the $p53$ locus), 91% of the time it is the mutant allele that is detected. In all colon carcinomas that express both $p53$ alleles, more than 70% of the time both alleles are mutant $p53$ genes. Thus, in colon cancer there is a strong selection for the inactivation or mutation of both $p53$ alleles, and when these cancer cells are examined, both wild type alleles are most often lost. That of course is one definition of a tumour suppressor gene.

Surprisingly, this is not the case in breast cancers. In these carcinomas, $p53$ missense mutations are found equally frequently (50% of the time) in tumours with or without a second wild type allele (Davidoff $et\ al$, 1991). In those breast carcinomas that express only one $p53$ allele, 60% express a mutant $p53$ and 40% a wild type $p53$. Here, a reduction to homozygosity would not be expected to uncover a wild type $p53$ allele 40% of the time, nor would the lack of selection (50% of the time) of second allele mutations be expected in the breast carcinomas. This is not a property of a tumour suppressor gene as classically defined. These results (Davidoff $et\ al$, 1991), if confirmed and extended, suggest some significant differences between the $p53$ gene and product in breast and colon cancers. It is too early to speculate what those differences might be.

THE PHENOTYPES OF WILD TYPE AND MUTANT $p53$ GENES

Mutant $p53$ Alleles

Because so many different tumours appear to select for a missense mutant $p53$ allele, it was of considerable interest to determine the cell growth promoting properties of these mutant alleles expressed in cell culture (Hinds $et\ al$, 1990).

When mutant *p53* cDNAs or hybrid cDNA/genomic clones are transfected into primary rat embryo fibroblasts in cell culture, the cells that take up these clones and express them have a sevenfold enhanced plating efficiency, ie the ability to form colonies in cell culture increases sevenfold (Finlay *et al*, 1989). When these colonies are selected and cloned, the cells derived from them produce immortalized cell lines that can grow forever, at a rate of about 50% (Levine *et al*, 1989), ie one in every two clones of cells give rise to a cell line. This is in contrast to 1 in 20 (5% efficiency) clones of cells of rat embryo fibroblasts (without mutant *p53*) producing permanent cell lines in culture. Thus, a mutant *p53* gene expressed in a rat embryo fibroblast cell line enhances its plating efficiency and its ability to produce an immortalized cell line in culture. Each of these cell lines was found to contain the original cDNA clone of mutant *p53* and express the altered *p53* protein in large amounts (Levine *et al*, 1989). The mutant p53 protein forms an oligomeric protein complex with the endogenous wild type p53 protein of the rat cell (Finlay *et al*, 1988; Martinez *et al*, 1991). It is hypothesized that such mutant proteins can act in a transdominant fashion (in a complex) to inactivate the growth regulatory effects of the endogenous wild type rat p53 protein (Finlay *et al*, 1989). Thus, mutant *p53* alleles promote immortality of cell lines in culture (Jenkins *et al*, 1984; Rovinski and Benchimol, 1988; Finlay *et al*, 1989).

In support of these ideas is a set of experiments in which 11 permanent cell lines were produced from primary mouse embryo fibroblasts (Harvey and Levine, 1991). These cell lines were passaged and propagated on a 3T3 schedule (Todaro and Green, 1963) (3×10^5 cells transferred every 3 days) so that they were immortalized but otherwise non-transformed. All of these cell lines suffered mutations in at least one *p53* allele during the establishment of these lines, and these mutations were selected for before and during the cloning of these cells. Five of the cell lines contained no wild type *p53*, and the remainder expressed wild type and mutant alleles. Thus, *p53* mutants are commonly selected for as cell lines established in culture, but variables such as species, passage schedule and cell or tissue type origins can all impact upon these results (Harvey and Levine, 1991).

When mutant *p53* alleles are introduced into non-tumorigenic cell lines in culture, the mutant or faulty protein enhances the tumorigenic potential of these cells (Wolf *et al*, 1984; Eliyahu *et al*, 1985). This is true even when the cells do not express any p53 protein (are deletion mutations for *p53*) before the introduction of the missense mutant *p53* clone (Wolf *et al*, 1984). This eliminates the notion that this mutant p53 protein confers enhanced tumorigenicity upon a cell by complexing with an endogenous wild type p53 protein and inactivates its function. Rather, this observation demonstrates that some mutant *p53* alleles produce a faulty protein with a true "gain of function" mutation, ie enhancement of cell growth in a tumour.

Mutant *p53* cDNAs cooperate with an activated *ras* oncogene and transform primary rat embryo fibroblasts in cell culture (Eliyahu *et al*, 1984; Parada *et al*, 1984). The transformed cells express very high levels of the mutant p53

TABLE 1. Properties of *p53* wild type and mutant alleles

Property	Wild type	Codon mutated			
		175	248	273	281
Relative transformation frequency	0	5.5	ND	2	1
Inhibition of transformed cell growth	+	–	–	–	–
Conformational alterations	WT	mutant	WT	WT	WT
Half life of the protein	20 min	3.6 hr	ND	7 hr	1.4 hr
Ability to *trans*-activate a test gene	+	–	ND	+	ND
Binding to SV40 T antigen	+	–	–	–	–

WT = wild-type
ND = not determined

protein, which is found in an oligomeric protein complex with the endogenous wild type p53 of the cell (Martinez *et al*, 1991). Unlike the enhanced tumorigenic potential in cells without *p53*, this appears to be a case where the mutant *p53* does act in a transdominant fashion to produce a transformed phenotype.

The different human mutant hot spot alleles have different efficiencies in promoting the transformation of primary rat embryo fibroblasts in cell culture. For example, the codon 175 mutant alleles are 5.5-fold more efficient transforming agents than codon 281 clones and 2.5-fold more efficient (number of transformed colonies produced) than codon 273 clones (Table 1). There are therefore some biological and biochemical distinctions between different human mutant hot spot alleles of *p53* (Table 1) (Hinds *et al*, 1990).

Wild Type *p53* Alleles

Unlike the mutant *p53* cDNA clones, the *p53* wild type cDNA or genomic clones will not immortalize or transform cells in culture even with the *ras* oncogene as a co-factor (Hinds *et al*, 1989). In fact, the wild type *p53* cDNA/genomic clones will suppress or inhibit a variety of oncogenes from transforming rat embryo fibroblasts in cell culture. Even in cases where a wild type *p53* cDNA/genomic clone was transfected into cells along with an oncogene and a transformed cell line resulted, in every case, it was shown that the *p53* gene selected for was a rare mutant *p53* allele producing either no protein at all or a missense faulty p53 protein (Finlay *et al*, 1989). The wild type p53 protein is incompatible with transformation in cell culture (Hinds *et al*, 1989; Mercer *et al*, 1990). On the other hand, the expression of wild type p53 protein in primary rat embryo fibroblasts (a normal cell) had no effect on the plating efficiency (number of colonies produced) of these cells (Finlay *et al*, 1989).

Wild type p53 is not acting as a toxic agent in these cells but is selectively blocking abnormal or transformed cell division (Michalovitz *et al*, 1990; Martinez *et al*, 1991). Similarly, the introduction of a wild type *p53* cDNA into a tumorigenic cell line in culture reduces the tumorigenic potential of these cells (Chen *et al*, 1990). In this case, the wild type *p53* gene acts as a tumour suppressor gene.

In a particularly clear demonstration of the impact of wild type *p53* upon abnormal cell division, a temperature sensitive *p53* mutant allele was employed (Michalovitz *et al*, 1990; Levine *et al*, 1991). The murine p53 protein containing valine instead of alanine at residue 135 produces a temperature sensitive p53 protein that acts like a wild type protein at 32°C and a mutant protein at 39.5°C. The monoclonal antibody PAb246 can react with the wild type p53 conformation but fails to bind to any known p53 mutant protein that transforms cells in culture (Tan *et al*, 1986; Yewdell *et al*, 1986). Conversely, the monoclonal antibody PAb240 binds to several different p53 missense mutant proteins but fails to react with the wild type p53 protein (Gannon *et al*, 1990). In cells harbouring the temperature sensitive p53 mutant, this protein reacts with PAb246 but not PAb240 when the cells are at 32°C, and the p53 protein from cells grown at 39.5°C reacts with PAb240 antibody but not PAb246. Thus, the conformation of p53 protein is different at 32°C and 39.5°C (Michalovitz *et al*, 1990; Martinez *et al*, 1991). At 37°C, about half the p53 is in the wild type conformation and half in the mutant form. The two conformers of p53 interact and form mixed oligomeric complexes expressing both PAb246 and PAb240 epitopes (Martinez *et al*, 1991).

When cells transformed by this temperature sensitive *p53* mutant plus *ras* are shifted to 32°C, the wild type p53 protein is detected in the cell nucleus and the cells stop dividing (Michalovitz *et al*, 1990; Martinez *et al*, 1991). At 39.5°C or at 37°C, the mutant p53 (or mutant-wild type complex) is found predominantly in the cytoplasm and the cells grow and divide with a rapid generation time (Martinez *et al*, 1991). At 32°C, the cells appear to be blocked at a specific stage of the cell cycle, in late G_1 (Michalovitz *et al*, 1990; Martinez *et al*, 1991). Thus, wild type p53, acting in the cell nucleus, negatively regulates cell division and does so some time in late G_1. When mixtures of wild type and mutant p53 proteins exist in a cell, they can form oligomeric complexes where the mutant form keeps the wild type p53 in the cytoplasm and it fails to act to stop cell division. Clearly, in transformed cells in culture, some p53 mutant proteins act in a transdominant fashion interfering with the proper function of the wild type protein. Although this has been observed in cell culture, no evidence yet exists that this type of process is observed in vivo or in tumours.

PROPERTIES OF THE p53 MUTANT AND WILD TYPE PROTEINS

The Wild Type *p53* Gene

The *p53* gene encompasses about 16–20 kb of DNA located on the short arm of human chromosome 17 at position 17p13.1 (Benchimol *et al*, 1985). In the mouse, the *p53* gene is found on chromosome 11 (Miller *et al*, 1986). Both human and mouse genes are composed of 11 exons. The first exon is non-coding, contains 213 base pairs and is found 8–10 kb away from exons 2–11. Thus, the first intron comprises about one-half of the gene. Northern blot analysis indicates a messenger RNA (mRNA) species of 2.2–2.5 kb. Little is known about the enhancer and promoter elements of this gene. A 400 base pair element 5′ to the first exon is sufficient to produce mRNA at the correct initiation site (termed P_1) in exon 1, and recently, a second promoter element start site (termed P_2) localized about 1 kb 3′ to the P_1 site has been identified (Harlow *et al*, 1985; Reisman *et al*, 1988). *p53* mRNA is expressed in all tissues of the body, and in the mouse, elevated levels of p53 mRNA are found in the spleen and thymus (Rogel *et al*, 1985). Promoter enhanced mutants and elements are only poorly characterized at this time, but at least one group has identified an expression element in intron 4 (Lozano and Levine, 1991), which has tissue preference for the spleen cells in transgenic mice.

The Wild Type and Mutant p53 Proteins

The aminoacid sequence of the p53 protein has been determined for several diverse species. Human and mouse sequences show 81% homology, and human and *Xenopus* show 56% homology (Soussi *et al*, 1987). A prediction of the structure of the p53 protein based on these primary sequences indicates three domains may be present. The first at the aminoterminus, encompassing aminoacid residues 1–75 or 80, is very acidic in charge and is predicted to be in a largely α-helical conformation. The next set of residues, at aminoacids 75–150, are quite hydrophobic and proline rich. The carboxyterminal domains consisting of residues 276–390 in the mouse and 319–393 in the human are very basic and could form an orderly amphipathic helix structure. This carboxyterminal domain appears to be important for the protein to form oligomeric complexes and for its binding to DNA (Pennica *et al*, 1984).

Several serine residues can be phosphorylated in p53. At the aminoterminus, casein kinase I phosphorylates several residues (serine 7, 9, 12, 18, 23, 37 and 58 are all candidates), adding to the acidic charge of this domain. It is therefore of some interest that the first 75 residues of p53 can be fused with the Gal-4 DNA binding domain from yeast, and this hybrid protein can promote transcription of a test gene regulated by a Gal-4 binding sequence. Thus, the first 75 residues can act as an "acidic blob" to promote the action of RNA polymerase on a gene. This is consistent with but does not prove that p53 could be a transcriptional activator. Phosphorylation of this domain could regulate that process. The aminoacid residues 316 and 317 (human) are serine-proline, a recognition site for cdc2 like protein kinase. Beach and colleagues (Bischoff *et al*, 1990) have shown that this serine can be phosphorylated by cdc2 kinase in vitro, and Jenkins and his colleagues (Sturzbecher *et al*, 1990) have demonstrated an association of cdc2 like kinases and p53 in cell extracts. This could link p53 to a cell cycle regulated kinase. The serine-proline site is quite close to a major nuclear localization signal (residues 319–323, proline-lysine-lysine-lysine-proline) in the p53 protein (Shaulsky *et al*, 1991), indicating a possible cell cycle regulation of cellular location with p53. Serine residue 389 (mouse) or 392 (human) is phosphorylated and resides one residue from the carboxyterminus of the protein. It appears that casein kinase II carries out this modification, and, as with the other phosphorylated proteins, the functional consequence of this is unclear.

As mentioned previously, several regions of the p53 protein retain very high conservation of aminoacid sequences (90–100%) even when human and *Xenopus* proteins are compared. These regions span residues 13–19, 117–142, 171–192, 236–258 and 270–286 (Soussi *et al*, 1987). The importance of these segments in the functioning of the protein is reinforced by the dramatic clustering of the p53 missense mutations found in human tumours to these regions (except residues 13–19) of the gene and protein (Levine, 1991).

The conformation of the p53 protein has been probed with a series of monoclonal antibodies that span the epitopes of this antigen. Monoclonal antibodies PAb242, residues 9–25; PAb246, residues 88–109; PAb248 and 2C2, residues 157–192; PAb240, residues 206–211 (212–217 human); and PAb421, residues 370–378 recognize an epitope localized to these aminoacid residues in the murine protein (Lane and Benchimol, 1990). As previously noted, PAb246 binds only to wild type proteins even when mutants span residues 120–300, demonstrating a loss of the available epitope to the antibody (residues 88–109) and a common conformational change in different mutant proteins. Similarly, several diverse mutant proteins gain a new epitope (residues 206–211) in the mouse or human (residues 212–217) p53 antigen, indicating a common conformational change in the faulty or altered proteins.

Several biochemical properties of the p53 proteins also change after the introduction of a missense mutation into the *p53* gene. The level of the wild type protein in most cells is quite low (Reich and Levine, 1984). The reason for this, in large measure, is the short half life of the protein, which is about 20 minutes in most tissues or cell types. Remarkably, all of the mutant p53 proteins examined to date have much longer half lives (in hours) (Finlay *et al*, 1988; Hinds *et al*, 1990) and are present at much higher concentrations in tumours or transformed cells (Iggo *et al*, 1990). This is one of the most consistent phenotypes of a mutant p53 protein.

A second common phenotype of the p53 mutant proteins is their reduced ability to bind to DNA (Kern *et al*, 1991a). The wild type p53 protein can bind specifically to the nucleotide sequence $TGCCT(X)_{5-8} TGCCT$, where X is any nucleotide (Kern *et al*, 1991b). This recognition of a nucleotide sequence is lost or altered upon mutation, although a large number of different mutant proteins have not been tested.

Similarly, *trans*-activation or the positive regulation of a promoter element has recently been reported using the murine muscle form of creatine phosphokinase gene (Weintraub *et al*, 1991). Here, the wild type *p53* gene product, but not a mutant p53 protein, could promote the transcription of a test gene regulated by this promoter. The muscle creatine phosphokinase promoter or enhancer element contains the sequence TGCCT-CTCTC-TGCCT (Zambetti G and Levine AJ, unpublished).

Similarly, several of the mutant *p53* alleles fail to *trans*-activate a test gene even when they are in a Gal-4 fusion protein. This would indicate that the conformational alterations in some mutant *p53* alleles could affect this biochemical function or assay in ways other than the loss of DNA binding potential.

FUNCTIONS OF THE *p53* GENE AND PROTEIN

In some tumours or transformed cell lines, especially osteogenic sarcomas, the *p53* gene has been deleted or rearranged in such a way as to eliminate the possibility of producing a *p53* gene product (Miller *et al*, 1990). Thus, it is clear that the p53 protein and its functions are not essential to the viability of a cell in culture or in a tumour. A mouse that has a similar set of rearranged *p53* genes (the knockout experiment) will indicate whether or not *p53* gene function is critical to a developmental pathway in vivo. What is clear from inherited alterations in the *p53* gene in vivo (both germline or somatic) is that the normal or wild type *p53* gene product controls a process central to regulating cell growth or division. It appears likely, on the basis of the transgenic mice containing mutant *p53* and individuals with the Li-Fraumeni syndrome, that additional mutational events are required to produce a tumour even if a mutant *p53* gene is present. Mutations of *p53* are necessary but not sufficient in the tumours observed to have such genetic alterations.

At present, two distinct but not mutually exclusive hypotheses have been advanced to explain the function of the p53 protein. The first suggests that the p53 protein is itself a transcriptional activator of gene expression. The p53 protein, acting in an oligomeric protein complex with itself or other proteins, could recognize specific DNA sequences in enhancer and/or promoter elements of a gene and positively or negatively regulate such a gene. In support of this idea are the primary sequence of p53 proteins and its predicted structure. This structure looks like that of a *trans*-activator protein (Soussi *et al*, 1988). The protein appears to bind to a specific DNA sequence (Kern *et al*, 1991b) and activates a promoter in a positive fashion (the creatine phosphokinase gene) (Weintraub *et al*, 1991) that contains that specific sequence (Zambetti G and Levine AJ, unpublished). When the aminoterminal domain of *p53*, an acidic blob, is fused to the yeast Gal-4 DNA binding domain, the hybrid gene promotes transcription of a test gene regulated by Gal-4 DNA binding sequences (Fields and Jang, 1990; Raycroft *et al*, 1990).

Mutant p53 proteins often fail to *trans*-activate directly or via Gal-4 DNA binding domain, indicating a genetic correlation with this biochemical assay. The wild type p53 protein has also been shown to have negative (repression) regulatory effects upon several test gene promoter elements (Santhanam *et al*, 1991). Although all of these data are consistent with the possibility that p53 is a transcription factor, the experiments do not prove that this is the case. We must await experiments that identify genes and products regulated by p53 at the enhancer-promoter element where DNA sequences, mutant enhancer elements and gene product regulation all are demonstrated.

A subset of this hypothesis is the suggestion that p53 is able to regulate, via its interactions, a transcription factor in the cell. Here, p53 itself may not participate directly in regulating a promoter but instead would positively or negatively regulate a protein that controls the expression of several genes important for the entry into the cell cycle. In this case, the "gain of function" ascribed to the missense mutant p53 protein could actually enhance the transcriptional activity of such a factor. The absence of the p53 protein would simply not regulate the transcription factor, and the wild type p53 protein would actively inhibit such a transcription factor. This hypothesis has the virtue of explaining several phenotypes.

The second major hypothesis for p53 function suggests that the p53 protein plays a part in the initiation of DNA replication or the assembly of the initiation replication complex. The SV40 large T antigen is required to initiate viral DNA at the origin of replication. The T antigen binds specifically to the SV40 origin of DNA replication where it acts as an ATP dependent helicase to unwind the DNA. The primase binding to T antigen synthesizes RNA primers near and at the origin of DNA replication. The alpha DNA polymerase binding to T antigen then utilizes these primers to initiate DNA synthesis extending the polynucleotide chains. When p53 is bound to T antigen, the alpha DNA polymerase fails to bind to this protein (Gannon and Lane, 1987) and the ATP dependent helicase functions poorly (Wang *et al*, 1989). Indeed, wild type but not mutant p53 proteins bind to the SV40 T antigen and inhibit viral DNA replication both in vivo and in vitro (Braithwaite *et al*, 1987; Wang *et al*, 1989). Viruses often encode proteins that have cellular homologues. The virus can then use its high affinity binding sites to deregulate the cellular control mechanisms. SV40 large T antigen binds to p53 (Lane and Crawford, 1979; Linzer and Levine, 1979) and RB proteins (DeCaprio *et al*, 1988) and could well dissociate these proteins from the T antigen homologue in a cell. If this reasoning is valid, then p53 might function in a cell by regulating the T antigen homologue, which in turn is involved in initiation of cellular DNA replication. T antigen would then bind to p53 so as to promote initiation of cellular DNA replication or entry into S phase. This would be critical for the virus because SV40 DNA replication and cellular histone synthesis (histones are used to package SV40 DNA) require a replicating cell.

The idea that p53 is or regulates a transcription factor is not mutually exclusive of the concept that it is also involved in the initiation of DNA replication. Some origins of replication are stimulated to duplicate DNA by the act of transcription near or at the origin. Transcription of a topologically constrained circular DNA template alters the superhelical density of the DNA and may result in altered base pairing at the origin. This could attract initiation proteins and promote the start of DNA replication. In this case, the DNA sequences recognized by p53 protein or the protein it regulates would be adjacent to or near the origins of DNA replication in a chromosome. This will shortly become a testable prediction.

CONCLUSIONS

It is now well accepted that the *p53* gene is best classified as a tumour suppressor gene. The wild type gene product negatively regulates cell growth or division. It is not essential for progression through the cell cycle, but it is critical as a checkpoint or stopping point that blocks uncontrolled cell division. It appears likely that the absence or loss of p53 function in the cell cycle is not in itself sufficient for uncontrolled cell division. Additional events are required. The p53 protein appears to act as a stop or checkpoint in the late G_1 phase of the cell cycle. Excessive wild type p53 at that time blocks progression into the S phase. It remains possible that normal levels of p53 also act at other times in the cell cycle to regulate cell division negatively.

Mutations of *p53* are the single most common somatic genetic alteration in human cancers. It appears that missense mutations are selected for in tumours, and this suggests that altered or missense proteins have an activity that promotes growth. The demonstration that the introduction of a missense mutation into a *p53* nullizygous cell line promotes enhanced tumour growth is in agreement with this concept. Different *p53* mutations produce p53 proteins with distinct biological and biochemical properties (ie conformational changes, transformation potential, *trans*-activating activities, see Table 1) (Hinds *et al*, 1990). There are, however, common phenotypes of *p53* missense mutations. Chief among these are an enhanced half-life of the mutant p53 protein and increased levels of the altered protein in tumours and transformed cells.

Both the mutant and wild type p53 proteins could function as transcription factors or regulatory subunits of *trans*-activators or could control directly the initiation of DNA replication. To improve our understanding of the nature of cancer, it is clear that we will have to understand the functions of tumour suppressor gene products such as p53.

References

Ahuja H, Bar-Eli M, Advani SH, Benchimol S and Cline MJ (1989) Alterations in the p53 gene and the clonal evolution of the blast crisis of chronic myelocytic leukemia. *Proceedings of the National Academy of Sciences of the USA* **86** 6783–6787

Arai N, Nomura D, Yokota K *et al* (1986) Immunologically distinct p53 molecules generated by alternative splicing. *Molecular and Cellular Biology* **6** 3232–3239

Baker SJ, Fearon ER, Nigro JM *et al* (1989) Chromosome 17 deletions and p53 gene mutations in colorectal carcinoma. *Science* **244** 217–221

Baker SJ, Preisinger AC, Jessup JM *et al* (1990) p53 gene mutations occur in combination with 17p allelic deletions or late events in colorectal tumorigenesis. *Cancer Research* **50** 7717–7722

Benchimol S, Pim D and Crawford L (1982) Radioimmunoassay of the cellular protein p53 in mouse and human cell lines. *EMBO Journal* **1** 1055–1062

Benchimol S, Lamb P, Crawford LV *et al* (1985) Transformation associated p53 protein is encoded by a gene on human chromosome 17. *Somatic Cell and Molecular Genetics* **11** 505–509

Bienz B, Zakut-Houri R, Givol D and Oren M (1984) Analysis of the gene coding for the murine cellular tumour antigen p53. *EMBO Journal* **3** 2179–2183

Bischoff JR, Friedman PN, Marshak DR, Prives C and Beach D (1990) Human p53 is phosphorylated by p60-cdc2 and cyclin B-cdc2. *Proceedings of the National Academy of Sciences of the USA* **87** 4766–4770

Braithwaite AW, Sturzbecher H-W, Addison C, Palmer C, Rudge K and Jenkins JR (1987) Mouse p53 inhibits SV40 origin-dependent DNA replication. *Nature* **329** 458–460

Bressac B, Kew M, Wands J and Ozturk M (1991) Selective G to T mutations of p53 gene in hepatocellular carcinoma from Southern Africa. *Nature* **350** 429–431

Chen P-L, Chen Y, Bookstein R and Lee W-H (1990) Genetic mechanisms of tumor suppression by the human p53 gene. *Science* **250** 1576–1579

Chiba I, Takahashi T, Nau MM *et al* (1990) Mutations in the p53 gene are frequent in primary resected non-small cell lung cancer. *Oncogene* **5** 1603–1610

Crawford LV, Pim DC and Bulbrook RD (1982) Detection of antibodies against the cellular protein p53 in sera from patients with breast cancer. *International Journal of Cancer* **30** 403–408

Crook T, Wrede D, Tidy J, Scholefield J, Crawford L and Vousden KH (1991) Status of c-myc, p53 and retinoblastoma genes in human papillomavirus positive and negative squamous cell carcinomas of the anus. *Oncogene* **6** 1251–1257

Davidoff AM, Humphrey PA, Iglehart JK and Marks JR (1991) Genetic basis for p53 overexpression in human breast cancer. *Proceedings of the National Academy of Sciences of the USA* **88** 5006–5010

DeCaprio JA, Ludlow JW, Figge J *et al* (1988) SV40 large tumor antigen forms a specific complex with the product of the retinoblastoma susceptibility gene. *Cell* **54** 275–283

DeLeo AB, Jay G, Appella E, Dubois GC, Law LW and Old LJ (1979) Detection of a transformation related antigen in chemically induced sarcomas and other transformed cells of the mouse. *Proceedings of the National Academy of Sciences of the USA* **76** 2420–2424

Eliyahu D, Raz A, Gruss P, Givol D and Oren M (1984) Participation of p53 cellular tumor antigen in transformation of normal embryonic cells. *Nature* **312** 646–649

Eliyahu D, Michalovitz D and Oren M (1985) Overproduction of p53 antigen makes established cells highly tumorigenic. *Nature* **316** 158–160

Eliyahu D, Goldfinger N, Pinhasi-Kimhi O *et al* (1988) Meth A fibrosarcoma cells express two transforming mutant p53 species. *Oncogene* **3** 313–321

Fields S and Jang SK (1990) Presence of a potent transcription activating sequence in the p53 protein. *Science* **249** 1046–1049

Finlay CA, Hinds PW, Tan T-H, Eliyahu D, Oren M and Levine AJ (1988) Activating mutations for transformation by p53 produce a gene product that forms an hsc70-p53 complex with an altered half-life. *Molecular and Cellular Biology* **8** 531–539

Finlay CA, Hinds PW and Levine AJ (1989) The p53 proto-oncogene can act as a suppressor of transformation. *Cell* **57** 1083–1093

Gaidano G, Ballerini P, Gong JZ *et al* (1991) p53 mutations in human lymphoid malignancies: association with Burkitt lymphoma and chronic lymphocytic leukemia. *Proceedings of the National Academy of Sciences of the USA* **88** 5413–5417

Gannon JV and Lane DP (1987) p53 and DNA polymerase α compete for binding to SV40 T antigen. *Nature* **329** 456–458

Gannon JV, Greaves R, Iggo R and Lane DP (1990) Activating mutations in p53 produce a common conformational effect: a monoclonal antibody specific for the mutant form. *EMBO Journal* **9** 1595–1602

Harlow E, Williamson NM, Ralston R, Halfman DM and Adams TE (1985) Molecular cloning and in vitro expression of a cDNA clone for human cellular tumor antigen p53. *Molecular and Cellular Biology* **5** 1601–1610

Harvey DM and Levine AJ, (1991) p53 alteration is a common event in the spontaneous immortalization of primary BALB/c murine embryo fibroblasts. *Genes and Development* **5** 2375–2385

Hensel CH, Xiang RH, Sakaguchi AY and Naylor SL (1991) Use of the single strand conformation polymorphism technique and PCR to detect p53 gene mutations in small cell lung cancer. *Oncogene* **6** 1067–1071

Hinds P, Finlay C and Levine AJ (1989) Mutation is required to activate the p53 gene for cooperation with the *ras* oncogene and transformation. *Journal of Virology* **63** 739–746

Hinds PW, Finlay CA, Quartin RS *et al* (1990) Mutant p53 cDNAs from human colorectal carcinomas can cooperate with *ras* in transformation of primary rat cells. *Cell Growth and Differentiation* **1** 571–580

Hollstein MC, Metcalf RA, Welsh JA, Montesano R and Harris CC (1990) Frequent mutation of the p53 gene in human esophageal cancer. *Proceedings of the National Academy of Sciences of the USA* **87** 9958–9961

Hollstein MC, Peri L, Mandard AM *et al* (1991) Genetic analysis of human esophageal tumors from two high incidence geographic areas: frequent p53 base substitutions and absence of *ras* mutations. *Cancer Research* **51** 4102–4106

Hsu IC, Metcalf RA, Sun T, Welsh JA, Wang NJ and Harris CC (1991) Mutational hotspot in the p53 gene in human hepatocellular carcinoma. *Nature* **350** 427–428

Iggo R, Gatter K, Bartek J, Lane D and Harris AL (1990) Increased expression of mutant forms of p53 oncogene in primary lung cancer. *Lancet* **335** 675–679

Isaacs WB, Carter BS and Ewing CM (1991) Wild-type p53 suppresses growth of human prostate cancer cells containing mutant p53 alleles. *Cancer Research* **51** 4716–4720

Jenkins JR, Rudge K and Currie GA (1984) Cellular immortalization by a cDNA clone encoding the transformation-associated phosphoprotein p53. *Nature* **312** 651–654

Kern SE, Kinzler KW, Baker SJ *et al* (1991a) Mutant p53 proteins bind DNA abnormally in vitro. *Oncogene* **6** 131–136

Kern SE, Kinzler KW, Bruskin A *et al* (1991b) Identification of p53 as a sequence-specific DNA-binding protein. *Science* **252** 1708–1711

Lane DP and Crawford LV (1979) T antigen is bound to a host protein in SV40-transformed cells. *Nature* **278** 261–263

Lane DP and Benchimol S (1990) p53: oncogene or anti-oncogene? *Genes and Development* **4** 1–8

Lavigueur A, Maltby V, Mock D, Rossant J, Pawson T and Bernstein A (1989) High incidence of lung, bone, and lymphoid tumors in transgenic mice overexpressing mutant alleles of the p53 oncogene. *Molecular and Cellular Biology* **9** 3982–3991

Levine AJ (1991) *Viruses* Scientific American Library Series, WH Freeman and Co, New York

Levine AJ, Finlay CA and Hinds PW (1989) The p53 proto-oncogene and its product, In: Villarreal LP (ed). *Common Mechanisms of Transformation by Small DNA Tumor Viruses,* Chapter 2, pp 21–37, ASM Publications, Washington, DC

Levine AJ and Momand J (1990) Tumor suppressor genes: the p53 and retinoblastoma sensitivity genes and gene products. *Biochimica et Biophysoca Acta* **1032** 119–136

Levine AJ, Momand J and Finlay CA (1991) The p53 tumor suppressor gene. *Nature* **351** 453–456

Li FP (1988) Cancer families: human models of susceptibility to neoplasia. *Cancer Research* **48**

5381–5386

Li FP, Fraumeni JF, Mulvihill JJ *et al* (1988) A cancer family syndrome in twenty-four kindreds. *Cancer Research* **48** 5358–5362

Linzer DIH and Levine AJ (1979) Characterization of a 54K dalton cellular SV40 tumor antigen in SV40 transformed cells. *Cell* **17** 43–52

Linzer DIH, Maltzman W and Levine AJ (1979) The SV40 A gene product is required for the production of a 54,000 MW cellular tumor antigen. *Virology* **98** 308–318

Lozano G and Levine AJ (1991) Tissue-specific expression of p53 in transgenic mice is regulated by intron sequences. *Molecular Carcinogenesis* **4** 3–9

Malkin D, Li FP, Strong LC *et al* (1990) Germ line p53 mutations in a familial syndrome of breast cancer, sarcomas, and other neoplasms. *Science* **250** 1233–1238

Marks JR, Davidoff AM, Kerns BJ *et al* (1991) Overexpression and mutation of p53 in epithelial ovarian cancer. *Cancer Research* **51** 2979–2984

Martinez J, Georgoff I, Martinez J and Levine AJ (1991) Cellular localization and cell cycle regulation by a temperature sensitive p53 protein. *Genes and Development* **5** 151–159

Mercer WE, Shields MT, Amin M *et al* (1990) Negative growth regulation in a glioblastoma tumor cell line that conditionally expresses human wild-type p53. *Proceedings of the National Academy of Sciences of the USA* **87** 6166–6170

Michalovitz D, Halevy O and Oren M (1990) Conditional inhibition of transformation and of cell proliferation by a temperature-sensitive mutant of p53. *Cell* **62** 671–680

Miller C, Mohandas T, Wolf D, Prokocimer M, Rotter V and Koeffler PH (1986) Human p53 localized to short arm of chromosome 17. *Nature* **319** 783–784

Miller CW, Aslo A, Tsay C *et al* (1990) Frequency and structure of p53 rearrangements in human osteosarcoma. *Cancer Research* **50** 7950–7954

Mowat M, Cheng A, Kimura N, Bernstein A and Benchimol S (1985) Rearrangements of the cellular p53 gene in erythroleukaemia cells transformed by Friend virus. *Nature* **314** 633–636

Mulligan LM, Matlashewski GJ, Scrable HJ and Cavenee WK (1990) Mechanisms of p53 loss in human sarcoma. *Proceedings of the National Academy of Sciences of the USA* **87** 5863–5867

Munroe DG, Rovinski B, Bernstein A and Benchimol S (1988) Loss of a highly conserved domain on p53 as a result of gene deletion during Friend-virus-induced erythroleukemia. *Oncogene* **2** 621–624

Nigro JM, Baker SJ, Preisinger AC *et al* (1989) Mutations in the p53 gene occur in diverse human tumour types. *Nature* **342** 705–708

Oren M, Maltzman W and Levine AJ (1981) Post-translational regulation of the 54K cellular tumor antigen in normal and transformed cells. *Molecular and Cellular Biology* **1** 101–110

Oren M, Bienz B, Givol D, Rechavi G and Zakut R (1983) Analysis of recombinant DNA clones specific for the murine p53 cellular tumor antigen. *EMBO Journal* **2** 1633–1639

Parada LF, Land H, Weinberg RA, Wolf D and Rotter V (1984) Cooperation between gene encoding p53 tumour antigen and *ras* in cellular transformation. *Nature* **312** 649–651

Pennica D, Goeddel DV, Hayflick JS, Reich NC, Anderson CW and Levine AJ (1984) The amino acid sequence of murine p53 determined from a cDNA clone. *Virology* **134** 477–483

Prosser J, Thompson AM, Cranston G and Evans HJ (1990) Evidence that p53 behaves as a tumor suppressor gene in sporadic breast tumors. *Oncogene* **5** 1573–1579

Raycroft L, Wu H and Lozano G (1990) Transcriptional activation by wild-type but not transforming mutants of the p53 anti-oncogene. *Science* **249** 1049–1051

Raycroft L, Schmidt JR, Yoas K and Lozano G p53 growth suppression correlates with transcriptional activation. *Molecular and Cellular Biology* (in press)

Reich NC and Levine AJ (1984) Growth regulation of a cellular tumor antigen, p53, in non-transformed cells. *Nature* **308** 199–201

Reich NC, Oren M and Levine AJ (1983) Two distinct mechanisms regulate the levels of a cellular tumor antigen, p53. *Molecular and Cellular Biology* **3** 2143–2150

Reisman D, Greenberg M and Rotter V (1988) Human p53 oncogene contains one promoter upstream of exon 1 and a second, stronger promoter within intron 1. *Proceedings of the National Academy of Sciences of the USA* **85** 5146–5150

Rogel A, Popliker M, Webb CG and Oren M (1985) p53 cellular tumor antigen: analysis of mRNA levels in normal adult tissues, embryos, and tumors. *Molecular and Cellular Biology* **5** 2851–2855

Rovinski B and Benchimol S (1988) Immortalization of rat embryo fibroblasts by the cellular p53 oncogene. *Oncogene* **2** 445–452

Rovinski B, Munroe D, Peacock J, Mowat M, Bernstein A and Benchimol S (1987) Deletion of 5′-coding sequences of the cellular p53 gene in mouse erythroleukemia: a novel mechanism of oncogene regulation. *Molecular and Cellular Biology* **7** 847–853

Santhanam U, Ray A and Sehgal PB (1991) Repression of the interleukin 6 gene promoter by p53 and the retinoblastoma susceptibility gene product. *Proceedings of the National Academy of Sciences of the USA* **88** 7605–7609

Shaulsky G, Goldfinger N, Tosky MS, Levine AJ and Rotter V (1991) Nuclear localization is essential for the activity of p53 protein. *Oncogene* **6** 2055–2065

Sidransky D, von Eschenbach A, Tsai YC *et al* (1991) Identification of p53 gene mutations in bladder cancers and urine samples. *Science* **252** 706–708

Soussi T, Caron de Fromental C, Mechali M, May P and Kress M (1987) Cloning and characterization of a cDNA from *Xenopus laevis* coding for a protein homologous to human and murine p53. *Oncogene* **1** 71–78

Soussi T, Caron de Fromentel C, Breugnot C and May E (1988) Nucleotide sequence of a cDNA encoding the rat p53 nuclear oncoprotein. *Nucleic Acids Research* **16** 11384

Srivastava S, Zou Z, Pirollo K, Blattner W and Chang EH (1990) Germ-line transmission of a mutated p53 gene in a cancer-prone family with Li-Fraumeni syndrome. *Nature* **348** 747–749

Sturzbecher HW, Maimets T, Chumakov P *et al* (1990) p53 interacts with p34cdc2 in mammalian cells: implication for cell cycle control and oncogenesis. *Oncogene* **5** 795–801

Takahashi T, Nau MM, Chiba I *et al* (1989) p53: a frequent target for genetic abnormalities in lung cancer. *Science* **246** 491–494

Tamura G, Kihana T, Nomura K, Terada M, Sugimura T and Hirohashi S (1991) Detection of frequent p53 gene mutations in primary gastric cancer by cell sorting and polymerase chain reaction single-strand conformation polymorphism analysis. *Cancer Research* **51** 3056–3058

Tan T-H, Wallis J and Levine AJ (1986) Identification of the p53 protein domain involved in formation of the simian virus 40 large T antigen-p53 protein complex. *Journal of Virology* **59** 574–583

Thomas R, Kaplan L, Reich N, Lane DP and Levine AJ (1983) Characterization of human p53 antigen employing primate specific monoclonal antibodies. *Virology* **131** 502–517

Todaro GJ and Green H (1963) Quantitative studies of the growth of mouse embryo cells in culture and their development into established lines. *Journal of Cellular Biology* **17** 299–313

Tooze J (ed) (1973) *Molecular Biology of the Tumor Viruses*, pp 350–403, Cold Spring Harbor Laboratory, Cold Spring Harbor, New York

Varley JM, Brammar WJ, Lane DP, Swallow JE, Dolan C and Walker RA (1991) Loss of chromosome 17p13 sequences and mutation of p53 in human breast carcinomas. *Oncogene* **6** 413–421

Wang EH, Friedman PN and Prives C (1989) The murine p53 protein blocks replication of SV40 DNA in vitro by inhibiting the initiation functions of SV40 large T-antigen. *Cell* **57** 379–392

Weintraub H, Hauschka S and Tapscott SJ (1991) The MCK enhancer contains a p53 responsive element. *Proceedings of the National Academy of Sciences of the USA* **88** 4570–4571

Wolf D, Harris N and Rotter V (1984) Reconstitution of p53 expression in a nonproducer Ab-MuLV-transformed cell line by transfection of a functional p53 gene. *Cell* **38** 119–126

Yewdell J, Gannon JV and Lane DP (1986) Monoclonal antibody analysis of p53 expression in normal and transformed cells. *Journal of Virology* **59** 444–452

The author is responsible for the accuracy of the references.

Transforming Growth Factor-β

J MASSAGUÉ • S CHEIFETZ • M LAIHO • D A RALPH
F M B WEIS • A ZENTELLA

Howard Hughes Medical Institute and Memorial Sloan-Kettering Cancer Center, New York, New York 10021

INTRODUCTION

The term transforming growth factor-β (TGF-β) applies to the members of a group of closely related paracrine factors distinguished by their ability to inhibit cell proliferation. The growth of cells from virtually every lineage can be reversibly inhibited by TGF-β, in some cases with a complete arrest of the cell cycle in late G_1 phase. One mechanism through which TGF-β inhibits cell entry into S phase appears to involve growth suppressor gene products including retinoblastoma (RB). However, TGF-β may also have important effects on cell growth and differentiation through indirect mechanisms such as perturbing the expression of autocrine growth promoting factors and their receptors, or altering the extracellular matrix environment of the cell. TGF-βs affect differentiation, adhesion and proliferation by acting through a common signalling receptor complex. The complex biology of TGF-βs is relevant to normal development and repair processes and to various human disease conditions that could result from either an excess or a loss of TGF-β function. This chapter reviews recent advances in these areas and some of the questions that they raise.

TGF-β AND RELATED FACTORS

Structure of TGF-β

TGF-βs are disulphide-linked polypeptide dimers (reviewed in Massagué 1990; Roberts and Sporn, 1990). Each mature chain is 112 aminoacids in length and is derived from a larger precursor. At least three genes encode TGF-β precursors in human and other mammalian genomes. They are known, respectively, as the TGF-β1, β2 and β3 genes. Although each TGF-β gene is located on a separate chromosome in human and mouse, the similarity of their seven-exon structure and the high degree of sequence conservation strongly suggest that they are derived from a common ancestor. Two additional genes, TGF-β4 and TGF-β5, have been identified in chicken and *Xenopus laevis* genomes, respectively, and several more may exist in these and other organisms.

The TGF-β precursors are approximately 400 aminoacids in length (Fig. 1). They contain potential N-linked glycosylation sites outside the bioactive domain and, with the exception of the TGF-β4 precursor, they contain an aminoterminal hydrophobic signal sequence for translocation into the lumen

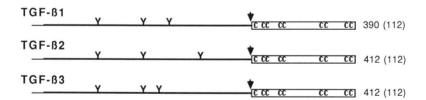

Bioactive Domains

Identity		Conservation	
β1:β2	71%	TGF-β1 (Human:Chick)	100%
β1:β3	72%	TGF-β2 (Human:Simian)	100%
β2:β3	76%	TGF-β3 (Human:Chick)	99%

Fig. 1. Precursor structure and homology of mammalian TGF-βs. TGF-β precursors are 390–412 aminoacids long with the 112 aminoacid bioactive domain (box) located at the carboxyterminus of the precursor. The precursors also contain an aminoterminal signal sequence (thin line), three potential N-linked glycosylation sites (Y) and a basic residue cleavage site (arrows). The approximate location of the nine cysteines in the bioactive domain is indicated (C). The degree of identity between the aminoacid sequences of different human TGF-β isoforms and between the same isoform from different species is indicated. Data are from references reviewed in Massagué 1990

of the endoplasmic reticulum to undergo exocytosis. The bioactive domain is located at the carboxyterminus of the precursor, preceded by a sequence of four basic aminoacids. Proteolytic cleavage at this site appears to occur intracellularly after dimerization of the precursors. The TGF-β dimers consist of two chains of the same type yielding the homodimers known as TGF-β1, β2 and β3. Heterodimeric TGF-βs are also found in cells that simultaneously express various TGF-β genes, as is the case in porcine megakaryocytes, which yield platelets containing TGF-β1, β2 and the heterodimer TGF-β1.2. Therefore, at least theoretically, mammalian cells can express as many as six distinct TGF-β isoforms. This diversity increases the specificity and regulatory flexibility of the TGF-β system. The degree of identity of the TGF-β1, β2 and β3 aminoacid sequences ranges from 64% to 82%. The mature TGF-β sequences contain nine cysteines with conserved spacing and all forming inter- or intrasubunit disulphide bonds.

Disulphide bonded dimer formation is required for biological activity. The aminoacid sequence of each TGF-β isoform is strictly conserved, being 98–100% identical between chicken and human. The evolutionary pressure to retain such a degree of conservation suggests that the functional differences of the various TGF-β isoforms, however limited, are critical for the biological role of this group of factors. The various TGF-β isoforms display a similar potency in many biological assays, but differ in others by as much as 100-fold. Systems in which such differences are observed include vascular endothelial cells and haematopoietic progenitor cells in which the potency of TGF-β2 as a growth inhibitor is only 1% of the potency of TGF-β1 or β3.

The TGF-β Family

TGF-βs are the prototype of a large family of growth, differentiation and morphogenesis paracrine factors which includes over 20 members (reviewed in Massagué, 1990). Structurally, the members of this family share with the TGF-βs a common precursor structure, a conserved positioning of seven or nine cysteines in the mature sequence, and a homodimeric or heterodimeric structure as bioactive factors. Aminoacid sequence identity between bioactive domains of individual family members ranges from 25% to 90%, whereas the proregions in the precursors of these factors show a more limited degree of similarity.

Besides the members of the TGF-β group, the family includes the activins and inhibins, which can act as regulators of pituitary, gonadal and placental hormone production, inducers of mesoderm in early amphibian embryos and inducers of mammalian erythroid cell differentiation. The Müllerian inhibiting substance (MIS) is expressed in male gonadal tissue early in mammalian development and induces regression of the female genital primordium, the Müllerian duct. The decapentaplegic (DPP) gene product controls dorsoventral development during embryogenesis and formation of epithelial structures during larval stages in *Drosophila*. The aminoacid sequence of mature DPP is, remarkably, up to 75% identical to the corresponding sequence of six mammalian bone morphogenesis proteins (BMPs) or various Vg-related products (Vgrs) and, to a lesser extent, the Vg1 gene. Maternal Vg1 transcripts are present in the vegetal pole of *Xenopus* oocytes, and their product is thought to participate in development of the frog embryo. The biology of the DPP/BMP/Vgr/Vg group of TGF-β related factors underscores the high degree of evolutionary conservation of this growth factor family, its multifunctional nature and its involvement in the guidance of critical developmental processes in a vast span of metazoan organisms.

TGF-β Activation, Distribution and Regulated Expression

The aminoterminal proregion in the biosynthetic precursors of TGF-β and related factors have important roles in the biology of these factors, some of which are unique when compared with other polypeptide hormone proregions. The proregion guides the correct folding and disulphide bonding of the bioactive domain during TGF-β synthesis (Gray and Mason, 1990). Unlike the proregions of other hormones, the TGF-β proregion remains noncovalently associated with the bioactive domain even after proteolytic cleavage of the precursor. When this complex is secreted, its activity remains latent because the factor cannot bind to cell surface receptors (Pircher *et al*, 1986). Thus, the latent TGF-β complex may function as a regulator of cell access to secreted TGF-β or as a mechanism to prevent rapid clearance of activated TGF-β.

In addition to these functions, the TGF-β proregion may actively participate in the intricate activation process of the latent complex. This process is still poorly understood. Latent TGF-β can be activated in vitro by extreme pH conditions or by deglycosylating agents (Pircher *et al*, 1986; Miyazono and Heldin, 1989). Evidence suggests that mannose-6-phosphate (man-6-P) residues in the TGF-β proregion may tether the complex to cell surface man-6-P receptors as a requisite for activation in vivo (Kovacina *et al*, 1989; Dennis and Rifkin, 1991). This event, however, is insufficient to activate latent TGF-β because many cells that express man-6-P receptors fail to activate latent TGF-β. Plasmin, acting as a protease, and the acidic pH of certain cellular microenvironments have also been implicated in physiological activation of latent TGF-β (Lyons *et al*, 1990). An additional complexity in this process stems from the fact that the TGF-β1 proregion in the latent complex is disulphide linked to a glycoprotein of 125–160 kDa. This protein, known as "latent TGF-β binding protein" (LTBP) contains multiple epidermal growth factor like repeats in tandem as the main distinctive feature (Kanzaki *et al*, 1990; Tsuji *et al*, 1990). LTBP does not bind TGF-β directly and its function is unknown at present (Kanzaki *et al*, 1990).

Despite its name and the fact that some transformed cells express it at higher levels than their normal counterparts, TGF-β production is not an exclusive attribute of oncogenically transformed cells. On the contrary, TGF-βs are expressed by many normal cell types (reviewed in Massagué, 1990; Roberts and Sporn, 1990). In vivo, TGF-βs are expressed in discrete locations in virtually all tissues during embryonic development. Expression of the various TGF-β isoforms during this process occurs with distinctive spatial and temporal patterns. Enhanced TGF-β expression occurs also during processes of tissue repair and recycling. TGF-β is stored at high levels in the alpha granules of blood platelets, which can deliver it to sites of tissue injury (Assoian and Sporn, 1986). A high level of TGF-β is also found in bone matrix and other interstitial matrices, possibly bound to specific matrix components (Seyedin et al, 1985; Thompson et al, 1989). At least two proteoglycans, betaglycan and decorin, as well as collagen have been shown to bind TGF-β and may represent important sources of retention TGF-β storage in extracellular matrices (Massagué, 1990; Yamaguchi et al, 1990).

The promoter region of each mammalian TGF-β gene displays distinct regulatory elements, suggesting that expression of each isoform can be independently regulated (Lafyatis et al, 1991). This is supported by the fact that each isoform has a distinct pattern of expression in vivo and can respond to cell stimulation by a specific set of agonists in vitro. TGF-β1 upregulates its own expression by increasing Jun and Fos, which in turn activate TGF-β1 transcription by binding to AP-1 sites in the TGF-β1 gene promoter (Kim et al, 1990). This autoinduction mechanism might be important in the establishment of TGF-β gradients during morphogenesis or accumulaton of TGF-β at sites of injury.

GROWTH CONTROL BY TGF-β

Multifunctional Nature of TGF-β

TGF-β is remarkable in that it can affect diverse cellular functions in cells from virtually every lineage. Furthermore, effects of TGF-β in vitro can be positive or negative depending on the cell type and culture conditions. The activity of TGF-β1, β2 and β3 on various cell types has been the subject of several recent comprehensive reviews (Massagué, 1990; Roberts and Sporn, 1990) and will be covered here only in an abbreviated form.

Although diverse, the cellular responses to TGF-β can be grouped into three main categories according to the aspect of cellular behaviour that they affect. These categories include: proliferative responses; effects on cell differerentiation and differentiated functions; and responses involving cell adhesion, migration and extracellular matrices. TGF-β affects the proliferation of many cell types. In most cases, the effect of TGF-β is inhibitory. Cases in which this factor acts as a growth promoter are relatively few, and in most of them, the effect of TGF-β may be indirect (see below). There is no clear evidence that TGF-β receptors can directly elicit mitogenic signals.

Cell differentiation is regulated by TGF-β in myoblasts, preadipocytes, osteoblasts, chondroblasts, haematopoietic progenitors and other cell types. Depending on the cell lineage or cell type, TGF-β either favors or reversibly inhibits differentiation. Cell types whose specialized activities are regulated by TGF-β include lymphocytes and hormone-producing adrenocortical, granulosa and pituitary cells. Most of the evidence for effects of TGF-β on cell differentiation is derived from in vitro experiments. However, it is known that TGF-β enhances induction of myogenic structures in developing embryos (Kimelman and Kirschner, 1987; Rosa *et al*, 1988; Potts *et al*, 1991), whereas it inhibits differentiation of skeletal muscle myoblast in culture. In vitro studies have shown that TGF-β could regulate cell differentiation, but the positive or negative nature of this effect must be interpreted with caution since cell differentiation systems in vitro cannot properly replicate many of the extracellular determinants that affect cell differentiation in vivo.

Direct and Indirect Effects

Some effects of TGF-β on cell proliferation and differentiation appear to be mediated entirely through intracellular mechanisms that alter the cell's ability to progress through the proliferative cycle or to commit to a more differentiated state. Other effects, however, are indirect in that they result from changes in extracellular matrix or autocrine cytokine production induced by TGF-β. These indirect effects are important because they are likely to have major roles in the physiological action of TGF-β in processes of tissue morphogenesis, remodelling and repair.

The ability of cell adhesion receptors and extracellular matrices to regulate various cellular functions is well documented. Cell migration, homing and positioning in tissues result directly from physical interactions between cell adhesion receptors and molecules that surround the cell. In addition, cell adhesion signals can affect cell proliferation or differentiation through as of yet unknown mechanisms. Furthermore, extracellular matrix components can also act as important reservoirs of peptide growth factors. These functions can be altered by factors, such as TGF-β, that regulate extracellular matrix and cell adhesion receptor levels.

TGF-β regulates expression of cell adhesion components in many normal and transformed cell lines (reviewed in Massagué, 1990). The integrins, a major class of cell adhesion receptors, are heterodimeric transmembrane proteins with affinity for extracellular matrix components and certain cell surface determinants. Cell adhesion molecules (CAM) mediate cell to cell adhesion through homophilic interactions. TGF-β increases expression of these adhesion molecules and of extracellular matrix components including fibronectins, interstitial collagens, small secretory proteoglycans, thrombospondin, tenascin, laminin and others. Raised transcription rate of the corresponding genes and, in some instances, increased stability of their mRNAs account for the effects of

TGF-β. Extracellular matrix production is further enhanced by the ability of TGF-β to inhibit matrix degradation; this is accomplished through decreased expression of collagenases as well as increased expression of plasminogen activator inhibitor and metalloproteinase inhibitors. Thus, the net effect of TGF-β is to upregulate cell adhesion. Exceptions in which this factor selectively decreases cell adhesion to certain matrix components are also known.

There are several cases that illustrate how TGF-β may affect cell proliferation and differentiation through changes in cell adhesion. For example, the growth promoting effect of TGF-β on NRK fibroblasts plated in soft agar medium appears to be the result of enhanced expression of fibronectin, type I collagen and proteoglycans, and increased integrin-mediated adhesion to these molecules (Ignotz and Massagué, 1986; 1987). Thus, anchorage dependent fibroblasts suspended in agar are able to proliferate in response to other mitogens in this medium because TGF-β induces these cells to produce an extracellular matrix for their own use. In contrast, monolayer cultures of NRK fibroblasts grow more slowly in response to TGF-β (Roberts *et al*, 1985) because of lengthening of G_1 phase (Shipley *et al*, 1985) or the negative effect of a collagen rich extracellular matrix under these conditions (Nugent and Newman, 1989). Furthermore, TGF-β inhibits skeletal muscle myoblast differentiation apparently through two parallel mechanisms: it inhibits expression of the differentiation promoting genes MyoD1 or myogenin (Vaijda *et al*, 1989; Heino and Massagué, 1990), and it induces a rich collagen matrix that impairs differentiation of certain myoblast cell lines such as L6E9 cells (Heino and Massagué, 1990).

Evidence that TGF-β can oppose mitogenic signals by acting at a level distal from growth factor receptors is provided by studies of lung epithelial cells and fibroblasts in which TGF-β arrests the cell cycle without downregulating epidermal growth factor receptor signal transduction (Like and Massagué, 1986; Chambard and Pouyssegur, 1988). However, in certain cases, TGF-β can affect cell proliferation by altering production of cytokines or regulating expression of their receptors. For example, certain fibroblasts and vascular smooth muscle cells, when kept in serum free medium, show a limited proliferative response to TGF-β due to induction of autocrine platelet derived growth factor production (Leof *et al*, 1986; Majack *et al*, 1990). Likewise, proliferation of certain cells may be inhibited by the ability of TGF-β to downregulate expression of receptors for various mitogens including platelet derived growth factor (Battegay *et al*, 1990).

In vivo, TGF-β is expressed in tissues undergoing rapid morphogenesis during normal development or repair. These processes are also characterized by the dynamic accumulation and turnover of extracellular matrices and multiple cytokines. It is reasonable to anticipate that TGF-β has a major role in tissue development and organization through its influence on the composition of extracellular matrices and cytokines produced in situ. Furthermore, excessive TGF-β activity may cause extracellular matrix overproduction in certain fibrotic disorders (Border *et al*, 1990).

TGF-β Inhibits G$_1$ Progression

All TGF-β isoforms tested display reversible growth inhibitory activity on normal as well as transformed epithelial, endothelial, fibroblast, neuronal, lymphoid and haematopoietic cells (Tucker *et al*, 1984; Moses *et al*, 1985; Roberts *et al*, 1985; Frater-Schröder *et al*, 1986; Kehrl *et al*, 1986; Shipley *et al*, 1986; Cheifetz *et al*, 1987; Knabbe *et al*, 1987; Ohta *et al*, 1987; Kimchi *et al*, 1988; Graycar *et al*, 1989). The extent of the growth inhibitory response to TGF-β varies with each cell type, reaching a virtual growth arrest in lung epithelial cells and keratinocytes (Tucker *et al*, 1984; Shipley *et al*, 1986).

Although the effects of TGF-β on the extracellular matrix and cytokine activity mentioned above may decrease the proliferative rate of some cells, the kinetics of these effects are too slow to easily explain the ability of TGF-β to rapidly arrest the cell cycle in other cells.

TGF-β inhibits cell proliferation induced by diverse mitogens. This and other evidence suggest that in many instances, TGF-β opposes the proliferative effect of mitogens by interfering at a level distal from mitogen receptors and their early signals in the pathway of mitogenic stimulation. Recent progress in identifying events involved in the TGF-β growth inhibitory response derives from the observation, made with several cell lines, that TGF-β lengthens or arrests the cell cycle in G$_1$ phase (Nakamura *et al*, 1985; Shipley *et al*, 1985; Heimark *et al*, 1986; Lin *et al*, 1987; Laiho *et al*, 1990a). Specifically, TGF-β interferes with the ability of cells to reach or traverse a stage in late G$_1$ close to the time point known as R (or W).

G$_1$ consists of a succession of stages through which the cell commits to DNA replication. Entry and progression through these stages require the continuous presence of growth promoting factors. Each cell type may require a distinct set of growth factors, but the common effect of their signals is similar in all cases. That is, mitogenic factors act in concert to bring cells to a certain point in G$_1$, after which the cells can progress into S phase without further mitogenic stimulation. This time point, termed the R (or W) arrest point, is located approximately 2 hours before entry into S phase (Pledger *et al*, 1978; Campisi *et al*, 1982). Since the converging effects of multiple mitogens lead a cell to the R point, the events in the late portion of G$_1$ appear to provide effective targets for negative regulation of cell commitment to DNA replication. This possibility is substantiated by the following results. TGF-β added to lung epithelial cells or keratinocytes in middle to late G$_1$ prevents cell entry into S phase (Laiho *et al*, 1990a; Pietenpol *et al*, 1990b). Furthermore, TGF-β added less than 2 hours before entry into S phase does not arrest cells until the next G$_1$ phase. Finally, TGF-β added to exponentially growing cells accumulates the entire population in G$_1$. Thus, cycle arrest by TGF-β and the R point are close to one another. They also map closely to the time point when the phosphorylation state of a growth suppressor gene product, RB, is regulated. The increased phosphorylation and presumed reduction in growth suppressive activity of RB at this point is a prerequisite for cell progression towards S phase. These observations led to the finding that TGF-β action prevents RB phosphorylation in late G_1, retaining RB in its putative growth suppressive state (Laiho *et al*, 1990a).

RB Kinase as a TGF-β Target

RB is a growth suppressor gene whose loss of function due to mutation or deletion of both alleles leads to oncogenic transformation that can be reverted, at least in some instances, by reintroduction of normal *RB* into the cell (see chapter by Weinberg RA, this issue). The gene product, RB, is a nuclear phosphoprotein, which is expressed throughout the cell cycle. Its phosphorylation level, however, oscillates in a cell cycle dependent manner (see chapters by Dyson N and Harlow E, Livingston D, and Munger K *et al*, this issue). Underphosphorylated RB prevails in G_0 and during G_1, is rapidly phosphorylated as cells approach S phase and remains phosphorylated until M phase. The transforming protein of SV40, T antigen, binds underphosphorylated RB (Ludlow *et al*, 1989) and other related cellular proteins (Dyson *et al*, 1989a; Ewen *et al*, 1989). This interaction is thought to perturb the growth suppressive function of RB. These observations favour the hypothesis that the form of RB that is actively involved in growth suppression is the underphosphorylated form.

In Mv1Lu lung epithelial cells, TGF-β interferes with the events that lead to RB phosphorylation in late G_1 (Laiho *et al*, 1990a). TGF-β acts by preventing the appearance of a specific RB kinase activity in middle G_1 rather than by inactivating this kinase once it has appeared, or by inducing dephosphorylation of RB. This conclusion is supported by the observation that if TGF-β is added during the last 2 hours of G_1 or during S, when RB is already phosphorylated, TGF-β does not cause RB dephosphorylation and does not prevent phosphorylation of RB molecules newly synthesized during that period.

Inhibition of RB phosphorylation by TGF-β1 thus retains RB in its presumed growth suppressive state (Fig. 2). Is this effect part of a sequence of events that lead to growth arrest or is it simply a consequence of an earlier cell cycle block imposed by TGF-β? Of these two possibilities, only the former is informative with regard to the mechanism of growth inhibitory signal transduction. To distinguish between the two possibilities, use has been made of cells that express a transfected SV40 T antigen gene. Mv1Lu and keratinocytes become resistant to growth inhibition by TGF-β if they express wild type T antigen but are inhibited if they express a T antigen variant that fails to bind RB because it carries point mutations in the RB binding region (Laiho *et al*, 1990a; Pietenpol *et al*, 1990b). Resistance of wild type T antigen expressing cells to growth inhibition by TGF-β may be due to interference of T antigen with the growth suppressive activity of RB or an RB like protein. However, although Mv1Lu cells expressing T antigen are no longer growth inhibited by TGF-β, they still respond to this factor by inhibiting RB phosphorylation (Laiho *et al*, 1990a). Thus, TGF-β does not arrest cells in order to inhibit RB phosphorylation, which argues that inhibition of RB phosphorylation is part of

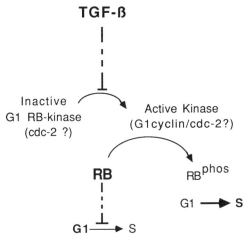

Fig. 2. A model for TGF-β inhibition of progression from G_1 to S phase in Mv1Lu lung epithelial cells. A G_1 specific RB kinase, which could be a cdc2 related protein kinase, is activated in middle G_1 phase, resulting in the phosphorylation of RB which is a prerequisite for cell progression through G_1 and into S phase TGF-β prevents RB phosphorylation, which can lead to cell cycle arrest in late G_1. Since TGF-β does not reverse the phosphorylation of RB or inhibit the G_1 specific RB kinase once it has been activated, TGF-β will not arrest cells at other points in the cell cycle

the sequence of events that lead to growth arrest by TGF-β rather than a consequence of growth arrest.

The exact identity of the serine-threonine kinase(s) that phosphorylates RB in G_1 is not clear. However, the cell cycle dependent nature of this phosphorylation suggests that a cell cycle regulated kinase(s) is involved. Cdc2 is a paradigm for such kinases. Cdc2 or a related enzyme (a large family of cdc2 related genes is being uncovered at present) are good candidates for the role discussed here. The RB aminoacid sequence contains multiple copies of the putative cdc2 consensus phosphorylation site (Lin *et al*, 1991). Furthermore, RB phosphorylated in vitro by cdc2 yields a phosphopeptide map that is remarkably similar to the map from RB phosphorylated in intact cells. The difficulty in definitely assigning a physiological role to cdc2 in this process stems in part from the uncertainties inherent in the analysis of multiphosphorylated substrates such as RB and in part from the fact that cdc2 may represent a vast family of members with overlapping substrate specificities.

These limitations notwithstanding, a connection between cdc2 related kinases and RB phosphorylation seems probable, which raises the question of how TGF-β may interfere with activation of this kinase system. What is known from the study of cdc2 in yeast, clams, frog oocytes and mammalian cells is that this enzyme becomes active when it associates with one of several cyclins which are proteins synthesized and degraded in a cell cycle dependent manner. Cyclin:cdc2 complexes that function during G_2/M are subject to a series of events that lead to activation of the cdc2 kinase activity. Any of these events could in principle be a target for regulation by exogenous factors. There is evidence that the cdc2 kinase is active at the G_1/S boundary and can be inhibited by TGF-β (Howe *et al*, 1991). Less is known about the presence of these types of complexes earlier in G_1. However, candidate G_1 cyclins have been identified recently (Matsushime *et al*, in press; Xiong *et al*, in press), and progress on this front may be forthcoming.

Also to be noted is the possibility that RB might be phosphorylated by multiple kinases throughout the cell cycle. In support of this possibility, the pattern of phosphorylated RB species changes as cells progress from late G_1 to M phase (DeCaprio J, personal communication). The enzymes involved could be multiple unrelated kinases or distinct forms of activated cdc2 that appear throughout the cell cycle. TGF-β might inhibit only G_1 specific RB phosphorylation(s). In the presence of T antigen, cells complete the cycle even though TGF-β may prevent the initial phosphorylation of RB in G_1. This might expose RB to TGF-β insensitive kinases later in the cell cycle, which would explain why TGF-β only partly inhibits RB phosphorylation in exponentially growing Mv1Lu cells that express T antigen.

Early TGF-β Response Genes

TGF-β1 regulates the expression of nuclear factors including c-*jun* and *junB* (Pertovaara *et al*, 1989; Kim *et al*, 1990; Heino and Massagué, 1990; Laiho *et al*, 1991a), c-*fos* (Kim *et al*, 1990) and c-*myc* (Fernandez-Pol *et al*, 1987; Takehara *et al*, 1987; Coffey *et al*, 1988; Pietenpol *et al*, 1990a), growth factors including TGF-β1, platelet derived growth factors A and B (Leof *et al*, 1986; Daniel *et al*, 1987), many components of the cell adhesion apparatus including extracellular matrix proteins and cell adhesion integrin receptors (Massagué, 1990) and various other genes and cellular activities. The promoter region in various TGF-β regulated genes may contain multiple TGF-β response elements that vary in different TGF-β regulated genes (Rossi *et al*, 1988; Kim *et al*, 1989, 1991). TGF-β response elements include NF1 binding sites, AP-1 binding sites, cyclic AMP response elements and others. Some of these responses, especially the increase of *junB* and plasminogen activator inhibitor-1 (*PAI-1*), or the decrease of c-*myc* transcription, are relatively rapid, being observed within 30 minutes after addition of TGF-β.

As progress is made in elucidating steps in the TGF-β mechanism of growth inhibition, it is important to determine how, at the molecular level, the diverse effects of TGF-β1 may relate to each other. The effect on *junB* and *PAI-1* expression is observed in various cell lines independently of whether or not they are growth inhibited by TGF-β (Pertovaara *et al*, 1989; Li *et al*, 1990; Laiho *et al*, 1991a). Downregulation of c-*myc* does appear to have an important role in the response of mouse keratinocytes to TGF-β because proliferation of these cells depends on a high level of c-*myc* expression (Pietenpol *et al*, 1990a). However, downregulation of c-*myc* expression is not observed in some cell lines that are growth inhibited by TGF-β (Chambard and Pouyssegur, 1988; Sorrentino and Bandyopadhyay, 1989).

Genetic and biochemical evidence suggests that the effects of TGF-β on gene expression originate by activation of the same TGF-β receptor complex that mediates suppression of RB phosphorylation and cell cycle arrest (see below). Since, directly or indirectly, RB may influence gene expression (Robbins *et al*, 1990; Kim *et al*, 1991), this has raised the question whether effects of TGF-β1 on expression of certain genes lie downstream from the TGF-β1 induced changes in RB function that lead to growth arrest. One approach to establish causal links between the various effects of TGF-β has been to use cells that express T antigen or related proteins (Laiho *et al*, 1990a, 1991a; Pietenpol *et al*, 1990b). Since T antigen and other DNA tumour virus transforming proteins bind RB and this is thought to perturb RB function (Ludlow *et al*, 1989; Whyte *et al*, 1988; Dyson *et al*, 1989b), the ability of these proteins to inhibit specific effects to TGF-β could be interpreted as evidence that such responses lie downstream from RB in a pathway leading to growth inhibition. Certain effects of TGF-β in Mv1Lu cells, including stimulation of *junB* and extracellular matrix gene expression, are not affected by the presence of T antigen, suggesting that these responses do not involve RB (Laiho *et al*, 1990a, 1991b). Downregulation of c-*myc* gene transcription by TGF-β is, however, lost in mouse keratinocytes transformed by T antigen or other related viral proteins (Pietenpol *et al*, 1990b). It has therefore been proposed that growth inhibition by TGF-β is caused by downregulation of c-*myc* expression through a mechanism that involves RB or a related protein (Pietenpol *et al*, 1990).

In considering this possibility, one may reason that if DNA tumour virus proteins interfere with c-*myc* regulation by inactivating the growth suppressive function of RB, it should be expected that inactivation of RB function by other means should also lead to loss of c-*myc* response to TGF-β1. Other approaches have been recently adopted to investigate the possible involvement of RB in the response of genes whose expression is rapidly modulated, positively or negatively, by TGF-β. One of these approaches has made use of S phase Mv1Lu cells (Zentella *et al*, in press). In S phase, these cells contain essentially all their RB protein in a highly phosphorylated state (Laiho *et al*, 1990a; Howe *et al*, 1991), a state of RB that is thought to be inactive as a growth suppressor (Buchkovich *et al*, 1989; DeCaprio *et al*, 1989; Ludlow *et al*, 1989). Yet, addition of TGF-β1 to S phase Mv1Lu cells alters c-*myc*, *junB* and *PAI-1* gene expression as effectively as it does in early G_1 cells (Zentella *et al*, in press). These results suggest that the underphosphorylated (growth suppressive) form of RB may not be required for regulation of c-*myc*, *junB* or *PAI-1* expression in Mv1Lu cells.

Furthermore, the TGF-β response has also been examined in DU-145 human prostate carcinoma cells (Zentella *et al*, in press). This cell line lacks RB function due to a deletion of exon 21 in the *RB* gene (Huang *et al*, 1990). DU-145 cells are not growth inhibited by TGF-β, which is consistent with the suggested involvement of RB in this response. However, these cells display functional TGF-β receptors and respond to TGF-β1 with downregulation of c-*myc* expression as well as increased *junB* and *PAI-1* expression (Zentella *et al*, in press). Furthermore, as in mouse keratinocytes (Pietenpol *et al*, 1990a), this effect is due to inhibition of c-*myc* transcription initiation by TGF-β1. These results indicate that the growth suppressive activity of RB is not required for inhibition of c-*myc* expression by TGF-β1 in DU-145 cells. In fact, transfection of an RB expression vector actually increases the transcriptional activity of a cotransfected c-*myc* promotor segment in MvlLu cells (Kim *et al*, 1991).

The discrepancy between this conclusion and previous ones implicating RB in the regulation of c-*myc* expression by TGF-β1 (Pietenpol *et al*, 1990b) could be bridged by the possibility that distinct mechanisms might mediate similar effects of TGF-β1 in different cell lines. The RB binding site of T antigen binds cellular components other than RB (see chapter by Livingston D, this issue). It is possible that T antigen binding components other than RB might be involved in the c-*myc* response to TGF-β1 in MvlLu cells. Additionally, T antigen could alter cell responsiveness to TGF-β secondarily to its ability to transform cells. Cellular transformation by T antigen is dependent on its ability to sequester RB but results in pleiotropic cell changes. It seems unlikely that RB directly controls every process in normal cells that becomes altered in T antigen transformed cells.

TGF-β SIGNAL TRANSDUCTION

Multiple Responses Mediated by a Common Receptor Complex

TGF-β1, β2 and β3, and the heterodimer TGF-β1.2, bind with high affinity to a set of cell surface proteins that include the type I receptor, the type II receptor and betaglycan (Massagué, 1990). Receptor types I and II are cell surface glycoproteins of 53 kDa and 70 kDa, respectively. They are expressed ubiquitously, but in low numbers, in most normal and transformed mammalian and avian cells (Massagué *et al*, 1990), and they display ligand binding properties that strikingly discriminate between the various TGF-β isoforms. Receptor types I and II are separate products based on differences in the peptide maps of their ligand binding domains (Cheifetz *et al*, 1986) and differences in their ability to bind various TGF-β isoforms (Cheifetz *et al*, 1990).

Betaglycan is a proteoglycan with chondroitin sulphate and heparan sulphate chains linked to a 110–130 kDa core protein that also contains the TGF-β binding site (Segarini and Seyedin, 1988; Cheifetz *et al*, 1988; Cheifetz and Massagué, 1989). The tissue distribution of betaglycan is more restricted than that of receptors I and II and is absent from myoblasts, haematopoietic cells and endothelial cells which, nevertheless, respond to TGF-β (Massagué *et al*, 1986; Ohta *et al*, 1987; Segarini *et al*, 1989). No evidence is presently available for a direct role of betaglycan in signal transduction. Its proteoglycan nature, secretion as soluble forms and presence in extracellular matrices and serum (Andres *et al*, 1989) have suggested that betaglycan may function as a TGF-β

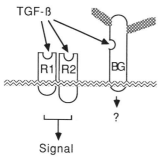

Fig. 3. TGF-β membrane binding proteins in Mv1Lu cells. Receptor components I and II (R1 and R2) are glycoproteins of 53 kDa and 70 kDa that bind TGF-β and are required for mediation of multiple responses to this factor. R1 requires R2 to reach the cell surface or to bind TGF-β. R2 requires R1 to signal but not to bind TGF-β. Thus, R1 and R2 cooperate as components of a signalling TGF-β receptor complex. TGF-β also binds to the core protein of the membrane proteoglycan, betaglycan (BG). There is no evidence that betaglycan is directly involved in signal transduction. The higher abundance and lower binding affinity of betaglycan suggest a role as a reservoir of activated TGF-β

storage protein or as a regulator of the availability of the bioactive ligand to the cell.

Identification of cell surface receptors involved in TGF-β signal transduction has been accomplished by isolation of mutant Mv1Lu clones resistant to the growth inhibitory action of TGF-β1 and β2 (Boyd and Massagué, 1989; Laiho *et al*, 1990b). Although these mutants were selected on the basis of their resistance to growth inhibition by TGF-β, they show a loss of all other known responses to TGF-β, including stimulation of fibronectin and PAI-1 production, inhibition of RB phosphorylation and morphological changes. Analysis of cell surface TGF-β binding proteins shows that the mutations frequently affected the expression of TGF-β receptors I and II but not betaglycan. Certain mutant clones present a decreased number or complete loss of detectable type I receptor. Others show concomitant loss of type I and type II receptors with evidence of structural alterations in the type II receptor, as determined by receptor affinity labelling assays (Laiho *et al*, 1990b).

This evidence has linked receptors I and II to mediation of the pleiotropic action of TGF-β in Mv1Lu cells (Fig. 3). Somatic cell hybrids demonstrate the recessive nature of these mutants with respect to the wild type phenotype and have defined various mutant complementation groups (Laiho *et al*, 1991b). Among these, hybrids between cells that express only type II receptor (R mutants) and cells that express neither receptor type (DRa mutants) rescu°e wild type expression of type I receptors. Moreover, these hybrids regain full responsiveness to TGF-β1, as measured by inhibition of DNA synthesis as well as stimulation of fibronectin and PAI-1 production. These results provide evidence for an interaction between TGF-β receptor components I and II and show that both receptor components are required for mediation of biological responses to TGF-β1 in Mv1Lu cells.

TGF-β Receptors in RB Defective Tumour Cells

TGF-β receptors in RB defective human tumour cells are an interesting subject. Each of several human retinoblastoma cell lines examined in one study lack detectable TGF-β receptors I and II and fail to respond to TGF-β, which contrasts with the presence of these receptors and responses in retinoblasts (Kimchi et al, 1988). Since absence of these receptors is very rare in other normal or tumour cells including human fetal retinoblasts (Massagué et al, 1990), this observation suggested that loss of the TGF-β growth inhibitory response in retinoblasts due to loss of TGF-β receptors might contribute to the escape of cells from normal growth control and lead to a more tumorigenic phenotype. The presence of TGF-β receptors in DU-145 cells (Zentella et al, in press) shows that RB function is not required for expression of functional TGF-β receptors. Rather, loss of TGF-β receptors appears to be an independent event that may confer a growth advantage to certain cells lacking RB. This is consistant with the possibility that TGF-β may cause growth inhibition through RB independent mechanisms like those mentioned in preceding sections.

Non-signalling Receptors and Other Binding Proteins

TGF-β has high affinity for betaglycan, a proteoglycan that exists in membrane anchored and released forms in various tissues and in many cultured cell lines (Andres et al, 1989). Betaglycan contains heparan sulphate and chondroitin sulphate GAG chains, and has lower affinity (K_d ~100 pmol/l) for TGF-β than the signalling TGF-β receptors (K_d ~10 pmol/l). In contrast to other growth factors such as the heparin binding members of the fibroblast growth factor family that bind to the heparan sulphate GAG chains of certain proteoglycans, TGF-β binds to the core protein of betaglycan (Cheifetz et al, 1988; Segarini and Seyedin, 1988; Cheifetz and Massagué, 1989). Experiments with cell mutants that fail to synthesize GAGs have shown that the GAG chains in betaglycan are dispensable for TGF-β binding (Cheifetz and Massagué, 1989). Also, in contrast to fibroblast growth factor binding proteoglycans, betaglycan does not appear to be required for TGF-β binding to signalling receptors since these receptors bind TGF-β with high affinity in several cell lines that lack detectable betaglycan. Betaglycan might serve as a cell surface reservoir of TGF-β by capturing this factor and preventing its rapid clearance after a local burst of TGF-β production or release from blood platelets (see Fig. 3). What is the role of GAGs in betaglycan? One possibility is that, by binding to extracellular matrices via the GAG chains, membrane anchored and released forms of betaglycan might function as TGF-β concentrators on the cell surface or reservoirs in the extracellular matrix.

Other proteoglycans that bind TGF-β are decorin and biglycan (Yamaguchi et al, 1990). These are major chondroitin sulphate proteoglycans found in extracellular matrices. Since the expression of decorin and biglycan is raised by TGF-β (Bassols and Massagué, 1988), it has been proposed that these proteoglycans may act as negative feedback regulators of the level of free TGF-β in tissues (Yamaguchi *et al*, 1990). Other proteins shown to bind TGF-β in vitro include α2-macroglobulin (O'Connor-McCourt and Wakefield, 1987), β-amyloid precursor protein (Bodmer *et al*, 1990), type IV collagen (Paralkar *et al*, 1990) and others. The physiological role of these interactions is unknown.

PHYSIOLOGY: IMPLICATIONS IN ONCOGENESIS

The effects of TGF-β in vitro are thought to be a reflection of its physiological roles. Its expression throughout embryogenic development and its ability to control cell proliferation, differentiation, adhesion and extracellular matrix layout suggest a broad role for TGF-β in the generation and modification of the signals that guide embryogenesis, tissue remodelling and repair. The expression of TGF-βs is indeed high in sites undergoing intense development and morphogenesis (reviewed in Roberts and Sporn, 1990). Addition of TGF-β stimulates mesodermal development in explants from *Xenopus laevis* embryonic ectoderm (Kimelman and Kirschner, 1987; Rosa *et al*, 1988).

The same applies to processes of tissue recycling and repair. TGF-βs stored at high levels in platelets (Assoian *et al*, 1983, Cheifetz *et al*, 1987) or expressed in activated monocytes and macrophages (Assoian *et al*, 1987, Tsunawaki *et al*, 1988) can be physiologically delivered to sites of injury or inflammation. As a potent chemoattractant for monocytes and fibroblasts (Postlethwaite *et al*, 1987; Wahl *et al*, 1987; Yang and Moses, 1990), TGF-β is thought to bring these cells to sites of inflammation and repair. Subcutaneous administration of TGF-β stimulates accumulation of granulation tissue and wound healing responses (Roberts *et al*, 1986, Mustoe *et al*, 1987). Likewise, bone remodelling and, when necessary, bone repair are responsive to control by TGF-βs that are abundant in this tissue (Seyedin *et al*, 1985; Thompson *et al*, 1989).

An excess of TGF-β activity could lead to unbalanced deposition of extracellular matrix and contribute to various fibrotic disorders. Evidence for such a role has been obtained in proliferative vitreoretinopathy that may occur after surgery for retinal detachment and which leads to excessive intraocular fibrosis and blindness (Connor *et al*, 1989). The intense deposition of extracellular matrix in kidney glomerulonephritis in humans and in experimental models has also been linked to an excess of TGF-β activity in renal glomeruli (Border *et al*, 1990). The presence of TGF-β may also contribute to certain forms of viral tumorigenesis and tumour cell invasion (Sieweke *et al*, 1990; Welch *et al*, 1990)

Antiproliferative effects have been observed with TGF-β1 implanted near the epithelial end buds of immature rat mammary glands (Silberstein and Daniel, 1987) or by intravenous injection of TGF-β which has a negative effect on the proliferative response of regenerating rat liver (Russell *et al*, 1988). The antiproliferative action of TGF-β on lymphocytes (Kehrl *et al*, 1986) and thymocytes (Ristow 1986) is one of the components of the immunosuppressive activity that these factors display in vitro and in vivo (Wrann *et al*, 1987; Carel *et al*, 1990; Torre-Amione *et al*, 1990; Kuruvilla *et al*, 1991).

Unrestricted cell growth due to lack of growth inhibitory activity appears as the most important of the possible consequences of a defect in TGF-β function. The possibility that loss of TGF-β activity may contribute to the development of oncogenic processes is of major interest. Just as many components of growth activating pathways can become oncogenes (Cantley *et al*, 1991), so growth inhibitors such as the TGF-βs, their receptors or their cytoplasmic and nuclear signal transducers might become loss of function or "recessive" oncogenes. Although proof is not yet available, the lack of TGF-β responsiveness in certain human tumour cells (McMahon *et al*, 1986), the absence of TGF-β receptors in human retinoblastoma cells (Kimchi *et al*, 1988) and the evidence of RB involvement in the TGF-β growth inhibitory pathway provide some preliminary signs of validity of this hypothesis.

SUMMARY

This chapter has described some of the most salient features of the biology of the TGF-βs. The TGF-βs are of great interest as growth inhibitors, regulators of cell phenotype and regulators of cell adhesion. The various TGF-β isoforms are highly conserved and display a complex pattern of interactions with multiple membrane receptor components. Activation of these receptors leads to inhibition of epithelial cell proliferation by a mechanism that may involve proteins related to the growth suppressor, RB. TGF-β receptors are also coupled to mechanisms that control expression of differentiation commitment genes and differentiated cell functions. TGF-β can affect cell proliferation and differentiation through indirect mechanisms involving regulation of expression of cytokines, extracellular matrix molecules and their respective receptors. These responses strongly influence the growth and phenotype of an array of cell types. Excess or reduced TGF-β activity may contribute to the pathogenesis of certain fibrotic disorders and certain hyperproliferative disorders including cancer, respectively.

Reference

Andres JL, Stanley K, Cheifetz S and Massagué J (1989) Membrane-anchored and soluble forms of betaglycan, a polymorphic proteoglycan that binds transforming growth factor-β. *Journal of Cell Biology* **109** 3137–3145

Assoian RK and Sporn MB (1986) Type-beta transforming growth factor in human platelets: release during platelet deregulation and action on vascular smooth muscle cells. *Journal of Cell Biology* **102** 1712–1733

Assoian RK, Komoriya A, Meyers CA, Miller DM and Sporn MB (1983) Transforming growth factor-beta in human platelets. *Journal of Biological Chemistry* **258** 7155–7160

Assoian RK, Fleurdelys BE, Stevenson HC *et al* (1987) Expression and secretion of type beta transforming growth factor by activated human macrophages. *Proceedings of the National Academy of Sciences of the USA* **84** 6020–6024

Bassols A and Massagué J (1988) Transforming growth factor-β regulates the expression and structure of extracellular matrix chondoitin/dermatan sulfate proteoglycans. *Journal of Biological Chemistry* **263** 3039–3045

Battegay EJ, Raines EW, Seifert RA, Bowen-Pope DF and Ross R (1990) TGF-β induces bimodal proliferation of connective tissue cells via complex control of an autocrine PDGF loop. *Cell* **63** 515–524

Bodmer S, Podlisny MB, Selkoe DJ, Heid I and Fontana A (1990) Transforming growth factor-beta bound to soluble derivatives of the beta amyloid precursor protein of Alzheimer's disease. *Biochemical and Biophysical Research Communications* **171** 890–897

Border WA, Okuda S, Languino LR, Sporn MB and Ruoslahti E (1990) Suppression of experimental glomerulonephritis by antiserum against transforming growth factor β1. *Nature* **346** 371–374

Boyd FT and Massagué J (1989) Transforming growth factor-β inhibition of epithelial cell proliferation linked to the expression of a 53-kD membrane receptor. *Journal of Biological Chemistry* **264** 2272–2278

Buchkovich K, Duffy LA and Harlow E (1989) The retinoblastoma protein is phosphorylated during specific phases of the cell cycle. *Cell* **58** 1097–1105

Campisi J, Medrano EE, Morreo G and Pardee AB (1982) Restriction point control of cell growth by a labile protein: evidence for increased stability in transformed cells. *Proceedings of the National Academy of Sciences of the USA* **79** 436–440

Cantley LC, Auger KR, Carpenter C *et al* (1991) Oncogenes and signal transduction. *Cell* **64** 281–302

Carel J, Schreiber RD, Falqui L and Lacy PE (1990) Transforming growth factor β decreases the immunogenicity of rat islet xenografts (rat to mouse) and prevents rejection in association with treatment of the recipient with a monoclonal antibody to interferon-gamma. *Proceedings of the National Academy of Sciences of the USA* **87** 1591–1595

Chambard JC and Pouyssegur J (1988) TGF-β inhibits growth factor-induced DNA synthesis in hamster fibroblasts without affecting the early mitogenic events. *Journal of Cell Physiology* **135** 101–107

Cheifetz S and Massagué J (1989) The TGF-β receptor proteoglycan: cell surface expression and ligand binding in the absence of glycosaminoglycan chains. *Journal of Biological Chemistry* **264** 12025–12028

Cheifetz S, Like B and Massagué J (1986) Cellular distribution of type I and type II receptors for transforming growth factor-β. *Journal of Biological Chemistry* **261** 9972–9978

Cheifetz S, Weatherbee JA, Tsang MLS *et al* (1987) The transforming growth factor-β system, a complex pattern of cross-reactive ligands and receptors. *Cell* **48** 409–415

Cheifetz S, Andres JL and Massagué J (1988) The transforming growth factor-β receptor type III is a membrane proteoglycan. *Journal of Biological Chemistry* **263** 16984–16991

Cheifetz S, Hernandez H, Laiho M, ten Dijke P, Iwata KK and Massagué J (1990) Distinct transforming growth factor-β (TGF-β) receptor subsets as determinants of cellular responsiveness to three TGF-β isoforms. *Journal of Biological Chemistry* **265** 20533–20538

Coffey RJ Jr, Bascom CC, Sipes NJ, Graves-Deal R, Weissman BE and Moses HL (1988) Selective inhbition of growth-related gene expression in murine keratinocytes by transforming growth factor β. *Molecular and Cellular Biology* **8** 3088–3093

Connor TB, Roberts AB, Sporn MB *et al* (1989) Correlation of fibrosis and transforming growth factor-β type 2 in the eye. *Journal of Clinical Investigation* **83** 1661–1666

Daniel TO, Gibbs VC, Milfay DF and Williams LT (1987) Agents that increase cAMP accumulation block endothelial c-*sis* induction by thrombin and transforming growth factor-β. *Journal of Biological Chemistry* **262** 11893–11896

DeCaprio JA, Ludlow JW, Lynch D *et al* (1989) The product of the retinoblastoma susceptibility gene has properties of a cell cycle regulatory element. *Cell* **58** 1085–1095

Dennis PA and Rifkin DB (1991) Cellular activation of latent transforming growth factor-β requires binding to the cation-independent mannose 6-phosphate/insulin-like growth factor type II receptor. *Proceedings of the National Academy of Sciences of the USA* **88** 580–584

Dyson N, Buchkovich K, Whyte P and Harlow E (1989a) The cellular 107 K protein that binds to adenovirus E1A also associates with the large T antigens of SV40 and JC virus. *Cell* **58** 249–255

Dyson N, Howley PM, Munger K and Harlow E (1989b) The human papilloma virus-16 E7 oncoprotein is able to bind to the retinoblastoma gene product. *Science* **243** 934–937

Ewen ME, Ludlow JW, Marsilio E *et al* (1989) An N-terminal transformation-governing sequence of SV40 large T antigen contributes to the binding of both p110RB and a second cellular protein, p120. *Cell* **58** 257–267

Fernandez-Pol JA, Talkad VD, Klos DJ and Hamilton PD (1987) Suppression of the EGF-dependent induction of c-myc protooncogene expression by transforming growth factor β in a human breast carcinoma cell line. *Biochemical and Biophysical Research Communications* **144** 1197–1205

Frater-Schröder M, Muller G, Birchmeier W and Bhlen P (1986) Transforming growth factor-β inhibits endothelial cell proliferation. *Biochemical and Biophysical Research Communications* **137** 295–302

Gray AM and Mason AV (1990) Requirement for activin A and transforming growth factor β1 proregions for homodimer assembly. *Science* **247** 1328–1330

Graycar JL, Miller DA, Arrick BA, Lyons RM, Moses HL and Derynck R (1989) Human transforming growth factor-β3: recombinant expression, purification and biological activities in comparison with transforming growth factors β1 and β2. *Molecular Endocrinology* **3** 1977–1986

Heimark RL, Twardzik DR and Schwarz SM (1986) Inhibition of endothelial cell regeneration by type-beta transforming growth factor from platelets. *Science* **233** 1078–1080

Heino J and Massagué J (1990) Cell adhesion to collagen and decreased myogenic gene expression implicated in the control of myogenesis by TGF-β. *Journal of Biological Chemistry* **265** 10181–10184

Howe PH, Draetta G and Leof EB (1991) Transforming growth factor β1 inhibition of p34^{cdc2} phosphorylation and histone H1 kinase activity is associated with G1/S-phase growth arrest. *Molecular and Cellular Biology* **11** 1185–1194

Huang S, Wang NP, Tseng BY, Lee WH and Lee EHHP (1990) Two distinct and frequently mutated regions of retinoblastoma protein are required for binding to SV40 T antigen. *EMBO Journal* **9** 1815–1822

Ignotz RA and Massagué J (1986) Transforming growth factor-β stimulates the expression of fibronectin and collagen and their incorporation into the extracellular matrix. *Journal of Biological Chemistry* **261** 4337–4345

Ignotz RA and Massagué J (1987) Cell adhesion receptors as targets for transforming growth factor-β action. *Cell* **51** 189–197

Kanzaki T, Olofsson A, Morén A *et al* (1990) TGF-β1 binding protein: a component of the large latent complex of TGF-β1 with multiple repeat sequences. *Cell* **61** 1051–1061

Kehrl JH, Wakefield LM, Roberts AB *et al* (1986) Production of transforming growth factor beta by human T lymphocytes and its potential role in the regulation of T cell growth. *Journal of Experimental Medicine* **163** 1037–1050

Kim SJ, Jeang KT, Glick A, Sporn MB and Roberts AB (1989) Promoter sequences of the human transforming growth factor-β1 gene responsive to transforming growth factor-β1 autoinduction. *Journal of Biological Chemistry* **264** 7041–7045

Kim SJ, Angel P, Lafyatis R *et al* (1990) Autoinduction of TGF-β1 is mediated by the AP-1 complex. *Molecular and Cellular Biology* **10** 1492–1497

Kim SJ, Lee H, Robbins PD, Busam K, Sporn MB and Roberts AB (1991) Regulation of transforming growth factor β1 gene expression by the product of the retinoblastoma-susceptibility gene. *Proceedings of the National Academy of Sciences of the USA* **88** 3052–

3056

Kimchi A, Wang XF, Weinberg RA, Cheifetz S and Massagué J (1988) Absence of TGF-β receptors and growth inhibitory responses in retinoblastoma cells. *Science* **240** 196–199

Kimelman D and Kirschner M (1987) Synergistic induction of mesoderm by FGF and TGF-β and the identification of an mRNA coding for EGF in the early Xenopus embryo. *Cell* **51** 869–877

Knabbe C, Lippman ME, Wakefield LM *et al* (1987) Evidence that transforming growth factor-β is a hormonally regulated negative growth factor in human breast cancer cells. *Cell* **48** 417–428

Kovacina KS, Steele-Perkins G, Purchio AF *et al* (1989) Interactions of recombinant and platelet transforming growth factor-β1 precursor with the insulin-like growth factor/mannose 6-phosphate receptor. *Biochemical and Biophysical Research Communications* **160** 393–403

Kuruvilla AP, Shah R, Hochwald GM, Liggitt HD, Palladino MA and Thorbecke GJ (1991) Protective effect of transforming growth factor β1 on experimental autoimmune diseases in mice. *Proceedings of t he National Academy of Sciences of the USA* **88** 2918–2921

Lafyatis R, Lechleider R, Kim SJ, Jakowlew S, Roberts AB and Sporn MB (1990) Structural and functional characterization of the transforming growth factor β3 promoter: a cAMP responsive element regulates basal and induced transcription. *Journal of Biological Chemistry* **265** 19128–19136

Laiho M, DeCaprio JA, Ludlow JW, Livingston DM and Massagué J (1990a) Growth inhibition by TGF-β linked to suppression of retinoblastoma protein phosphorylation. *Cell* **62** 175–185

Laiho M, Weis FMB and Massagué J (1990b) Concomitant loss of transforming growth factor (TGF)-receptor types I and II in TGF-β-resistant cell mutants implicates both receptor types in signal transduction. *Journal of Biological Chemistry* **265** 18518–18524

Laiho M, Ronnstrand L, Heino J *et al* (1991a) Control of JunB and extracellular matrix protein expression by transforming growth factor-β1 is independent of simian virus 40 T antigen-sensitive growth-inhibitory events. *Molecular and Cellular Biology* **11** 972–978

Laiho M, Weis FMB, Boyd FT, Ignotz RA and Massagué J (1991b) Responsiveness to transforming growth factor-β (TGF-β) restored by genetic complementation between cells defective in TGF-β receptors I and II. *Journal of Biological Chemistry* **266** 9108–9112

Leof EB, Proper JA, Goustin AS, Shipley GD, DiCorleto PE and Moses HL (1986) Induction of c-sis mRNA and activity similar to platelet-derived growth factor by transforming growth factor β: a proposed model for indirect mitogenesis involving autocrine activity. *Proceedings of the National Academy of Sciences of the USA* **83** 2453–2457

Li L, Hu JS and Olson EN (1990) Different members of the jun proto-oncogene family exhibit distinct patterns of expression in response to type β transforming growth factor. *Journal of Biological Chemistry* **265** 1556–1562

Like B and Massagué J (1986) The antiproliferative effect of type β transforming growth factor occurs at a level distal from receptors for growth-activating factors. *Journal of Biological Chemistry* **261** 13426–13429

Lin BTY, Gruenwald S, Morla AO, Lee WH and Wang JYJ (1991) Retinoblastoma cancer suppressor gene product is a substrate of the cell cycle regulator cdc2 kinase. *EMBO Journal* **10** 857–864

Lin P, Liu C, Tsao MS and Grisham JW (1987) Inhibition of proliferation of cultured rat liver epithelial cells at specific cell cycle stages by transforming growth factor-β. *Biochemical and Biophysical Research Communications* **143** 26–30

Ludlow JW, DeCaprio JA, Huang CM, Lee WH, Paucha E and Livingston DM (1989) SV40 large T antigen binds preferentially to an underphosphorylated member of the retinoblastoma susceptibility gene product family. *Cell* **56** 57–65

Lyons RM, Gentry LE, Purchio AF and Moses HL (1990) Mechanism of activation of latent recombinant transforming growth factor β1 by plasmin. *Journal of Cell Biology* **110** 1361–

1367

Majack RA, Majesky MW and Goodman LV (1990) Role of PDGF-A expression in the control of vascular smooth muscle cell growth by transforming growth factor-β. *Journal of Cell Biology* **111** 239–247

Massagué J (1990) The transforming growth factor-β family. *Annual Review of Cell Biology* **6** 597–641

Massagué J, Cheifetz S, Endo T and Nadal-Ginard B (1986) Type β transforming growth factor is an inhibitor of myogenic differentiation. *Proceedings of the National Academy of Sciences of the USA* **83** 8206–8210

Massagué J, Boyd FT, Andres JL and Cheifetz S (1990) Mediators of TGF-β action: TGF-β receptors and TGF-β-binding proteoglycans. *Annals of the New York Academy of Sciences* **593** 59–72

Matsushime H, Roussel MF, Ashmun RA and Sherr CJ Colony-stimulating factor 1 regulates a novel gene (*CYL1*) with properties of a mammalian G1 cyclin. *Cell* (in press)

McMahon JB, Richards WL, del Campo CC, Song M-K and Thorgiersson SS (1986) Differential effects of transforming growth factor-β on proliferation of normal and malignant rat liver epithelial cells in culture. *Cancer Research* **46** 4665–4671

Miyazono K and Heldin CH (1989) Interaction between TGF-β1 and carbohydrate structures in its precursor renders TGF-β1 latent. *Nature* **388** 158–160

Moses HL, Tucker RF, Leof EB, Coffey RJJ, Halper J and Shipley GD (1985) Type β transforming growth factor is a growth stimulator and growth inhibitor, In: Feramisco J, Ozanne B, and Stiles C, (eds). *Cancer Cells*, p3, Cold Spring Harbor Laboratory, Cold Spring Harbor, New York

Mustoe TA, Pierce GF, Thomason A, Gramates P, Sporn MB and Deuel TF (1987) Transforming growth factor beta induces accelerated healing of incisional wounds in rats. *Science* **237** 1333–1336

Nakamura T, Tomita Y, Hirai R, Yamaoka K, Kaji K and Ichihara A (1985) Inhibitory effect of transforming growth factor-β on DNA synthesis of adult rat hepatocytes in primary culture. *Biochemical and Biophysical Research Communications* **133** 1042–1050

Nugent MA and Newman MJ (1989) Inhibition of normal rat kidney cell growth by transforming growth factor-β is mediated by collagen. *Journal of Biological Chemistry* **264** 18060–18067

O'Connor-McCourt MD and Wakefield LM (1987) Latent transforming growth factor-β in serum. *Journal of Biological Chemistry* **262** 14090–14099

Ohta M, Greenberger JS, Anklesaria P, Bassols A and Massagué J (1987) Two forms of transforming growth factor-β distinguished by multipotential haematopoietic progenitor cells. *Nature* **329** 539–541

Paralkar VM, Vukicevic S and Reddi AH (1991) Transforming growth factor β type 1 binds to collagen IV of basement membrane matrix: implications for development. *Developmental Biology* **143** 303–308

Pertovaara L, Sistonen L, Bos TJ, Vogt PK, Keski-Oja J and Alitalo K (1989) Enhanced jun gene expression is an early genomic response to transforming growth factor β stimulation. *Molecular and Cellular Biology* **9** 1255–1262

Pietenpol JA, Holt JT, Stein RW and Moses HL (1990a) Transforming growth factor β-1 suppression of c-myc gene transcription: role in inhibition of keratinocyte proliferation. *Proceedings of the National Academy of Sciences of the USA* **87** 3758–3762

Pietenpol JA, Stein RW, Moran E *et al* (1990b) TGF-β1 inhibition of c-myc transcription and growth in keratinocytes is abrogated by viral transforming protein with pRB binding domains. *Cell* **61** 777–785

Pircher R, Jullien P and Lawrence DA (1986) β-Transforming growth factor is stored in human blood platelets as a latent high molecular weight complex. *Biochemical and Biophysical Research Communications* **136** 30–37

Pledger WJ, Stiles CD, Antoniades HN and Cher CD (1978) An ordered sequence of events is required before BALB/c-3T3 cells become commited to DNA synthesis. *Proceedings of the National Academy of Sciences of the USA* **75** 2839–2843

Postlewaite AE, Keski-Oja J, Moses HL and Kang AH (1987) Stimulation of the chemotactic migration of human fibroblasts by transforming growth factor beta. *Journal of Experimental Medicine* **165** 251–256

Potts JD, Dagle JM, Walder JA, Weeks DL and Runyan RB (1991) Epithelial-mesenchymal transformation of embryonic cardiac endothelial cells is inhibited by a modified antisense oligodeoxynucleotide to transforming growth factor β3. *Proceedings of the National Academy of Sciences of the USA* **88** 1516–1520

Ristow HJ (1986) BSC-1 growth inhibitor type β transforming growth factor is a strong inhibitor of thymocyte proliferation. *Proceedings of the National Academy of Sciences of the USA* **83** 5531–5534

Robbins PD, Horowitz JM and Mulligan RC (1990) Negative regulation of human c-fos expression by the retinoblastoma gene product. *Nature* **346** 668–671

Roberts AB and Sporn MB (1990) The transforming growth factor-betas, In: Sporn MB and Roberts AB (eds). *Peptide Growth Factors and Their Receptors*, pp 419–472, Springer-Verlag, Heidelberg

Roberts AB, Anzano MA, Wakefield LM, Roche NS, Stern DF and Sporn MB (1985) Type-β transforming growth factor: a bifunctional regulator of cellular growth. *Proceedings of the National Academy of Sciences of the USA* **82** 119–123

Roberts AB, Sporn MB, Assoian RK *et al* (1986) Transforming growth factor type β: rapid induction of fibrosis and angiogenesis in vivo and stimulation of collagen formation in vitro. *Proceedings of the National Academy of Sciences of the USA* **83** 4167–4171

Rosa F, Roberts AB, Danielpour D, Dart LL, Sporn MB and David IB (1988) Mesoderm induction in amphibians: the role of TGF-β2-like factors. *Science* **236** 783–786

Rossi P, Karsenty G, Roberts AB, Roche NS, Sporn MB and de Crombrugghe B (1988) A nuclear factor 1 binding site mediates the transcriptional activation of a type I collagen promoter by transforming growth factor-β. *Cell* **52** 405–414

Russell WE, Coffey RJ, Ouellette AJ and Moses HL (1988) Transforming growth factor beta reversibly inhibits the early proliferative response to partial hepatectomy in the rat. *Proceedings of the National Academy of Sciences of the USA* **85** 5126–5130

Segarini PR and Seyedin SM (1988) The high molecular weight receptor to transforming growth factor-β contains glycosaminoglycan chains. *Journal of Biological Chemistry* **263** 8366–8370

Segarini PR, Rosen DM and Seyedin SM (1989) Binding of TGF-β to cell surface proteins varies with cell type. *Molecular Endocrinology* **3** 261–272

Seyedin SM, Thomas TC, Thompson AY, Rosen DM and Piez KA (1985) Purification and characterization of two cartilage-inducing factors from bovine demineralized bone. *Proceedings of the National Academy of Sciences of the USA* **82** 2267–2271

Shipley GD, Tucker RF and Moses HL (1985) Type β-transforming growth factor/growth inhibitor stimulates entry of monolayer cultures of AKR-2B cells into S-phase after prolonged prereplicative interval. *Proceedings of the National Academy of Sciences of the USA* **82** 4147–4151

Shipley GD, Pittelkow MR, Wille JJ Jr, Scott RE and Moses HL (1986) Reversible inhibition of normal human prokeratinocyte proliferation by type β transforming growth factor-growth inhibitor in serum-free medium. *Cancer Research* **46** 2068–2071

Sieweke MH, Thompson NL, Sporn MB and Bissell MJ (1990) Mediation of wound-related rous sarcoma virus tumorigenesis by TGF-β. *Science* **248** 1656–1660

Silberstein GB and Daniel CW (1987) Reversible inhibition of mammary gland growth by transforming growth factor-β. *Science* **237** 291–293

Sorrentino V and Bandyopadhyay S (1989) TGFβ inhibits G0/S-phase transition in primary fibroblasts: loss of response to the antigrowth effect of TGFβ is observed after immortalization. *Oncogene* **4** 569–574

Takehara K, LeRoy EC and Grotendorst GR (1987) TGF-β inhibition of endothelial cell proliferation: alteration of EGF binding and EGF-induced growth-regulatory (competence) gene expression. *Cell* **49** 415–422

Thompson NL, Flanders KC, Smith M, Ellingsworth LR, Roberts AB and Sporn MB (1989) Expression of transforming growth factor-β1 in specific cells and tissues of adult and neonatal mice. *Journal of Cell Biology* **108** 661–669

Torre-Amione G, Beauchamp RD, Koeppen H *et al* (1990) A highly immunogenic tumor transfected with a murine transforming growth factor type β1 cDNA escapes immune surveillance. *Proceedings of the National Academy of Sciences of the USA* **87** 1486–1490

Tsuji T, Okada F, Yamaguchi K and Nakamura T (1990) Molecular cloning of the large subunit of transforming growth factor type β masking protein and expression of the mRNA in various rat tissues. *Proceedings of the National Academy of Sciences of the USA* **87** 8835–8839

Tsunawaki S, Sporn MB, Ding A and Nathan C (1988) Deactivation of macrophages by transforming growth factor-β. *Nature* **334** 260–262

Tucker RF, Shipley GD, Moses HL and Holley RW (1984) Growth inhibitor from BSC-1 cells is closely related to the platelet type β transforming growth factor. *Science* **226** 705–707

Vaidya TB, Rhodes SJ, Taparowsky EJ and Konieczny SF (1989) Fibroblast growth factor and transforming growth factor-β repress transcription of the myogenic regulatory gene MyoD1. *Molecular and Cellular Biology* **9** 3576–3579

Wahl SM, Hunt DA, Wakefield LM *et al* (1987) Transforming growth-factor beta (TGF-β) induces monocyte chemotaxis and growth factor production. *Proceedings of the National Academy of Sciences of the USA* **84** 5788–5792

Welch DR, Fabra A and Nakajima M (1990) Transforming growth factor β stimulates mammary adenocarcinoma cell invasion and metastatic potential. *Proceedings of the National Academy of Sciences of the USA* **87** 7678–7682

Whyte P, Buchkovich KJ, Horowitz JM *et al* (1988) Association between an oncogene and an antioncogene: the adenovirus E1A proteins bind to the retinoblastoma gene product. *Nature* **334** 124–129

Wrann M, Bodmer S, de Martin R *et al* (1987) T cell supressor factor from human glioblastoma cells is a 12.5 kd protein closely related to transforming growth factor-β. *EMBO Journal* **6** 1633–1636

Xiong Y, Connolly T, Futcher B and Beach D Identification of human cyclin D1: overexpression in a glioblastoma cell line. *Cell* (in press)

Yamaguchi Y, Mann DM and Ruoslahti E (1990) Negative regulation of transforming growth factor-β by the proteoglycan decorin. *Nature* **346** 281–283

Yang EY and Moses HL (1990) Transforming growth factor β1-induced changes in cell migration, proliferation, and angiogenesis in the chicken chorioallantoic membrane. *Journal of Cell Biology* **111** 731–741

Zentella A, Weis FMB, Ralph DA, Laiho M and Massagué J Early gene responses to transforming growth factor-β in cells lacking growth suppressive RB function. *Molecular Cellular Biology* (in press)

The authors are responsible for the accuracy of the references.

Role of the *WT1* Gene in Wilms' Tumour

D A HABER[1,2] • **D E HOUSMAN**[1]

[1]*Center for Cancer Research, Massachusetts Institute of Technology, Cambridge, Massachusetts 02139;* [2]*Massachusetts General Hospital Cancer Center, Charlestown, Massachusetts 02115*

INTRODUCTION

Wilms' tumour or nephroblastoma is a relatively common paediatric solid tumour, occurring in 1 in 10 000 children. The tumour arises in the kidney and is noted for its histological complexity. The characteristic morphology is often described as triphasic, including undifferentiated or blastemal cells, as well as stromal and epithelial elements (see Fig. 1). The relative proportion of these cell types varies among individual tumours, with some showing additional histological subtypes. In addition, preneoplastic lesions or nephrogenic rests have also been described in association with Wilms' tumour, particularly in individuals who have bilateral tumours or other genetic evidence of tumour susceptibility (Beckwith *et al*, 1990). These suggest an inherent abnormality in kidney development in these individuals, which enhances the likelihood of tumour formation. Indeed, the histology of Wilms' tumour points to a defect in the early precursor cells that give rise to the normal kidney, and it is the genetic analysis of individuals predisposed to this tumour that led to the identification of a gene specifically involved in kidney development.

THE KNUDSON MODEL

The conceptual framework for the analysis of susceptibility to Wilms' tumour was established by Knudson and Strong in their prophetic model of childhood malignancies (Knudson 1971, Knudson and Strong, 1972). Using an epidemiological analysis of the incidence of paediatric cancers, namely retinoblastoma, Wilms' tumour and neuroblastoma, these authors sought to predict the num-

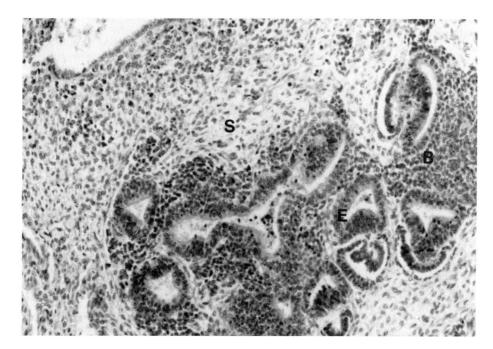

Fig. 1. Triphasic histology of Wilms' tumour. Three cellular components are found characteristically in Wilms' tumours; the blastemal (B) cells thought to be undifferentiated, the epidermal (E) cells which form tubular structures, and the stromal (S) cells. In addition, some tumours may contain regions of cellular differentiation including neural or muscle elements. Photomicrograph provided by Dr Tom Glaser and Dr Druscilla Roberts, Harvard Medical School

ber of rate limiting steps required for tumorigenesis. Wilms' tumour, like retinoblastoma, has a high frequency of synchronous bilateral cancers, estimated at 10% of cases (Matsunaga, 1981). These tumours occur a mean of 2 years earlier than the more common unilateral cases and in retinoblastoma, often arise within a family. Knudson speculated that bilateral tumours therefore represented an inherited genetic lesion that conferred a predisposition to tumorigenesis in a specific organ. Using Poisson statistics, he analysed the relative incidence of unilateral versus bilateral tumours in susceptible individuals and calculated that only one rate limiting step was required for tumour formation in these individuals. The Knudson model thus predicted that susceptible individuals carried an initial first hit in their germline, and only required one additional genetic event for a tumour to develop. The relatively frequent second somatic event accounts for the incidence of multiple cancers and their early presentation. Sporadic tumours, on the other hand, were assumed to require two independent rare events and are hence unilateral and slower to develop.

LOCALIZATION OF A WILMS' TUMOUR GENE

The genetic analysis of Wilms' tumours has begun to fulfill the predictions of Knudson and Strong, although some questions remain unanswered. Although bilateral tumours are common, accounting for some 10% of Wilms' tumours, familial transmission is documented in less than 1% of cases (Matsunaga, 1981). This is in contrast with the relatively frequent familial inheritance of susceptibility to retinoblastoma and suggests that in the case of Wilms' tumour, new germline mutations are primarily responsible for the development of bilateral tumours. In very rare cases, individuals with such apparent predisposition to Wilms' tumours have also demonstrated specific congenital abnormalities. These observations proved to be the key to the mapping of the Wilms' tumour loci. An early observation was that of a genetic link between the development of Wilms' tumour and a congenital abnormality of the eye, known as aniridia (Miller *et al*, 1964). Although both aniridia and Wilms' tumour occur in isolation, the presence of one was found to enhance greatly the probability of the other, suggesting that the responsible genes might be physically linked. Of particular importance was the observation that individuals with Wilms' tumour very rarely manifested a constellation of congenital abnormalities, including aniridia, genitourinary abnormalities and mental retardation (so-called WAGR syndrome). These congenital defects, among the earliest contiguous gene syndromes, were associated with a gross constitutional chromosome deletion on the short arm of chromosome 11, at band p13 (Riccardi *et al*, 1978; Francke *et al*, 1979).

One of the major insights provided by Knudson's hypothesis was the link between an inherited genetic lesion and a later somatic second event. Solid tumours tend to show a high degree of genomic instability, but consistent chromosomal abnormalities are suggestive of important steps in tumorigenesis. Sporadic Wilms' tumours were seen to have lost heterozygosity at polymorphic markers on chromosome 11p13, thus demonstrating loss of genetic material at that locus (Fearon et al, 1984; Koufos *et al*, 1984; Orkin *et al*, 1984; Reeve *et al*, 1984). The somatic loss of genetic material at a site previously associated with inherited tumour susceptibility points to a gene whose inactivation is critical to tumour formation. As demonstrated by the retinoblastoma gene *RB*, the rate limiting steps predicted by Knudson reflect the inactivation of the two alleles of a tumour suppressor gene, the first in the germline and the second in somatic tissues (Dunn *et al*, 1988; Yandell *et al*, 1989).

ISOLATION OF *WT1*

The search for the Wilms' tumour gene at chromosome 11p13 began with the construction of a detailed genetic linkage map of that region (Compton et al, 1988; Gessler and Bruns, 1989; Glaser *et al*, 1989; Rose *et al*, 1990). Of particular importance was the development of hybrid cell lines, consisting of a single abnormal chromosome 11 from a patient with WAGR syndrome in a rodent cell background (Glaser *et al*, 1987). The WAGR 11p13 deletion was found to be flanked by the genes for catalase and follicle stimulating hormone, and genetic markers within the deletion were identified (Glaser *et al*, 1986; Porteous *et al*, 1987; Davis *et al*, 1988). By characterizing a number of unequal but over-

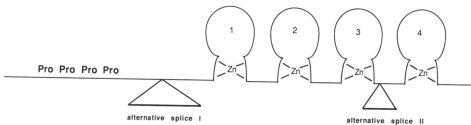

Fig. 2. Schematic representation of the *WT1* functional domains. The *WT1* gene product contains four Cys-His zinc finger domains at the carboxyterminus, which are thought to mediate DNA-binding. A proline and glutamine-rich stretch is found at the aminoterminus. Two alternative splices are found in the *WT1* transcript, resulting in a combination of four distinct mRNA species. Splice I contains 17 aminoacids inserted between the proline rich domain and the zinc finger region, whereas splice II encodes 3 aminoacids inserted in the knuckle between zinc fingers three and four

lapping WAGR deletions, as well as a Wilms' cell line with a small chromosomal deletion, the smallest region of overlap was established to be some 400 kilobases (kb) in length (Rose *et al*, 1990). Within this region a genomic DNA clone was identified, showing cross-species hybridization, implying a conserved transcription unit, and leading to the isolation of a transcript, which we now call the *WT1* gene (Call *et al*, 1990). This gene was also cloned by another group of investigators, using the presence of rare restriction enzyme recognition sites known to occur at the 5′ end of transcription units (Gessler *et al*, 1990).

The *WT1* gene contains ten exons spanning 50 kb of DNA and encoding a transcript of 3 kb (Call *et al*, 1990; Haber *et al*, in press). The predicted protein is 46–49 kDa (reflecting the presence of alternative splices), and analysis of the nucleotide sequence suggests two functional domains (Fig. 2). The carboxyterminus contains four cysteine-histidine type zinc finger motifs, consensus sequences that have been identified in a number of transcription factors and are thought to mediate DNA binding (Evans and Hollenberg, 1988). The *WT1* zinc finger domains share extensive aminoacid homology with those of the early growth response (*EGR*) genes 1 and 2 (Joseph *et al*, 1988; Sukhatme *et al*, 1988), and a construct of the *WT1* domains has been shown to bind the *EGR1* DNA recognition site (Rauscher *et al*, 1990). The yeast gene *MIG1*, involved in regulating genes involved in sugar metabolism, also shares homology with the *WT1* zinc finger region (Nehlin and Ronne, 1990). A second recognizable domain is seen in the aminoterminus of the *WT1* gene. This region is very rich in prolines and glutamines, a finding also described in a number of transcription factors (Mitchell and Tijan, 1989). The aminoterminus may be involved in the *trans*-activation signal mediated by *WT1*.

WT1 EXPRESSION AND ALTERNATIVE SPLICING

Two alternative splices are present in the *WT1* transcript, resulting in a combination of four distinct mRNA species (Haber *et al*, in press). Splice I inserts

17 aminoacids between the proline rich aminoterminus and the zinc finger domains. The aminoacids encoded by this alternative splice are rich in serines and threonines, potential sites for phosphorylation of the protein. Splice II inserts 3 aminoacids (lysine, threonine, serine) between zinc fingers three and four. The presence of the splice II insertion in a *WT1* zinc finger construct greatly reduces binding to the *EGR1* DNA recognition site (Rauscher *et al*, 1991). However, it is unclear whether this splicing variant has a distinct DNA recognition site or whether it acts to block DNA binding by the other splicing variant that is missing the splice II insertion. All four possible *WT1* mRNA transcripts, reflecting presence or absence of each alternative splice, are found in tissues expressing this gene. The relative ratio appears to be virtually constant in tissues that express *WT1*, both in humans and in mice, with the prevalent form being that which contains both alternative splices, and the least common form being that which lacks both splices (Haber *et al*, in press). These observations suggest that each alternative splicing variant contributes to the normal function of the *WT1* gene function.

An initial understanding of the normal function of the *WT1* gene can be derived from its pattern of expression. The best studied tumour suppressor gene, *RB*, is expressed ubiquitously (Friend *et al*, 1986; Lee *et al*, 1987; Bernards *et al*, 1989) and appears to be involved in the control of such basic cellular mechanisms as progression through the cell cycle (Buchkovich *et al*, 1989; Chen et al, 1989; DeCaprio *et al*, 1989; Ludlow *et al*, 1989). In contrast, *WT1* is expressed in a very restricted number of tissues, with a striking pattern of developmental regulation. In the mouse and in the baboon, *WT1* mRNA is readily detectable in kidney, spleen, gonads and uterus (Call *et al*, 1990; Buckler *et al*, 1991; Pelletier *et al*, in press). It is in the kidney that developmental control of expression is most dramatic. In the mouse, *WT1* levels are detectable at day 8 of gestation, peak sharply at day 17 and then rapidly decline to the low adult levels by day 3 after birth (see Fig. 3) (Buckler *et al*, 1991). In situ hybridization studies show that *WT1* expression is restricted to the internal surface of the S-shaped bodies of the fetal renal cortex, structures thought to be precursors to the podocytes of the developing glomerulus (Pritchard-Jones *et al*, 1990). In other tissues, *WT1* expression is also confined to specific cell types. In the male gonads, *WT1* mRNA is found in the Sertoli cells, whereas in the ovary, expression is limited to the epithelial lining of the follicles (Pelletier *et al*, in press). In those tissues, however, *WT1* expression increases during fetal development and then remains raised during adult life, rather than peaking sharply as it does during kidney development.

INACTIVATION OF *WT1* IN WILMS' TUMOURS

The role of *WT1* in tumorigenesis may reflect its normal function as a regulator of cell proliferation, within the context of kidney-specific developmental pathways in which it has a role. A striking observation in the case of retinoblastoma is that *RB* is expressed in all tissues and many different

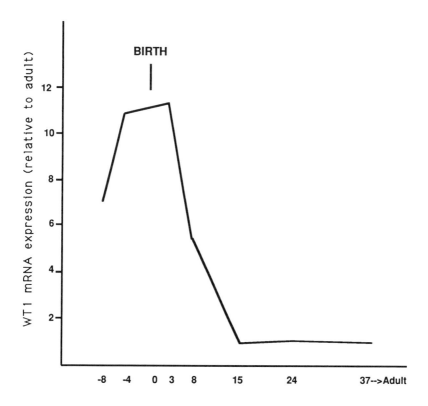

Fig. 3. Developmental time course of *WT1* expression in mouse kidney. Expression of *WT1* mRNA in mouse kidney at various stages of development. Data are derived from quantitative analysis of northern blots (from Buckler *et al*, 1991)

tumours contain *RB* mutations, yet a germline *RB* mutation predisposes an individual to only two specific types of cancer, namely retinoblastoma and osteosarcoma. Such an observation suggests that *RB* mutations are rate limiting steps in tumorigenesis in the retina and in osteoblasts, yet are only contributory to the malignant process in other tissues (see Haber and Housman, 1991). So far, *WT1* mutations have only been detected in Wilms' tumours, and patients with germline inactivation of this gene (eg WAGR patients) do not have an increased incidence of other forms of cancer. Nonetheless, *WT1* is expressed in some tissues other than kidney, and it is possible that it is also involved in tumorigenesis in these organs.

Most Wilms' tumours express high levels of *WT1* mRNA, consistent with their presumed tissue of origin, fetal kidney (Haber *et al*, 1990). Gross deletions or rearrangements of the gene have been described, but they appear to be infrequent. More common are small deletions internal to the gene, resulting in its inactivation (Haber *et al*, 1990; Cowell *et al*, 1991; Ton *et al*, 1991).

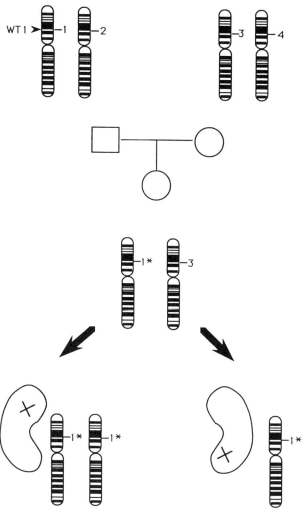

Fig. 4. Homozygous inactivation of *WT1* in Wilms' tumours. Schematic representation of *WT1* inactivation as predicted by the Knudson model. A heterozygous germline mutation is present in an affected individual with bilateral Wilms' tumours. On the basis of the low incidence of familial transmission, this appears to be a new germline event in most cases of Wilms' tumour. The second hit, representing the loss of the remaining normal *WT1* allele, is sufficiently frequent to result in a high incidence of bilateral tumours. Loss of the normal allele can occur by a recombinational event (left tumour) or by chromosomal non-disjunction (right tumour), or by deletion or mutational events. Two cases of bilateral Wilms' tumour have been found to fulfill these postulates of the Knudson hypothesis (from Huff *et al*, 1991; Pelletier *et al*, unpublished)

As predicted by the Knudson model, individuals with bilateral Wilms' tumours have been shown to have a heterozygous *WT1* mutation in the germline, with subsequent loss of the normal gene in each tumour (see Fig. 4) (Huff *et al*, 1991; Pelletier *et al*, unpublished). Such homozygous gene inactivation, however, appears not to be strictly necessary for Wilms' tumorigenesis. For instance, one sporadic tumour was found to contain a deletion in only one of the two *WT1* alleles (Haber *et al*, 1990). This mutation consists of a deletion of 25 base pairs, spanning an exon/intron junction. The resultant transcript is missing exon eight of *WT1*, consisting of the third zinc finger domain and alternative splice II, yet it maintains an open reading frame distal to the mutation, thus encoding a possibly functional protein. This observation suggested the possibility that an altered *WT1* gene product might be able to suppress normal function of the wild type allele, the so-called trans-dominant or dominant suppressor effect (Herskowitz *et al*, 1987). If such a mechanism were confirmed by in vitro functional studies, it would imply that a single mutational hit could be sufficient to inactivate *WT1* function. Such a specific mutation, however, would be more infrequent than the simple inactivating mutations that are the basis of Knudson's two-hit model.

OTHER WILMS' TUMOUR GENES

Unlike retinoblastoma, which appears to be associated with a single tumour suppressor gene, *RB*, Wilms' tumour presents a more complex genetic picture. Inactivation of the *WT1* gene at the 11p13 locus can be demonstrated in Wilms' tumours by the presence of gross chromosomal deletions, the loss of heterozygous markers mapping to that region or the characterization of small internal mutations in *WT1* with polymerase chain reaction amplification. However, some Wilms' tumours show loss of heterozygosity at a different locus on chromosome 11, namely band p15, rather than 11p13 (Raizis *et al*, 1985; Mannens *et al*, 1987; Henry *et al*, 1989; Reeve *et al*, 1989). In addition, patients with the rare constellation of symptoms known as Beckwith-Wiedemann syndrome (Wilms' tumour and hemi-hypertrophy) show constitutional chromosome abnormalities involving 11p15, especially duplications of this band (Waziri *et al*, 1983; Turleau *et al*, 1984; Koufos *et al*, 1989). These observations point to a second Wilms' tumour locus involved in the genesis of these tumours. It is possible that Wilms' tumours are heterogeneous, with mutations at distinct genetic loci responsible for different subpopulations of tumours. Alternatively, inactivation of both *WT1* and the putative 11p15 gene might contribute to tumorigenesis within the same cancer. Tumours arising in patients with WAGR syndrome, which are hemizygous for *WT1* at 11p13, have been shown to have loss of heterozygosity within 11p15, but not 11p13 (Henry *et al*, 1989). Similarly, a sporadic Wilms' tumour with a *WT1* mutation has been shown to have a chromosomal non-disjunction and reduplication event affecting both 11p13 and 11p15 that preceded the *WT1* mutation (Haber *et al*, 1990). These observations suggest potential interactions between different tumour suppressor genes involved in the development of Wilms' tumour.

In addition to the two Wilms' tumour genes residing on chromosome 11, a third locus has been implicated based on linkage analyses of three families with an inherited predisposition to Wilms' tumour (Grundy *et al*, 1988; Huff *et al*, 1988; Schwartz *et al*, 1991). Unlike retinoblastoma in which the number of patients with bilateral tumours is consistent with the incidence of a positive family history, familial Wilms' tumour is very rare, estimated at less than 1% of cases (Matsunaga, 1981). However, in familial Wilms' tumours, unassociated with WAGR or Beckwith-Wiedemann syndromes, analysis using polymorphic markers has excluded both 11p13 and 11p15 from transmission of disease susceptibility. These observations suggest the existence of a third Wilms' tumour locus, as yet unmapped, which is responsible for hereditary susceptibility to this tumour.

The apparent genetic complexity of Wilms' tumour is confirmed in a mouse model that has been characterized recently. The Sey/Dey mouse strain has been found to carry a heterozygous deletion on mouse chromosome 2 that is homologous to the WAGR deletion in humans (Glaser *et al*, 1990). These mice have a defect in eye development, which may be analogous to aniridia in WAGR patients. However, unlike WAGR patients, Sey/Dey mice do not appear to have an increased incidence of nephroblastoma. Several hypotheses have been suggested to explain this discrepancy. It is possible that the smaller number of target cells in the mouse kidney makes it unlikely for an affected mouse to acquire a second hit at the *WT1* gene. Alternatively, *WT1* function may not be as critical in the mouse kidney developmental pathway as it appears to be in humans. An intriguing observation is that in humans, the 11p13 and 11p15 loci are on the same arm of a single chromosome, making it possible for a single chromosomal recombinational event to cause loss of both genes. However, in the mouse, these two homologous regions are on different chromosomes, thus making it necessary to invoke two different and rare genetic events (Glaser *et al*, 1990).

CONCLUSIONS

The involvement of multiple genes in the development of Wilms' tumour points to the complex pathways that regulate the growth and differentiation of nephroblasts. Some tumours show evidence of involvement of more than one locus, suggesting potential interactions between the different Wilms' tumour genes. However, these genes may act at different points in the differentiation pathway, with their inactivation leading to distinct abnormalities in kidney development. These are best studied in individuals with a genetic susceptibility to Wilms' tumour, associated with constitutional chromosomal abnormalities at the 11p13 or 11p15 loci. Nephroblastosis, the presence of multiple premalignant lesions or nephrogenic rests, is frequently seen in the kidneys of such individuals (Beckwith *et al*, 1990). These developmental abnormalities may reflect the reduction in gene dosage associated with a heterozygous constitutional chromosomal defect. As observed by Beckwith, patients with aniridia or Drash syndrome, which are associated with 11p13 abnormalities, show a particular localization of nephrogenic rests within kidney lobules (intralobar). By contrast, individuals with Beckwith-Wiedemann syndrome, which is associated with abnormalities at the chromosome 11p15 locus, show nephrogenic rests surrounding kidney lobules (perilobar) (Beckwith *et al*, 1990). On the basis of studies of the morphological development of the kidney, Beckwith has proposed that intralobar rests represent an earlier developmental abnormality than perilobar rests, perhaps associated with a gene defect at a distinct stage in kidney development. In this context, it is noteworthy that *WT1* expression in Wilms' tumours is not homogeneous, but appears to be localized within the blastemal and epithelial components (Pritchard-Jones *et al*, 1990). The morphological heterogeneity of Wilms' tumour itself implies the arrest of cells within distinct pathways of differentiation.

A complete understanding of Wilms' tumorigenesis will require the identification of all members of the Wilms' tumour gene family. The *WT1* gene itself has been shown to play a key role in this process, as evidenced by its inactivation in Wilms' tumours. In some tumours, *WT1* inactivation appears to be the rate limiting step in tumorigenesis, whereas in others it may be a contributory event. Understanding the mechanism whereby functional loss of the *WT1* gene leads to tumour formation will require an appreciation of its normal role in cell growth and differentiation.

SUMMARY

Wilms' tumour is a paediatric kidney cancer which, in a substantial number of cases, has been associated with a genetic predisposition. Susceptibility to Wilms' tumour can be manifested by the presence of bilateral tumours, and in rare cases by a family history of this tumour or by associated congenital malformations. Like retinoblastoma, Wilms' tumour has been postulated to result from the inactivation of a tumour suppressor gene, although genetic studies implicate more than a single genetic locus. The recent isolation of the *WT1* gene, which maps to chromosome 11, band p13, has provided the first molecular clue to Wilms' tumorigenesis. *WT1* is specifically inactivated in a number of Wilms' tumours, and mutations have been found in the germline of susceptible individuals. This gene appears to encode a transcription factor with complex alternative splices, whose expression is strictly regulated in the developing kidney. Functional studies will be required to elucidate the role of *WT1* in normal kidney development and in tumorigenesis.

References

Beckwith JB, Kiviat NB and Bonadio JF (1990) Nephrogenic rests, nephroblastomatosis and the pathogenesis of Wilms' tumor. *Pediatric Pathology* **10** 1–36

Bernards R, Schackleford F, Gerber M *et al* (1989) Structure and expression of the murine retinoblastoma gene and characterization of its encoded protein. *Proceedings of the National Academy of Sciences of the USA* **86** 6474–6478

Buchkovich K, Duffy LA and Harlow E (1989) The retinoblastoma protein is phosphorylated during specific phases of the cell cycle. *Cell* **58** 1097–1105

Buckler AJ, Pelletier J, Haber DA, Glaser T and Housman DE (1991) Isolation, characterization and expression of the murine Wilms' tumor gene (WT1) during kidney development.

Molecular and Cellular Biology **11** 1707–1712

Call KM, Glaser T, Ito CY *et al* (1990) Isolation and characterization of a zinc finger polypeptide gene at the human chromosome 11 Wilms' tumor locus. *Cell* **60** 509–520

Chen P-L, Scully P, Shew J-Y, Wang JYJ and Lee W-H (1989) Phosphorylation of the retinoblastoma gene product is modulated during the cell cycle and cellular differentiation. *Cell* **58** 1193–1198

Compton DA, Weil MM, Jones CA, Riccardi VM, Strong LC and Saunders GF (1988) Long range physical map of the Wilms' tumor-aniridia region on human chromosome 11 *Cell* **55** 827–836

Cowell JK, Wadey RB, Haber DA, Call KM, Housman DE and Pritchard J (1991) Structural rearrangements of the WT1 gene in Wilms' tumour cells. *Oncogene* **6** 595–599

Davis LM, Byers MG, Fukushima Y *et al* (1988) Four new DNA markers are assigned to the WAGR region of 11p13: isolation and regional assignment of 112 chromosome 11 anonymous DNA segments. *Genomics* **3** 264–272

DeCaprio JA, Ludlow JW, Lynch D *et al* (1989) The product of the retinoblastoma susceptibility gene has properties of a cell cycle regulatory element. *Cell* **58** 1085–1095

Dunn J, Phillips R, Becker A and Gallie B (1988) Identification of germline and somatic mutations affecting the retinoblastoma gene. *Science* **241** 1797–1800

Evans R and Hollenberg S (1988) Zinc fingers: gilt by association. *Cell* **52** 1–3

Fearon E, Vogelstein B and Feinberg A (1984) Somatic deletion and duplication of genes on chromosome 11 in Wilms' tumours. *Nature* **309** 176–178

Francke U, Holmes LB, Atkins L and Riccardi VM (1979) Aniridia-Wilms' tumor association: evidence for specific deletion of 11p13. *Cytogenetics and Cell Genetics* **24** 185–192

Friend SH, Bernards HR, Rogelj S *et al* (1986) A human DNA segment with properties of the gene that predisposes to retinoblastoma and osteosarcoma. *Nature* **323** 643–646

Gessler M and Bruns GAP (1989) A physical map around the WAGR complex on the short arm of chromosome 11. *Genomics* **5** 43–55

Gessler M, Poustka A, Cavenee W, Neve RL, Orkin SH and Bruns GAP (1990) Homozygous deletion in Wilms tumours of a zinc-finger gene identified by chromosome jumping. *Nature* **343** 774–778

Glaser T, Lewis WH, Bruns GAP *et al* (1986) The B-subunit of follicle-stimulating hormone is deleted in patients with aniridia and Wilms' tumour, allowing a further definition of the WAGR locus. *Nature* **321** 882–887

Glaser T, Jones C, Call KM *et al* (1987) Mapping the WAGR region of chromosome 11p: somatic cell hybrids provide a fine-structure map. *Cytogenetics and Cell Genetics* **46** 620

Glaser T, Jones C, Douglass EC and Housman DE (1989) Constitutional and somatic mutations of chromosome 11p in Wilms' tumor. *Molecular Diagnostics of Human Cancer*, pp 253–277, Cold Spring Harbor Laboratory, Cold Spring Harbor

Glaser T, Lane J and Housman DE (1990) A mouse model of the aniridia-Wilms' tumor deletion syndrome. *Science* **250** 823–827

Grundy P, Kougos A, Morgan K, Li FP, Meadows A and Cavenee WK (1988) Familial predisposition to Wilms' tumor does not map to the short arm of chromosome 11. *Nature* **336** 374–376

Haber DA and Housman DE (1991) Rate-limiting steps: the genetics of pediatric cancers. *Cell* **64** 5–8

Haber DA, Buckler AJ, Glaser T *et al* (1990) An internal deletion within an 11p13 zinc finger gene contributes to the development of Wilms' tumor. *Cell* **61** 1257–1269

Haber DA, Sohn RL, Buckler AJ, Pelletier J, Call KM and Housman DE Alternative splicing and genomic structure of the Wilms' tumour gene, WT1. *Proceedings of the National Academy of Sciences of the USA* (in press)

Henry I, Grandjouan S, Couillin P *et al* (1989) Tumor-specific loss of 11p15.5 alleles in del 11p13 Wilms' tumor and in familial adrenocortical carcinoma. *Proceedings of the National Academy of Sciences of the USA* **86** 3247–3251

Herskowitz I (1987) Functional inactivation of genes by dominant negative mutations. *Nature* **329** 219–222

Huff V, Compton D, Chao L, Strong L, Geiser C and Saunders G (1988) Lack of linkage of familial Wilms' tumour to chromosomal band 11p13. *Nature* **336** 377–378

Huff V, Miwa H, Haber DA *et al* (1991) Evidence for WT1 as a Wilms' tumor (WT) gene: intragenic germinal deletion in bilateral WT. *American Journal of Human Genetics* **48** 997–1003

Joseph LJ, LeBeau MM, Jamieson GA *et al* (1988) Molecular cloning, sequencing and mapping of EGR2, a human early growth response gene encoding a protein with zinc-binding finger structure. *Proceedings of the National Academy of Sciences of the USA* **85** 7164–7168

Knudson AG (1971) Mutation and cancer: a statistical study. *Proceedings of the National Academy of Sciences of the USA* **68** 820–823

Knudson AG and Strong LC (1972) Mutation and cancer: a model for Wilms' tumor of the kidney. *Journal of the National Cancer Institute* **48** 313–324

Koufos A, Hansen MF, Lampkin BC *et al* (1984) Loss of alleles on human chromosome 11 during genesis of Wilms' tumour. *Nature* **309** 170–172

Koufos A, Grundy P, Morgan K *et al* (1989) Familial Wiedemann-Beckwith syndrome and a second Wilms' tumor locus map to 11p15.5. *American Journal of Human Genetics* **44** 711–719

Lee W-H, Bookstein R, Hong F, Young L-J, Shew J-Y and Lee EY-H (1987) Human retinoblastoma susceptibility gene: cloning, identification, and sequence. *Science* **235** 1394–1399

Ludlow JW, DeCaprio JA, Huang C-M, Lee W-H, Paucha E and Livingston DM (1989) SV40 large T antigen binds preferentially to an underphosphorylated member of the retinoblastoma susceptibility gene product family. *Cell* **56** 57–65

Mannens M, Slater RM, Heyting C *et al* (1987) Chromosome 11 Wilms' tumour and associated congenital diseases. *Cytogenetics and Cell Genetics* **46** 655

Matsunaga E (1981) Genetics of Wilms' tumor. *Human Genetics* **57** 231–246

Miller RW, Fraumeni JF and Manning MD (1964) Association of Wilms' tumor with aniridia, hemihypertrophy and other congenital abnormalities. *New England Journal of Medicine* **270** 922

Mitchell PJ and Tijan T (1989) Transcriptional regulation in mammalian cells by sequence-specific DNA binding proteins. *Science* **245** 371–378

Nehlin JO and Ronne H (1990) Yeast repressor is related to the mammalian early growth response and Wilms' tumor finger proteins. *EMBO Journal* **9** 2891–2898

Orkin SH, Goldman DS and Sallan SE (1984) Development of homozygosity for chromosome 11p markers in Wilms' tumour. *Nature* **309** 172–174

Pelletier J, Schalling M, Buckler A, Rogers A, Haber D and Housman D The Wilms' tumor gene (WT1) is involved in genitourinary development. *Genes and Development* (in press)

Porteous DJ, Bickmore W, Christie S *et al* (1987) HRAS1-selected chromosome transfer generates markers that colocalize aniridia- and genitourinary dysplasia-associated translocation breakpoints and the Wilms' tumor gene within 11p13. *Proceedings of the National Academy of Sciences of the USA* **84** 5355–5359

Pritchard-Jones K, Fleming S, Davidson D *et al* (1990) The candidate Wilms' tumour gene is involved in genitourinary development. *Nature* **346** 194–197

Raizis AM, Becroft DM, Shaw RL and Reeve AE (1985) A mitotic recombination in Wilms' tumor occurs between the parathyroid hormone locus and 11p13. *Human Genetics* **70** 344

Reeve AE, Housiaux PJ, Gardner RJ, Chewing WE, Grindley RM and Millow LJ (1984) Loss of a Harvey ras allele in sporadic Wilms' tumour. *Nature* **309** 174–176

Reeve AE, Sih SA, Raizis AM and Feinberg AP (1989) Loss of allelic heterozygosity at a second locus on chromosome 11 in Wilms' tumor cells. *Molecular and Cellular Biology* **9** 1799–1803

Riccardi VM, Sujansky E, Smith AC and Francke U (1978) Chromosomal imbalance in the aniridia-Wilms' tumor association: 11p interstitial deletion. *Pediatrics* **61** 604–610

Rauscher III FJ, Morris JF, Tournay OE, Cook DM and Curran T (1990) Binding of the Wilms' tumor locus zinc finger protein to the EGR1 consensus sequence. *Science* **250** 1259–1262

Rose EA, Glaser T, Jones C *et al* (1990) Complete physical map of the WAGR region of 11p13 localizes a candidate Wilms' tumor gene. *Cell* **60** 495–508

Schwartz CE, Haber DA, Stanton VP, Strong LC, Skolnick MH and Housman DE (1991) Familial predisposition to Wilms' tumor does not segregate with the WT1 gene. *Genomics* **10** 927–930

Sukhatme VP, Cao X, Chang LC *et al* (1988) A zinc finger encoding gene coregulated with c-fos during growth and differentiation and after cellular depolarization. *Cell* **53** 37–43

Ton CCT, Huff V, Call KM *et al* (1991) Smallest region of overlap in Wilms' tumor deletions uniquely implicates an 11p13 zinc finger gene as the disease locus. *Genomics* **10** 293–297

Turleau C, de Grouchy J, Nihoul-Fekete C, Chavin-Colin F, and Junien C (1984) Del 11p13/nephroblastoma without aniridia. *Human Genetics* **67** 455–456

Waziri M, Patil S, Hanson J and Bartley SA (1983) Abnormality of chromosome 11 in patients with features of Beckwith-Wiedemann syndrome. *Journal of Pediatrics* **102** 873–876

Yandell DW, Campbell TA, Dayton SH *et al* (1989) Oncogenic point mutations in the human retinoblastoma gene: their application to genetic counseling. *New England Journal of Medicine* **321** 1689–1695

The authors are responsible for the accuracy of the references.

Genetic Alterations Underlying Colorectal Tumorigenesis

ERIC R FEARON

Johns Hopkins University School of Medicine, Baltimore, Maryland 21205

INTRODUCTION

The development of common human cancers, such as those of the colon and rectum, is undoubtedly a highly complex process with many potential causes, including environmental factors and both inherited and somatic mutations. The proposal that a genetic component for the development of cancer exists is not novel. A genetic basis for cancer has been hypothesized for over 100 years, and a variety of familial, epidemiological and cytogenetic studies have provided substantial support for this hypothesis (reviewed in Hansen and Cavenee, 1987). Only in the past decade, however, have recombinant DNA based techniques been used to demonstrate directly that cancer is indeed a genetic disease, through the identification of some of the inherited and somatic mutations that underlie tumorigenesis. A current view is that human cancer results, at least in part, from mutations in two classes of genes—oncogenes and tumour suppressor genes (Weinberg, 1989). At the cellular level, oncogenic alleles may be defined as alleles that, when mutated or dysregulated in expression act in a dominant (positive) fashion to promote tumorigenesis. In contrast, wild type alleles of tumour suppressor genes normally regulate growth or differentiation and directly or, perhaps more likely, indirectly suppress tumorigenesis. Either inherited or somatic mutations in tumour suppressor alleles can result in the inactivation of normal gene function.

This chapter focuses on recent studies of genetic alterations involved in colorectal tumour development and progression. Specifically, I will discuss aspects of the natural history and genetics of colorectal tumour development; then, I will review studies that have led to the identification of alterations in both oncogenes and multiple tumour suppressor genes in various stages of colorectal tumour development. These mutations and their relative time of occurrence will be considered in terms of a genetic model for the development of colorectal cancer. Throughout this chapter, I will highlight some of the many remaining questions concerning the means by which the multiple genetic alterations detected in the majority of colorectal tumours may contribute to the development and progression of colorectal cancer.

NATURAL HISTORY OF INHERITED AND SPORADIC COLORECTAL CANCER

Colorectal tumours offer an excellent experimental system for the study of genetic alterations underlying the development and progression of a common human tumour. Indeed, colorectal cancer is an extremely common tumour type with over 150 000 new cases per year in the USA (Silverberg *et al*, 1990). It is estimated that a 50 year old person has about a 5% risk for the development of colorectal cancer by age 80 (Seidman *et al*, 1985). A widely held view is that many, if not the majority, of colorectal cancers are the end result of a rather orderly process of tumour progression occurring over a period of years to decades (Muto *et al*, 1975). In this neoplastic process, a small benign tumour (adenoma) arises from the colonic mucosa. Subsequent progression to a larger adenoma with an increased malignant potential may then occur in some cases, and finally some tumours progress to advanced and metastatic cancer (carcinoma). In reality, this biological process is likely to represent a continuum, with some discrete histopathological and clinical stages. Unlike many other common human cancers, colorectal tumours of all various stages of development from very small adenomas to large metastatic carcinomas can be easily obtained for study. In addition, because several inherited syndromes predispose strongly to the development of colorectal adenomas and cancers, both inherited and somatic mutations involved in colorectal tumorigenesis can be studied.

Inherited genetic factors are thought to contribute substantially to the development of about 10% of colorectal cancer cases. Although there may be significant heterogeneity in the genetics of inherited predisposition to colorectal cancer, several of the inherited syndromes leading to colorectal cancer development can be readily distinguished. Familial adenomatous polyposis (FAP) is an autosomal dominant disease that affects nearly 0.01% of the US, UK and Japanese populations (Utsunomiya and Lynch, 1990). Patients affected usually have hundreds to several thousand visible adenomatous polyps in the colon by the end of the second or third decade of life (Bussey, 1975; Burt and Samowitz, 1988). A relatively small proportion of the polyps will ultimately progress to carcinoma. Gardner syndrome (GS) is a variant of FAP in which desmoid tumours, osteomas and other neoplasms occur together with the colorectal tumours. The gene(s) that causes adenoma formation in FAP and GS was mapped to chromosome 5 (Bodmer *et al*, 1987; Leppert *et al*, 1987), and the recent identification of the FAP gene and its role in both inherited and sporadic cases will be discussed below.

At least two other inherited syndromes that predispose to the development of cancer of the colon and rectum can be identified. A large number of pedigrees have been identified that have inherited colorectal cancer without the features of typical polyposis (Utsunomiya and Lynch, 1990). Cancer is inherited in these families in an autosomal dominant pattern with high penetrance; in fact, two types of non-polyposis cancer can be distinguished by the inheritance of colorectal cancer solely (Lynch syndrome type I) or its inheritance with other cancers, including endometrial and gastric (Lynch syndrome type II). In some families, the locus predisposing to the Lynch type II syndrome has been reported to be linked to chromosome 18 (Lynch *et al*, 1985).

Several investigators have also noted that common or "sporadic" colorectal cancer often has a less clear-cut, yet identifiable, familial component. In addition, recent studies have suggested that colorectal cancer in general may be attributed, in part, to a genetic predisposition to the development of small numbers of adenomas (Cannon-Albright, 1988), a proportion of which progress to cancer. Identification of alleles that have a low phenotypic expressivity (relative to that seen in the polyposis syndromes) and that, in affected individuals, may predispose only weakly to the development of adenomas and cancers will undoubtedly prove interesting and useful. Nevertheless, in the majority of cases of colorectal cancer, no obvious inherited genetic component can be identified. Furthermore, the vast majority of cases of colorectal cancer occur after the sixth decade of life (Silverberg *et al*, 1990). This observation is consistent with the hypothesis that additional somatic genetic alterations are necessary, besides any mutations that may be inherited, for colorectal tumour development.

It has been proposed that somatic mutations are necessary for adenoma formation, regardless of the patient's genotype. Evidence to support this hypothesis has been obtained from the study of the clonal composition of such early stage tumours (Fearon *et al*, 1987). Although the normal colonic epithelium of patients both with and without polyposis has arisen from numerous stem cells, and has been shown to be polyclonal, all colorectal tumours examined to date have been found to have a monoclonal composition. Study of multiple adenomas from individual patients with polyposis revealed that each adenoma arose independently. Thus, adenomas appear to arise from a single stem cell or pocket of stem cells, and this is consistent with the notion that one cell or a small number of cells from within this pocket initiate the process of clonal expansion, perhaps as the result of a somatic mutation (Ponder and Wilkinson, 1986).

SOMATIC GENETIC ALTERATIONS UNDERLYING TUMOUR DEVELOPMENT AND PROGRESSION

Rationale for Their Study

In an effort to understand the molecular basis for the clonal expansion and clonal evolution presumed to occur during tumour initiation and progression, studies have been carried out to identify somatic genetic alterations present in colorectal tumours of various stages. Of greatest interest are those somatic mutations that are clonal, ie present in all or virtually all of the neoplastic cells of the primary tumour. The basis for inferring that such alterations might have a causal role in tumour initiation or progression is that mutations can only arise and become clonal by a limited number of mechanisms. The genetic alteration itself might be selected for by providing the cell with a growth advantage and allowing it to outgrow other progeny to become the predominant cell type in the tumour (clonal expansion) (Foulds, 1958; Nowell, 1976). Alternatively, the genetic alteration detected might have arisen coincidentally with another, perhaps undetected, change that actually provided the growth advantage. When somatic genetic alterations at the same locus are observed in tumours from many patients, the former explanation is more likely.

Somatic Mutations in Oncogenes

In colorectal tumours, alterations in the alleles of the cellular oncogenes have been studied with a variety of techniques, which vary in their sensitivity of detection or the nature of the oncogenic alleles that can be detected. Mutations in *ras* genes were first detected in colorectal tumours using transfection assays; when transfected into appropriate recipient cells, mutated alleles of *ras* genes confer neoplastic properties (Barbacid, 1987). Subsequent studies using hybridization with allele specific oligonucleotides have detected mutated *ras* alleles in about 50% of colorectal carcinomas (Bos *et al*, 1987; Forrester *et al*, 1987) and in a similar percentage of adenomas over 1 cm (Vogelstein *et al*, 1988). Adenomas of this size are thought to have an increased risk of malignant transformation (Muto *et al*, 1975). In contrast, such *ras* mutations were identified in fewer than 10% of adenomas under 1 cm. Over 85% of the mutations were detected at codons 12 or 13 of the Ki-*ras* gene, with the remainder of the mutations detected at codon 61 of Ki-*ras* and codons 12, 13 and 61 of N-*ras* (Vogelstein *et al*, 1988). The relative timing of *ras* gene mutations with respect to the various stages of colorectal tumour development suggests two alternative hypotheses for the means by which the mutated alleles may contribute to tumorigenesis. Mutation of the *ras* gene may be an early/initiating event in only a subset of adenomas, and those adenomas with *ras* gene mutations may be more likely to grow than adenomas without *ras* mutations. Alternatively, the *ras* mutations may usually arise only in one cell of a small pre-existing adenoma. Subsequent clonal expansion of this cell results in the conversion of a small adenoma to an adenoma with greater malignant potential. The study of classical or transgenic animal tumour models of colorectal cancer may help to distinguish between these two hypotheses for the role of *ras* gene mutations in colorectal tumour initiation, progression or both. In addition, whether the 50% of colorectal tumours in which no mutated *ras* alleles were detected with the allele specific hybridization assay contain mutations in regions of the *ras* genes not studied, or perhaps in other genes encoding products that interact with *ras* to regulate cell growth, remains to be determined.

In contrast to *ras* gene mutations, mutations in alleles of other cellular oncogenes have been detected much less frequently in colorectal tumours. A few cases of gene amplification of cellular oncogenes in primary tumours or cell lines have been observed; these include examples of *neu*, c-*myc* or *myb* amplification (Alitalo *et al*, 1983, 1984; D'Emilia *et al*, 1989). Similarly, although chromosomal translocation is a well documented mechanism of deregulating oncogene expression (Bishop, 1987) and chromosomal translocations can readily be detected in cytogenetic studies of many colorectal tumours (Reichmann *et al*, 1981), only one such rearrangement has been identified and characterized at the molecular level. In this case, sequences from the *trk* gene, which normally encodes a component of the nerve growth factor receptor, were rearranged (Martin-Zanca *et al*, 1986). The rearrangement generated a chimaeric protein in which the tyrosine kinase domain of *trk* was fused to tropomyosin sequences. Perhaps the failure to detect oncogenic alleles, other than *ras* alleles, in the vast majority of cases of colorectal tumours may be simply due to the inadequacies of the assays carried out to date, rather than the non-existence of such alleles.

In addition to specific mutations and structural alterations of the alleles of cellular oncogenes, a number of studies have reported consistent differences in the expression or activity of cellular oncogenes, despite the absence of concomitant mutations in the oncogenes themselves. For example, the c-*myc* gene and protein are expressed at high levels in most colorectal tumours (Rothberg *et al*, 1985; Stewart *et al*, 1986; Astrin and Costanzi, 1989); yet, as noted above, the gene has very rarely been found to be altered in colon tumours. These studies have led to the hypothesis that dysregulation of c-*myc* gene expression might not result from a defect at the c-*myc* locus but rather from a defect in a *trans*-acting factor or regulatory pathway (Erisman *et al*, 1989). Similarly, tyrosine kinase activities of several proteins, including c-*src*, are also elevated in many colorectal carcinomas, despite the absence of detectable genetic alterations at the corresponding locus or changes in total protein (Bolen *et al*, 1987). Thus, deregulation of the normal expression or activity of cellular oncogenes by mutations acting in *trans* may be an important alternative mechanism underlying tumour development in many common human cancers, including those of the colon and rectum. However, it should be noted that the significance of increased or decreased expression or activity of any gene product remains in question when the gene encoding the product is not demonstrably altered by mutation. In fact, many genes simply associated with cellular proliferation, and not demonstrated to have any oncogenic property, are much more highly expressed in colorectal primary tumours and tumour cell lines than in normal colonic mucosa (Calabretta *et al*, 1985).

Loss of Heterozygosity Mapping Reveals Candidate Tumour Suppressor Genes

Loss of specific chromosomal regions can be detected very frequently in many colorectal carcinomas, using either cytogenetic or molecular techniques. These chromosomal losses usually involve only one of the two parental chromosome sets present in normal cells. The losses can be readily detected, regardless of the mechanism of loss, by using restriction fragment length polymorphisms (RFLPs) to distinguish the two parental chromosomes from one another in the cells of the patient's normal and tumour tissues. Comparison of the RFLP pattern observed in normal tissue with that seen in the tumour tissue allows the identification of allelic losses or loss of heterozygosity (LOH) events that are clonal in the tumour cells. Although in many cases the LOH events result in a change in allele dosage for the chromosome region affected, in other cases they are not associated with a change in dosage, because the remaining alleles are duplicated (Fearon *et al*, 1987; Vogelstein *et al*, 1989). Thus, the importance of the change appears to be a qualitative one rather than a quantitative one; ie the alleles lost during tumorigenesis must differ in some way from the alleles retained. Previous studies of allelic losses in several childhood tumours, such as retinoblastoma and Wilms' tumour, have shown allelic losses to be one of the crucial mechanisms by which recessive mutations in tumour suppressor genes may be unmasked (reviewed in Hansen and Cavenee, 1987; Stanbridge and Cavenee, 1989). It was therefore inferred that the LOH events detected in colorectal and other common adult tumours might have been selected for during tumorigenesis by the unmasking of either somatic or inherited mutations in novel tumour suppressor genes (Knudson, 1985).

Chromosome 17p and the p53 gene   The chromosomal region identified as most frequently affected by these LOH events in colorectal carcinomas is chromosome 17p, which is affected in over 75% of these carcinomas (Fearon *et al*, 1987; Vogelstein *et al*, 1989). In contrast, LOH on 17p is detected infrequently in adenomas of any stage, including even very large, high grade adenomas with foci of carcinoma (Vogelstein *et al*, 1988). In addition, in several patients, the allelic losses on 17p were found to be associated with the progression of individual tumours from adenoma to carcinoma. Similar LOH events involving 17p can also be detected frequently in many other tumour types, including lung, breast, bladder and brain carcinomas, leukaemias and a number of paediatric bone and soft tissue tumours (Stanbridge and Cavenee, 1989). In colorectal tumours, the common region of allelic loss includes the *p53* gene (Baker *et al*, 1989).

Sequence analysis of a large number of *p53* alleles from colorectal carcinomas that had suffered LOH for 17p alleles revealed that in 20 of the 22 cases studied, a single missense mutation could be detected in the remaining *p53* allele (Baker *et al*, 1990a). In two of three cases in which no LOH for 17p was detected, both a wild type and a mutated *p53* allele were found in carcinoma cells; in the third case, the two *p53* alleles contained different missense mutations. Preliminary studies of *p53* alleles from adenomas suggest that, in general, mutated *p53* alleles are infrequently detected before the carcinoma stage (Baker *et al*, 1990a). In a study of 66 adenomas, only seven cases had LOH for 17p. Six of these were studied for *p53* mutations by DNA sequencing, and in four cases, missense mutations were found. DNA sequencing studies of 19 adenomas with no LOH on 17p detected mutated *p53* alleles in only two cases. The *p53* mutations in colorectal cancer detected to date have been found predominantly in the most highly conserved regions of the gene, similar to the findings in other common human cancers. In particular, codons 175, 248 and 273 have been found to be mutated at a very high frequency in colorectal tumours (Baker *et al*, 1990a; Hollstein *et al*, 1991).

Point mutation of one *p53* allele coupled with loss of the remaining wild type allele thus appears to occur very frequently during the development of colorectal carcinoma. The order of these changes at the *p53* locus in the majority of cases is not known. However, at least one colorectal tumour has been found in which both wild type and mutated *p53* alleles are expressed in all tumour cells (Nigro *et al*, 1989). (Note that the studies reviewed above suggest that a number of tumours may be heterozygous for expression of *p53* alleles, but in most cases, definitive evidence has not been obtained, since only genomic DNA was studied.) This observation suggests that a mutated *p53* allele in a colorectal tumour cell could provide a selective growth advantage, leading to clonal outgrowth, even in the presence of a wild type *p53* allele.

With further growth and progression, the remaining wild type allele is selectively lost in the majority of cases. This notion is consistent with several lines of experimental evidence which have established that mutated *p53* alleles can function in a dominant fashion to participate in transformation (Hinds *et al*, 1989; Lane and Benchimol, 1990). Moreover, it has been proposed that mutated *p53* alleles might function in a dominant negative fashion by binding the wild type gene product and preventing its normal association with other cellular constituents, or perhaps by altering the conformation of the wild type protein (Herskowitz, 1987; Lane and Benchimol, 1990). Nevertheless, it appears that the balance between mutated and wild type p53 protein, in at least some cell types, may be critical in determining whether transformation or suppression results. This hypothesis is based on the finding that high level expression of an exogenous wild type *p53* gene in colorectal tumour cells with mutated *p53* alleles results in complete cessation of cell growth (Baker *et al*, 1990b).

Many crucial questions still remain to be answered regarding the role of *p53* mutations and allelic losses in colorectal tumour development: (a) Why is expression of a mutated gene product, rather than complete inactivation of the gene, selected for during colorectal carcinoma development? (b) What is the explanation for the mutational spectrum in *p53* alleles of colorectal tumours, in particular the high frequency of *p53* mutations at CpG sites and the particular aminoacids affected in colon tumours compared with other tumour types (Hollstein *et al*, 1991)? (c) How do mutated *p53* alleles interact with other mutated alleles of oncogenes and tumour suppressor genes, such as mutated *ras* alleles? (d) What is the explanation for the apparent selection of mutated *p53* alleles only in late stages of colorectal tumour development, as suggested by studies of primary colorectal tumours and also by the apparently infrequent occurrence of colorectal tumours in both animals and humans with germline mutations of *p53* (see discussion below)? (e) Do allelic losses of 17p in colorectal tumours result in the unmasking of mutations at other tumour suppressor loci on 17p, in addition to those at the *p53* gene?

Chromosome 18q and the **DCC** *Gene*   Allelic losses involving chromosome 18q can be observed in over 70% of colorectal carcinomas, in almost 50% of late adenomas and very infrequently in early stage adenomas (Vogelstein *et al*, 1988). Initially, a common region of allelic loss was mapped to the 18q21-qter region, and subsequent studies identified a more defined region of 18q suspected to contain a tumour suppressor gene. A contiguous stretch of DNA consisting of about 370 kb was cloned, and a candidate tumour suppressor gene from this region has been identified (Fearon *et al*, 1990). This gene, termed *DCC* (deleted in colorectal carcinoma), encodes a protein that has significant homology with the neural cell adhesion molecule (NCAM) family (Edelman, 1988). The *DCC* cDNAs identified to date encode a putative transmembrane gene product with four immunoglobulin like domains, multiple repeats of fibronectin type III related domain and a cytoplasmic domain not highly related to any previously identified gene product (Fearon *et al*, 1990; Cho KR and Vogelstein B, personal communication). Although nothing is known of the normal function of the *DCC* gene and its product, it is intriguing that a gene considered to be a candidate tumour suppressor gene is very similar to genes thought to be involved in cell-cell or cell-extracellular matrix interactions. Alterations or inactivation of the *DCC* gene might account, at least in part, for some of the altered properties of adhesion and invasion noted in colorectal tumour cells.

Several observations support the hypothesis that the *DCC* gene may be inactivated during colorectal tumorigenesis and thus should be considered as a candidate tumour suppressor gene (Fearon *et al*, 1990). Firstly, as noted above, allelic losses involving the *DCC* gene can be detected in over 70% of colorectal carcinomas. Secondly, although the gene is expressed at low levels in most normal tissues, including normal colonic mucosa, *DCC* expression was found to be greatly reduced or absent in over 85% of the colorectal tumour cell lines studied. Thirdly, on Southern blot analysis, somatic mutations of the *DCC* gene were observed in about 15% of colorectal carcinomas. These somatic mutations included homozygous deletion of the 5′ region of the gene in one case, a point mutation within an intron in another case and multiple alleles in tumours in which insertions were present immediately downstream from an exon. Studies to identify somatic mutations localized solely to coding regions of the gene are in progress, and a few examples of point mutations within or flanking *DCC* exons have been obtained (Simons JW and Vogelstein B, personal communication). Although such a demonstration provides further proof that the gene is a target for somatic mutation, it cannot formally establish that the *DCC* gene is a suppressor of colorectal tumorigenesis. Confirmation of this hypothesis will require demonstration that a cDNA copy of the *DCC* gene functions to suppress some aspect of the tumorigenic phenotype when introduced into colorectal tumour cells with defects in endogenous *DCC* alleles. Further rationale for carrying out this proposed experiment has been provided by studies of Tanaka *et al*, who have carried out single chromosome transfer experiments with chromosome 18 in a colorectal tumour cell line. Clones retaining a copy of the transferred chromosome 18 were suppressed for growth in soft agar and for tumour formation in immunocompromised mice (Tanaka *et al*, 1991).

The localization of the *DCC* gene on chromosome 18q is interesting with respect to one of the hereditary non-polyposis colorectal cancer syndromes noted above (Lynch type II), in which affected individuals are predisposed to cancers of the colon and other organs. In several pedigrees affected by this syndrome, evidence for linkage of the predisposition gene to the Kidd blood group on chromosome 18q11.1-q21.1 was obtained (Lynch *et al*, 1985). Thus, the *DCC* gene could potentially be altered in the germline of individuals with this syndrome. However, in preliminary studies of a number of kindreds, no evidence for linkage of the disease predisposition to the *DCC* gene has been obtained (Peltomaki *et al*, 1991). At this time, the data to implicate the *DCC* gene in colorectal tumorigenesis include a rather limited number of somatic genetic alterations affecting the gene and frequent alterations in its expression pattern in colorectal tumours, compared with normal colonic mucosa. They do not yet include any germline alterations of the gene in individuals predisposed to colorectal tumour development.

Chromosome 5q and the* MCC *and* FAP *Genes As noted above, the FAP syndrome and its variant, Gardner syndrome (GS), predispose affected individuals to the development of hundreds of adenomas. Localization of the *FAP* gene was aided by the identification of a constitutional deletion of chromosomal band 5q21 in a patient with FAP (Herrera *et al*, 1986). Subsequent linkage studies established that several chromosome 5q21 markers were tightly linked to the development of adenomas in both the FAP and GS syndromes (Bodmer *et al*, 1987; Leppert *et al*, 1987). Additional studies suggested that the same chromosomal region might contain a gene involved in tumorigenesis in kindreds affected with variant forms of FAP that exhibit marked variation in expression of the disease phenotype even within a single pedigree (Leppert *et al*, 1990). Moreover, although the FAP and related syndromes are relatively uncommon, the potential importance of 5q21 genes in the majority of colorectal cancers was highlighted by the demonstration that LOH events affecting 5q21 alleles were observed in 35–45% of the tumours of patients with no obvious inherited tendency to colorectal cancer (Solomon *et al*, 1987; Vogelstein *et al*, 1988; Ashton-Rickardt *et al*, 1989). Although allelic losses involving 5q are rarely noted in adenomas from patients with polyposis, they are the most common genetic alteration so far described in small, early adenomas from patients without polyposis, occurring at almost the same frequency as 5q allelic losses in carcinomas from non-polyposis patients (Vogelstein *et al*, 1988). Taken together, these data strongly suggested that chromosomal band 5q21 contained a gene or genes with several of the properties expected of a tumour suppressor gene. The gene or genes might be inactivated by germline mutations in some cases of colorectal cancer and by somatic mutations in the majority.

In an effort to identify the *FAP* gene or genes, cloning of a large portion of of 5q21 was undertaken by two groups using yeast artificial chromosome (YAC) vectors and chromosome walking techniques (Joslyn *et al*, 1991; Kinzler *et al*, 1991a). Several candidate cDNAs from the region were isolated and examined either for germline mutations in DNA from patients with FAP or for somatic mutations in DNA from tumours of patients with sporadic colorectal cancer. The first candidate tumour suppressor gene identified in the region was termed *MCC* (mutated in colorectal cancer) (Kinzler et. al, 1991b). The *MCC* gene was found to be somatically mutated in tumour DNA of three patients with sporadic colorectal cancer; in one case, the gene was grossly rearranged or deleted, and in the other two cases, point mutations resulting in aminoacid substitutions were found. Further studies have identified four additional somatic mutations in the *MCC* gene in sporadic colorectal cancers, including missense mutations and splice site mutations (Nishisho *et al*, 1991). However, although the *MCC* gene is a target for somatic mutation in colorectal cancers, subsequent studies of DNA from FAP patients have failed to detect any germline mutations in the *MCC* gene in the studies to date (Groden *et al*, 1991; Nishisho *et al*, 1991).

Coincidentally with these observations, it was found that constitutional deletions at chromosomal band 5q21 in two unrelated patients with FAP, involving only about 100 kb in one patient and about 260 kb in another, did not include *MCC* sequences (Joslyn *et al*, 1991). It was believed that these deletions removed segments of the *FAP* gene. On this basis, cDNAs from three genes were identified that mapped within the DNA sequences deleted in the smaller of the two deletions. Point mutations in germline DNAs of FAP patients were detected in one of these genes, the *APC* (adenomatous polyposis coli) gene, using strategies based on the polymerase chain reaction to detect mutations. Subsequent sequence analysis confirmed that the germline mutations altered coding sequences within the *APC* gene, creating frameshifts, stop codons or missense mutations in the studies reported on nine FAP or GS patients (Groden *et al*, 1991; Nishisho *et al*, 1991). The mutation present in the *APC* gene does not appear to determine whether a patient will manifest solely colonic adenomas (FAP) or both colonic and extracolonic neoplasms (GS), since idential mutations were detected in one patient with FAP and one patient with GS (Nishisho *et al*, 1991). Further studies of DNAs from carcinomas of patients with sporadic colorectal cancer have revealed somatic mutations in the *APC* gene (Nishisho *et al*, 1991). Examples include mutations that alter the gene by creating missense mutations, stop codons and frameshifts or altered splice sites. Thus, the data firmly establish that the *APC* gene is mutated in the germline of patients with the polyposis syndromes. In addition, this gene also is a target for somatic mutations in sporadic colorectal cancer.

Although the studies on the *MCC* and *APC* genes are still rather preliminary at this time, a number of interesting questions have emerged concerning the relationship between mutations in these genes and colorectal tumour development. Firstly, although the data establish the importance of germline alterations of the *APC* gene in adenoma formation in individuals with inherited polyposis, the significance of somatic mutations in either the *MCC* or *APC* genes remains to be established. As noted above, mutations can arise and become clonal (present in all tumour cells) through a limited number of mechanisms. Either the specific mutation detected has a causal role in clonal outgrowth or it is a coincidental epiphenomenon that arises in concert with another undetected alteration for which selection occurs. As noted by Nishisho *et al* and others (see Nishisho *et al*, 1991 and references within), clonal mutations in tumours have previously been described only in genes suspected of being important in tumour formation. In accord with this proposal, somatic mutations in the *MCC* and *APC* genes in colorectal cancers are much more prevalent than the estimated prevalence of mutations in anonymous DNA sequences in such tumours (Vogelstein *et al*, 1989; Nishisho *et al*, 1991). Lastly, if the *MCC* and *APC* genes were mutational hot spots for random somatic mutations (ie mutations that do not provide a growth advantage to the cells in which they occur), then a high percentage of the mutations would be expected to result in silent changes. This hypothesis is not supported by the findings to date, since all ten of the somatic mutations identified in the *MCC* and *APC* genes would be expected to alter aminoacid sequence or affect splice site elements.

At present, the aminoacid sequences predicted from the cDNA sequences of both the *APC* and *MCC* genes shed little light on the possible function of the genes and gene products. The *APC* gene encodes a predicted product of 2843 aminoacids (Joslyn *et al*, 1991; Kinzler *et al*, 1991a), and the predicted product of the *MCC* gene is 829 aminoacids (Kinzler *et al*, 1991b). Both predicted protein products show only weak homology with other proteins or genes identified to date. The absence of a number of otherwise characteristic sequence features suggests a cytoplasmic localization for both proteins. Of interest is the identification of heptad repeat motifs in the predicted products of both the *APC* and *MCC* genes. These heptad repeats have been hypothesized to be capable of mediating protein-protein interactions (Cohen and Perry, 1986; Bourne, 1991). Thus, because of this observation, and also given the physical proximity of the genes, the potential involvement of both genes in colonic tumorigenesis and some short regions of sequence identity between the two genes, it has been speculated that perhaps the *APC* and *MCC* gene products physically interact or function in the same growth regulatory pathways. In addition, although little is known about the pattern of expression or developmental regulation of the genes, preliminary studies suggest that expression of both genes is ubiquitous in adult tissues, rather than confined to colonic epithelium (Groden *et al*, 1991; Kinzler *et al*, 1991a,b).

A GENETIC MODEL FOR COLORECTAL TUMORIGENESIS

Outline of the Model and Unanswered Questions

Clearly, significant progress at identifying the genetic basis for colorectal tumour development has been achieved in the recent past. One of the genes involved in an inherited predisposition to colorectal tumour development has been identified, as have several genes and/or chromosomal regions that have undergone frequent somatic mutation during tumour development. In addition, studies have been undertaken to address the relative timing of these somatic genetic alterations in colorectal tumour development and progression. Mutations involving at least four to five different loci can be identified in many colorectal cancers, and fewer mutations are generally noted in colonic adenomas.

A possible view is that the majority of colorectal cancers arise as the result of these multiple genetic alterations, including mutational activation of oncogene alleles and mutational inactivation of tumour suppressor gene alleles. Furthermore, the mutations that result in clonal expansion tend to arise in a certain order, although this is not invariable. Thus, the accumulation and interaction of the multiple genetic alterations within a tumour cell may determine its phenotype. These findings have been summarized in detail and advanced as support for a genetic model for colorectal tumorigenesis (Fearon and Vogelstein, 1990). Indeed, this model for tumorigenesis accurately reflects many of the data obtained to date, and it may serve as a useful framework, or first approximation, for further studies of genetic changes in human colorectal tumours. Similarly, the model makes predictions that can be tested in models of tumorigenesis in vitro or in studies of transgenic or homozygous mutant animal model systems of colonic tumours. Undoubtedly, however, this genetic model for colorectal tumorigenesis is likely to be incomplete and overly simplified. Moreover, many crucial questions remain concerning the relative contribution of the inherited and somatic mutations identified thus far to colorectal tumour development. For example, which, if any, of the mutations identified are rate limiting for tumour formation? Which mutations are sufficient for adenoma development and for carcinoma development? Similarly, are any of the genetic alterations necessary for colorectal tumour development?

Inherited Cancer Syndromes and Rate Limiting Mutations

The inherited cancer syndromes can offer important insights into the genes that function to determine the rate of tumour formation in various tissues. Germline inactivation of one retinoblastoma allele appears to influence significantly only the rate of retinoblastoma development, and less markedly the rate of osteosarcoma and soft tissue sarcoma development in affected individuals (Gordon, 1974; Abramson *et al*, 1984). Although the retinoblastoma predisposition gene (*RB*) and its protein product are ubiquitously expressed, the frequency of other tumour types, including colorectal tumours, in individuals with germline *RB* mutations is not significantly different from that in the general population. This finding is, perhaps, a result of greater redundancy in the *RB* regulated growth pathways in cell types other than retinoblasts and osteoblasts. Similarly, as noted above, somatic mutations in the *p53* gene are thought to contribute to later stages of colorectal tumour development. Yet, patients with the Li-Fraumeni syndrome have inherited mutated *p53* alleles, and colorectal cancers rarely develop in these individuals (Malkin *et al*, 1990; Vogelstein, 1990). Although this observation may be attributed to tissue specific differences in the oncogenic potential of different mutated *p53* alleles, these findings suggest that mutational inactivation of the *p53* gene may not be a rate determining event in colorectal tumour development. Also consistent with this hypothesis is the observation that *p53* mutations appear to be selected for only at late stages of colorectal tumour development. Taken together, the findings suggest that other genes may modify significantly the effect of a mutated *p53* allele in colonic epithelial cells. Perhaps these interacting or modifying genes may need to be inactivated before mutated *p53* alleles can exert a phenotypic effect.

The present data suggest that inactivation of the *APC* gene may be a rate determining event for adenoma formation. Germline mutations in the *APC* gene predispose affected individuals to the development of hundreds of colonic adenomas. Yet, a single defective allele presumably is not sufficient for adenoma development, since only a very small proportion of the colonic epithelial cells will subsequently undergo transformation and develop clonally into adenomas. Inactivation of the remaining wild type *APC* allele is a genetic event that might cause the conversion to adenoma of a predisposed colonic epithelial cell in a polyposis patient. Indeed, in some other inherited tumour syndromes, LOH events serve to unmask inherited recessive mutations. Frequent LOH events affecting chromosomes 13q and 22q have been observed in retinoblastoma and neurofibromatosis type II, respectively (Hansen and Cavenee, 1987; Seizinger et al, 1987; Stanbridge and Cavenee, 1989). However, previous studies of 5q allelic losses in small adenomas from patients with FAP have failed to detect LOH involving 5q (Vogelstein et al, 1988; Sasaki et al, 1989; Fearon and Vogelstein, 1990). This finding contrasts with the observation of LOH of 5q alleles detected in some carcinomas from FAP patients and in a high percentage of adenomas and carcinomas from patients with sporadic colorectal tumours. Thus, although the inherited or somatic mutations identified thus far in the APC and MCC genes appear to be inactivating (deletions, truncated proteins and presumably the missense proteins as well), further detailed molecular studies of the APC and MCC alleles present in adenomas and carcinomas, from patients both with and without polyposis, are necessary to clarify whether mutated alleles of these genes are dominant or recessive at the cellular level for various stages of tumour development.

Necessary, Sufficient or Neither?

The data at present argue that no single mutation at the cellular level is sufficient for carcinoma formation, and, as reviewed above, no single inherited mutation appears to suffice for the development of an adenoma. Preliminary estimates of the number of genetic alterations present in various stages of colorectal tumorigenesis, however, can be made. Four genetic alterations (ras gene mutations and LOH of chromosomes 5q, 17p and 18q) were studied in colorectal tumours of various stages, predominantly from patients without polyposis (Vogelstein et al, 1988). More than 90% of the carcinomas had two or more of the four alterations. In contrast, of the adenomas measuring less than 1 cm, about 20% had one of the four alterations detected and only 7% had two or more. In general, the number of genetic alterations detected was found to increase as the adenomas increased in size and malignant potential. In several advanced adenomas, all four genetic alterations were detected. This observation suggests that alterations in perhaps as many as four genes in some cases might not be sufficient for conversion to carcinoma. Additional studies of allelic losses have revealed that most carcinomas had, on average, four to five allelic losses per tumour (Sasaki et al, 1989; Vogelstein et al, 1989). Results from similar studies of a sizeable number of adenomas and carcinomas from patients with FAP were consistent with the findings for sporadic colorectal tumours reviewed above (Miyaki et al, 1990; Shirasawa et al, 1991). Together, the data suggest that approximately the same total number and frequency of each somatic mutation are observed regardless of the genotype of the patient.

Although it is possible that some of the clonal mutations identified in colorectal tumours may be epiphenomena, multiple, independent lines of evidence have been obtained in previous studies to support the likely functional importance of mutated *ras* and *p53* alleles in neoplasia (Weinberg, 1989; Lane and Benchimol, 1990). Each of these genes is altered in a large proportion of colorectal tumours: mutated *ras* alleles have been detected in over 50% and mutated *p53* alleles may be present in as many as 85% (Baker *et al*, 1990a). Yet, are mutations in either of these genes necessary for carcinoma development? The extremely high frequency of *p53* mutation in cancers argues for the possibility of a necessary role for mutated *p53* alleles at some (perhaps often relatively late) stage of colorectal carcinoma formation. Nevertheless, the present data suggest that some carcinomas arise despite the presence of wild type *p53* alleles, and thus it cannot be concluded that *p53* gene mutation is necessary for colorectal cancer development. It is interesting to speculate, however, that mutation in any one of several target genes in the growth pathways in which the *p53* and *ras* genes function is, in fact, necessary for tumour development. Thus, the growth pathway and not a particular gene would be the necessary target for mutation. Future studies may begin to address the many important questions on the role in normal growth regulation of *ras, p53* and other oncogenes and tumour suppressor genes implicated in colorectal tumorigenesis. In addition, these studies may help to illuminate the means by which deregulation of these genes and their growth pathways contributes to human cancer.

SUMMARY

Colorectal tumours have proven to be an excellent system in which to identify and study the genetic alterations involved in the development of a common human neoplasm. A prevalent view is that colorectal tumours appear to arise as the result of multiple genetic alterations in the alleles of both oncogenes and tumour suppressor genes. The accumulation of genetic alterations appears to accompany the clinical and biological progression of the tumours and may determine the phenotype of the tumour cells. In addition to the many somatic alterations identified at various stages of colorectal tumour development, recent studies have led to the identification of the adenomatous polyposis coli (*APC*) gene, which, when mutated in the germline, predisposes to the development of colorectal tumours. On the basis of studies of inherited and somatic mutations in colorectal tumours, a genetic model for colorectal cancer development has been proposed. Although the model is undoubtedly incomplete, it nevertheless provides a useful framework for further studies of the multiple events that underlie human tumour initiation and progression. Numerous questions remain to be answered, including identification of the normal function of the genes implicated in tumorigenesis, how mutations in these genes arise and are selected for and what the relative contribution of the altered genes is to various stages of the neoplastic process. Nevertheless, an optimistic outlook is that fundamental insights into the pathogenesis of human cancer are within our reach.

References

Abramson DH, Ellsworth RM, Kitchin FD and Tung G (1984) Second nonocular tumors in retinoblastoma survivors: are they radiation-induced? *Ophthamology* 91 1351–1355

Astrin SM and Costanzi C (1989) The molecular genetics of colon cancer. *Seminars in Oncology* 16 138–147

Alitalo K, Schwab M, Lin CC, Varmus HE and Bishop JM (1983) Homogeneously staining chromosomal regions contain amplified copies of an abundantly expressed cellular oncogene (c-*myc*) in malignant neuroendocrine cells from a human colon carcinoma. *Proceedings of the National Academy of Sciences of the USA* 80 1707–1711

Alitalo K, Winqvist, Lin CC, de la Chapelle A, Schwab M and Bishop JM (1984) Aberrant expression of an amplified c-*myb* oncogene in two cell lines from a colon carcinoma. *Proceedings of the National Academy of Sciences of the USA* 81 4535–4538

Ashton-Rickardt PG, Dunlop MG, Nakamura Y *et al* (1989) High frequency of APC loss in sporadic colorectal carcinoma due to breaks clustered in 5q21-22. *Oncogene* 4 1169–1174

Baker SJ, Fearon ER, Nigro JM *et al* (1989) Chromosome 17 deletions and p53 gene mutations in colorectal carcinomas. *Science* 244 217–221

Baker SJ, Preisinger AC, Jessup JM *et al* (1990a) p53 gene mutations occur in combination with 17p allelic deletions as late events in colorectal tumorigenesis. *Cancer Research* 50 7717–7722

Baker SJ, Markowitz S, Fearon ER, Willson JKV and Vogelstein B (1990b) Suppression of human colorectal carcinoma cell growth by wild-type p53. *Science* 249 217–221

Barbacid M (1987) *ras* genes. *Annual Reviews in Biochemistry* 56 779–827

Bishop JM (1987) The molecular genetics of cancer. *Science* 235 305–311

Bodmer WF, Bailey C, Bodmer J *et al* (1987) Localization of the gene for familial polyposis on chromosome 5. *Nature* 328 614–616

Bolen JB, Veillette A, Schwartz AM, DeSeau V and Rosen N (1987) Activation of pp60[c-src] protein kinase activity in human colon carcinoma. *Proceedings of the National Academy of Sciences of the USA* 84 2251–2255

Bos JL, Fearon ER, Hamilton SR *et al* (1987) Prevalence of *ras* gene mutations in human colorectal cancer. *Nature* 327 293–297

Bourne H (1991) Consider the coiled coil. *Nature* 351 188–190

Burt RW and Samowitz WS (1988) The adenomatous polyp and the hereditary polyposis syndromes. *Gastroenterology Clinics of North America* 17 657–678

Bussey HJR (1975) *Familial Polyposis Coli: Family Studies, Histopathology, Differential Diagnosis, and Results of Treatment*, Johns Hopkins University Press, Baltimore

Calabretta B, Kaczmarek L, Ming PL, Au F and Ming S (1985) Expression of c-*myc* and other cell cycle-dependent genes in human colon neoplasia. *Cancer Research* 45 6000–6004

Cannon-Albright LA, Skolnick MH, Bishop DT, Lee RG and Burt RW (1988) Common inheritance of susceptibility to colonic adenomatous polyps and associated colorectal cancers. *New England Journal of Medicine* 319 533–537

Cavenee WK, Dryja TP, Phillips RA *et al* (1983) Expression of recessive alleles by chromosomal mechanisms in retinoblastoma. *Nature* 305 779–784

Cohen C and Perry D (1986) Alpha-helical coiled coils - a widespread motif in proteins. *Trends in Biochemical Sciences* 11 245–248

D'Emilia J, Bulovas K, D'Erole D, Wolf B, Steele G and Summerhayes IC (1989) Expression of the c-erbB-2 gene product (P185) at different stages of neoplastic progression in the colon. *Oncogene* 4 1233–1239

Edelman GM (1988) Morphoregulatory molecules. *Biochemistry* 27 3533–3543

Erisman MD, Scott JK and Astrin SM (1989) Evidence that the FAP gene is involved in a subset of colon cancers with a complementable defect in c-myc regulation. *Proceedings of the National Academy of Sciences of the USA* 86 4264–4268

Fearon ER and Vogelstein B (1990) A genetic model for colorectal tumorigenesis. *Cell* 61 759–767

Fearon ER, Hamilton SR and Vogelstein B (1987) Clonal analysis of human colorectal tumors. *Science* **238** 193–197

Fearon ER, Cho KR, Nigro JM *et al* (1990) Identification of a chromosome 18q gene that is altered in colorectal cancers. *Science* **247** 49–56

Forrester K, Almoguera C, Han K, Grizzle WE and Perucho M (1987) Detection of high incidence of K-*ras* oncogenes during human colon tumorigenesis. *Nature* **327** 298–303

Foulds L (1958) The natural history of cancer. *Journal of Chronic Disease* **8** 2–37

Gordon H (1974) Family studies in retinoblastoma. *Birth Defects* **10** 185–190

Groden J, Thliveris A, Samowitz W *et al* (1991) Identification and characterization of the familial adenomatous polyposis coli gene. *Cell* **66** 589–600

Hansen MF and Cavenee WK (1987) Genetics of cancer predisposition. *Cancer Research* **47** 5518–5527

Herkowitz I (1987) Functional inactivation of genes by dominant negative mutations. *Nature* **329** 219–222

Herrera L, Kakati S, Gibas L, Pietrzak E and Sandberg A (1986) Brief clinical report: Gardner syndrome in a man with an interstitial deletion of 5q. *American Journal of Medical Genetics* **25** 473–476

Hinds PW, Finlay C and Levine AJ (1989) Mutation is required to activate the p53 gene for cooperation with the *ras* oncogene and transformation. *Journal of Virology* **63** 739–746

Hollstein M, Sidransky D, Vogelstein B and Harris CC (1991) p53 mutations in human cancers. *Science* **253** 49–53

Joslyn G, Carlson M, Thliveris A *et al* (1991) Identification of deletion mutations and three new genes at the familial polyposis locus. *Cell* **66** 601–613

Kinzler KW, Nilbert MC, Su L-K *et al* (1991a) Identification of FAP locus genes from chromosome 5q21. *Science* **253** 661–665

Kinzler KW, Nilbert MC, Vogelstein B *et al* (1991b) Identification of a gene located at chromosome 5q21 that is mutated in colorectal cancers. *Science* **251** 1366–1370

Knudson AG Jr (1985) Hereditary cancer, oncogenes, and anti-oncogenes. *Cancer Research* **45** 1437–1443

Lane DP and Benchimol S (1990) p53: oncogene or anti-oncogene? *Genes and Development* **4** 1–8

Leppert M, Dobbs M, Scambler P *et al* (1987) The gene for familial polyposis coli maps to the long arm of chromosome 5. *Science* **238** 1411–1413

Leppert M, Burt R, Hughes JP *et al* (1990) Genetic analysis of an inherited predisposition to colon cancer in a family with a variable number of adenomatous polyps. *New England Journal of Medicine* **322** 904–908

Lynch HT, Schuelke GS, Kimberling WJ *et al* (1985) Hereditary nonpolyposis colorectal cancer (Lynch syndromes I and II). Biomarker studies. *Cancer* **56** 939–951

Malkin D, Li F, Strong LC *et al* (1990) Germ line p53 mutations in a familial syndrome of breast cancer, sarcomas, and other neoplasms. *Science* **250** 1233–1238

Martin-Zanca D, Hughes SH and Barbacid M (1986) A human oncogene formed by the fusion of truncated tropomyosin and protein tyrosine kinase sequences. *Nature* **319** 743–748

Miyaki M, Seki M, Okamoto M *et al* (1990) Genetic changes and histopathological types in colorectal tumors from patients with familial adenomatous polyposis. *Cancer Research* **50** 7166–7173

Muto T, Bussey HJR and Morson BC (1975) The evolution of cancer of the colon and rectum. *Cancer* **36** 2251–2270

Nigro JM, Baker SJ, Preisinger AC *et al* (1989) Mutations in the p53 gene occur in diverse human tumour types. *Nature* **342** 705–707

Nishisho I, Nakamura Y, Miyoshi Y *et al* (1991) Mutations of chromosome 5q21 genes in FAP and colorectal cancer patients. *Science* **253** 665–669

Nowell P (1976) The clonal evolution of tumor cell populations. *Science* **194** 23–28

Peltomaki P, Sistonen P, Mecklin J *et al* (1991) Evidence supporting exclusion of the DCC gene and a portion of chromosome 18q as the locus for susceptibility to hereditary non-polyposis colorectal cancer in 5 kindreds. *Cancer Research* **51** 4135–4140

Ponder BAJ and Wilkinson MM (1986) Direct examination of the clonality of carcinogen-induced colonic epithelial dysplasia in chimeric mice. *Journal of the National Cancer Institute* **77** 967–976

Reichmann A, Martin P and Levin B (1981) Chromosomal banding patterns in human large bowel cancer. *International Journal of Cancer* **28** 431–440

Rothberg PG, Spandorfer HM, Erisman MD *et al* (1985) Evidence that c-*myc* expression defines two genetically distinct forms of colorectal adenocarcinoma. *British Journal of Cancer* **52** 629–632

Sasaki M, Okamoto M, Sato C *et al* (1989) Loss of constitutional heterozygosity in colorectal tumors from patients with familial polyposis coli and those with non-polyposis colorectal carcinoma. *Cancer Research* **49** 4402–4406

Seidman H, Mushinski MH, Gelb and Silverberg E (1985) Probabilities of eventually developing or dying of cancer - United States, 1985. *CA* **35** 36–56

Seizinger BR, Rouleau G, Ozelius LJ *et al* (1987) Common pathogenetic mechanism for three tumor types in bilateral acoustic neurofibromatosis. *Science* **236** 317–319

Shirasawa S, Urabe K, Yanagawa Y, Toshitani K, Iwama T and Sasazuki T (1991) p53 gene mutations in colorectal tumors from patients with familial polyposis coli. *Cancer Research* **51** 2874–2878

Silverberg E, Boring CE and Squires TS (1990) Cancer statistics, 1990. *CA* **40** 9–26

Solomon E, Voss R, Hall V *et al* (1987) Chromosome 5 allele loss in human colorectal carcinomas. *Nature* **328** 616–619

Stanbridge EJ and Cavenee WK (1989) Heritable cancer and tumor suppressor genes: a tentative connection, In: Weinberg RA (ed). *Oncogenes and the Molecular Origins of Cancer*, pp 281–306, Cold Spring Harbor Laboratory Press, Cold Spring Harbor, New York

Stewart J, Evan G, Watson J and Wikora K (1986) Detection of the c-*myc* oncogene product in colonic polyps and carcinomas. *British Journal of Cancer* **53** 1–6

Tanaka K, Oshimura M, Kikuchi R, Seki M, Hayashi T and Miyaki M (1991) Suppression of tumorigenicity in human colon carcinoma cells by introduction of normal chromosome 5 or 18. *Nature* **349** 340–342

Utsunomiya J and Lynch HT (eds) (1990) *Hereditary Colorectal Cancer*, Springer-Verlag, New York

Vogelstein B, Fearon ER, Hamilton SR *et al* (1988) Genetic alterations during colorectal-tumor development. *New England Journal of Medicine* **319** 525–532

Vogelstein B (1990) A deadly inheritance. *Nature* **348** 681–682

Vogelstein B, Fearon ER, Kern SE *et al* (1989) Allelotype of colorectal carcinomas. *Science* **244** 207–211

Weinberg RA (1989) Oncogenes, antioncogenes, and the molecular bases of multistep carcinogenesis. *Cancer Research* **49** 3713–3721

The author is responsible for the accuracy of the references.

Friend Virus Induced Murine Erythroleukaemia: The $p53$ Locus

P JOHNSON • S BENCHIMOL

Ontario Cancer Institute and Department of Medical Biophysics, University of Toronto, 500 Sherbourne Street, Toronto, Ontario M4X 1K9, Canada

INTRODUCTION: FRIEND VIRUS INDUCED ERYTHROLEUKAEMIA

The original strain of Friend leukaemia virus, isolated in 1957, induced a rapid erythroleukaemia associated with anaemia in susceptible mice (Friend, 1957). Strains derived from the original isolate fell into two classes depending on whether they induced a similar erythroleukaemia associated with anaemia (FV-A strains) or one that was associated with polycythaemia (FV-P strains). Both FV-A and FV-P are viral complexes consisting of a replication defective spleen focus forming virus ($SFFV_A$ and $SFFV_P$, respectively) and a replication competent helper Friend murine leukaemia virus (Fr-MLV) (Friend and Pogo, 1985). There is good evidence that the SFFV genome, and in particular the unique envelope glycoprotein encoded by SFFV, is required for the pathological properties of the virus complex (Ruscetti and Wolff, 1984). The role of Fr-MLV may not be entirely ancillary, since infection of newborn Balb/c or Swiss mice by Fr-MLV alone induces splenomegaly, anaemia and erythroleukaemia (Troxler and Scolnick, 1978).

Friend virus induced erythroleukaemia is regarded as a multistage disease (Tambourin *et al*, 1979). Infection of mice with FV-A or FV-P leads to a rapid, polyclonal proliferation of hyperbasophilic proerythroblast like cells in the spleen. An increase in the number of erythroid progenitor cells is detected by in vitro colony assays. Whereas haematopoietic cells from normal mice and from FV-A infected mice form erythroid colonies in culture only in the presence of erythropoietin (EPO), cells from FV-P infected mice give rise to erythroid colonies in the absence of exogenously added EPO. Infected spleen cells in the initial stage of the disease have limited self renewal capacity, are not tumorigenic and cannot be established as permanent cell lines in culture. Late after infection (3–4 weeks), however, truly malignant cells are detected in the spleen. These cells, which arise from one or few malignant precursors, are tumorigenic upon transplantation into recipient mice, form macroscopic colonies in methylcellulose culture medium and give rise to established erythroleukaemia cell lines in culture (Mager et al, 1981a). FV-P transformed cells can be identified, moreover, by their ability to form spleen colonies in genetically anaemic Sl/Sl^d mice (Mager et al, 1980). It is not clear whether the proerythroblast like cells present early after infection give rise, through a process of clonal evolution, to the malignant cells present late in the disease or whether the two populations of cells arise independently from different infected target cells (Mager et al, 1981b). Although viral infection is necessary to initiate the erythroleukaemia, it appears to be insufficient for the full development of the disease. The latency period and the clonality of the disease indicate an involvement of cellular genetic changes. This chapter considers certain cellular genes, primarily the p53 tumour suppressor gene, whose aberrant expression contributes to Friend erythroleukaemia. The involvement of two other cellular genes, Spi-1/PU.1 and Fli 1, and of the SFFV envelope (env) gene in this disease will be also be discussed.

GENETIC EVENTS IN FRIEND DISEASE

SFFV env Gene

SFFV is believed to have arisen by recombination between Fr-MLV and endogenous viral sequences, related to mink cell focus inducing virus (MCF), present in mouse DNA (Clark and Mak, 1983). Comparison of the nucleotide sequences of SFFV$_A$ with SFFV$_P$ shows that most of the differences reside in the 3' half of the env gene (Wolff et al, 1985). The env genes of SFFV$_A$ and SFFV$_P$ encode proteins of about 55 000 daltons (gp55) that are related to MCF env sequences at their 5' ends and to Fr-MLV env sequences at their 3' ends. The SFFV env genes are essential for the erythroleukaemia induced by FV-A and FV-P (Wolff and Ruscetti, 1988; Aizawa et al, 1990). Moreover, it is this region that determines the biological and biochemical differences between the two strains (Ruscetti and Wolff, 1985). The env genes of MLVs typically encode a polyprotein precursor that is processed to generate a glycoprotein of approximately 70 000 daltons (gp70) and a non-glycosylated protein of 15 000 daltons (p15E). gp70 env-encoded proteins normally localize to the cell surface, where they reside until budding progeny virions become enveloped in host derived components from the cell membrane and viral gp70 molecules. gp70 molecules constitute the major surface component of viral particles. The SFFV *env* gene is missing sequences required for cleavage, and consequently the encoded gp55 protein contains the aminoterminal portion of gp70 covalently linked to the carboxyterminal portion of p15E. In addition, a single frameshift mutation in the carboxyterminus results in the presence of unique aminoacid residues and premature termination (Clark and Mak, 1983). gp55 encoded by SFFV$_P$ is poorly transported to the cell surface, and most of it accumulates in the endoplasmic reticulum. gp55 encoded by SFFV$_A$ cannot be detected on the cell surface.

gp55 encoded by SFFV$_P$ has been shown to bind to the erythropoietin receptor (EPO-R) (Li *et al*, 1990). The significance of this interaction was examined in an interleukin 3 (IL-3) dependent cell line that was rendered EPO dependent after transfection with EPO-R cDNA. Coexpression of the EPO-R and gp55 allowed these cells to grow autonomously in the complete absence of growth factors (Hoatlin *et al*, 1990; Li *et al*, 1990). In a separate study, superinfection of an EPO dependent, Fr-MLV induced erythroleukaemia cell with FV-P readily generated EPO independent clones (Ruscetti *et al*, 1990). Physical interaction between the EPO-R and gp55 occurred intracellularly in the endoplasmic reticulum (Yoshimura *et al*, 1990). It is therefore likely that an intracellular mitogenic interaction between gp55 and the EPO-R occurs in FV-P infected erythroid cells serving to bypass the normal requirement of erythroid cells for EPO. This view was strengthened by the recent observation that mice infected with a mixture of recombinant EPO containing retroviruses and helper MLV developed a disease characterized by splenomegaly, polycythaemia and mortality that was similar to the Friend disease induced by FV-P (Hoatlin *et al*, 1990).

Spi-1/PU.1

The occurrence of common proviral integration sites in the DNA of virus transformed cells serves to identify adjacent cellular genes that may be involved in the generation of malignant clones. The cellular *Spi-1* gene resides downstream from a common SFFV proviral integration site detected in erythroleukaemias induced by FV-P (Moreau-Gachelin *et al*, 1988), FV-A (Ben-David *et al*, 1990a) and helper free SFFV$_P$ (Paul *et al*, 1989). In normal mouse spleen, *Spi-1* mRNA is expressed at low levels. Insertion of the SFFV proviral genome results in transcriptional activation of *Spi-1*, probably through the action of the viral long terminal repeat (LTR) enhancer (Moreau-Gachelin *et al*, 1989). Cloning and sequence analysis of the 1.5-kb *Spi-1* mRNA revealed that it was identical to the macrophage and B cell specific transcription factor *PU.1* (Goebl, 1990; Klemsz *et al*, 1990; Moreau-Gachelin *et al*, 1990; Paul *et al*, 1991). The PU.1 protein binds to a purine rich sequence, 5'-GAGGAA-3' (known as a PU box), and is related to proteins belonging to the *ets* oncogene family. Constitutive overexpression of *Spi-1/PU.1* may therefore activate inappropriate expression of cellular genes that contribute to the neoplastic transformation of erythroid cells during Friend disease.

Fli-1

Fr-MLV induces a variety of haematopoietic neoplasms in mice, including lymphoma, myeloblastic leukaemia and erythroleukaemia. The type of disease is influenced by the mouse genetic background and by the age of the mouse at the time of virus inoculation. In the erythroleukaemias induced in neonatal mice by Fr-MLV alone, a distinct locus termed *Fli-1* was a frequent integration site for the virus (Ben-David *et al*, 1990a). This locus was not rearranged in FV-P or FV-A induced erythroleukaemias nor in Fr-MLV induced myeloid or lymphoid leukaemia cell lines. Aberrant expression of the *Fli-1* gene is likely to have an important role during development of erythroleukaemias induced by Fr-MLV.

p53

In an early series of experiments with Alan Bernstein and Michael Mowat, we demonstrated that the *p53* locus was a common target for mutation in Friend erythroleukaemias. In Friend cell lines (FCLs) derived from the spleens of mice infected with FV-P, FV-A or Fr-MLV alone, several failed to express any detectable p53 protein as a result of gross structural alterations in the *p53* gene. Some clones with rearranged *p53* alleles expressed truncated *p53* related polypeptides, whereas other clones without DNA rearrangement synthesized very high levels of p53 protein with an altered antigenic phenotype. Rearrangement of one *p53* allele was frequently accompanied by loss of the remaining wild type allele. Importantly, we demonstrated that the rearrangements and loss of heterozygosity occurred in vivo. Thus, it appeared that loss of normal *p53* expression conferred a selective advantage on infected cells during the natural progression of Friend erythroleukaemia in mice (Mowat *et al*, 1985; Chow *et al*, 1987).

The isolation and partial sequencing of several rearranged *p53* alleles indicated that the structural alterations resulted from internal deletions or proviral insertions (Fig. 1). Several FCLs had insertions of SFFV$_A$, SFFV$_P$ or Fr-MLV proviruses within the *p53* gene and failed to express p53 protein (Ben-David *et al*, 1988, 1990b; Hicks and Mowat, 1988). Disruption of the *p53* gene by proviral integration, followed by a reduction to homozygosity, therefore represents a frequent event in the generation of malignant Friend cell clones. Internal deletions occurred less frequently. In two of three cell lines that sustained internal deletions of the *p53* gene, the deleted alleles retained the capacity to encode truncated and presumably functionally compromised polypeptides (Rovinski *et al*, 1987; Ben-David *et al*, 1988; Munroe *et al*, 1988). The deleted allele in DA22-1 cells, for example, was missing all of exon 7, a region that encodes a highly conserved domain of the p53 protein (Soussi *et al*, 1990).

Rearranged *p53* alleles were also detected by Aizawa *et al* (1990) in a small number of primary erythroleukaemic spleens from transgenic mice harbouring the entire SFFV$_P$ proviral genome. These erythroleukaemias arose in the absence of helper virus and in the absence of viral production. *p53* gene rearrangements were more frequently found in transplanted tumours and cell lines

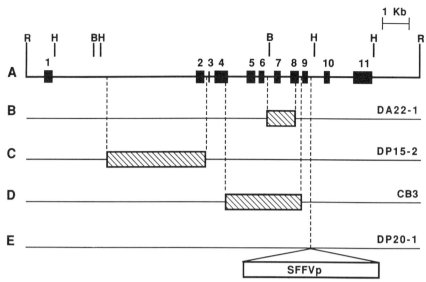

Fig. 1. Physical map of the mouse *p53* gene (A) showing the approximate positions of exons (depicted as black boxes) and cleavage sites for the restriction enzymes *Eco*RI (R), *Bam*HI (B) and *Hin*dlll (H). Panels B, C and D show the approximate positions and extent of the *p53* gene deletions in cell lines DA22-1, DP15-2 and CB3, respectively. Panel E shows the approximate position of the SFFV$_p$ insertion in cell line DP20-1. DA22-1 and DP15-2 encode truncated polypeptides of 46 000 and 44 000 daltons, respectively (adapted from Benchimol *et al*, 1989b)

derived from the primary erythroleukaemic spleens, suggesting that they may be associated with the later stages of erythroleukaemia. In a separate study, Dreyfus *et al* (1990) detected *p53* gene rearrangements in transplanted tumours or cell lines derived from the erythroleukaemic spleens of mice infected with Fr-MLV. Of 17 erythroid tumours, 6 showed *p53* gene rearrangements. In contrast, no rearrangement of the *p53* gene was found in 60 Fr-MLV induced lymphoid or myeloid leukaemias.

As noted above, numerous erythroleukaemia cell lines with an intact *p53* gene express p53 protein (Ruscetti and Scolnick, 1983; Shen *et al*, 1983; Mowat *et al*, 1985; Khochbin *et al*, 1988). However, five out of six independently derived *p53* producing Friend cell clones were shown to synthesize an immunologically aberrant form of p53 protein that was not recognized by PAb246 monoclonal antibodies (Munroe *et al*, 1990). These antibodies bind to a conformation sensitive epitope on p53 protein molecules (Milner and Cook, 1986; Yewdell *et al*, 1986). The possibility that these cells were expressing a mutant form of p53 was confirmed by sequence analysis of cDNA clones. Three of three cell lines examined, including the one line that expressed PAb246 positive p53 protein, contained single missense mutations in the *p53* coding sequence. Failure to detect the homologous wild type allele or its transcript in these cells indicated a loss of heterozygosity and again demonstrated the strong selection against wild type *p53* expression, even in the presence of a mutated *p53* allele, in Friend cells (Munroe *et al*, 1990).

Together, these data indicate that mutation of the *p53* gene may be necessary for the development of Friend erythroleukaemia. At least three genetic mechanisms—deletion, proviral insertion and missense mutation—target the *p53* gene in Friend cells. Recessive mutations in both *p53* alleles often abrogate expression. If the selection against wild type *p53* expression is satisfied equally by these diverse genetic mechanisms, then missense mutations in *p53* might be comparable to complete loss of *p53*, resulting in functional inactivation of the *p53* gene. These data provide strong experimental evidence that the wild type *p53* gene is a tumour suppressor gene whose expression interferes with the development of malignancy.

EXPRESSION OF EXOGENOUS *p53* ALLELES IN FRIEND CELL LINES

Introduction of *p53* Into *p53* Negative Tumour Cell Lines

Friend cell lines that fail to produce p53 protein as the result of mutations in the *p53* gene provide an attractive experimental model to examine the consequences of restoring *p53* expression after gene transfer. DP16-1 cells were chosen as recipients since both *p53* alleles are rearranged and endogenous *p53* is not expressed. *p53* expression vectors encoding mutant or wild type *p53* were transferred into these cells by electroporation along with a plasmid encoding a dominant selectable marker (pSV2neo encoding resistances to the analogue G418, or pHMR272, encoding resistance to hygromycin). Stable, drug resistant clones were picked from methylcellulose culture 2 weeks after gene transfer and expanded in suspension culture for analysis of *p53* expression. The results from this study were published previously (Johnson *et al*, 1991) and are summarized in Table 1.

pMR53 contains a mutant *p53* allele with a G to C transversion at codon 193 (Munroe *et al*, 1990) that changes an arginine to proline. This mutant allele was isolated from a *p53* positive FCL, CB-7 (Mowat *et al*, 1985), and was previously shown to immortalize early passage rat embryo fibroblasts (REFs)

TABLE 1. Exogenous *p53* expression in Friend cell lines

| Cell line | Plasmid | No of positive clones/No of clones examined | |
		DNA	protein
DP16-1	pEW53-6 (wt gene)	3/15	0/3
	pECM53 (wt cDNA)	0/9	
	p11-4[a] (wt cDNA)	0/5	
	pMR53 (mutant gene)	18/18	18/18
DP16-1 1.7	pβw (wt cDNA)	6/6[b]	0/6
DP15-1	pEW53-6	4/11	0/4

[a]11-4 (Tan *et al*, 1986); all other plasmid vectors are described in Johnson *et al* (1991)
[b]pβw carries the mouse wild type *p53* cDNA and sequences conferring resistance to G418; 3/6 clones had lost the *p53* cDNA but retained G418 resistance coding sequence

and to cooperate with activated *ras* in REF transformation assays, presumably through a dominant negative mechanism (Rovinski and Benchimol, 1988; Munroe *et al*, 1990). Examination of 18 independent clones resulting from electroporation with this mutant *p53* gene showed that all expressed abundant levels of the exogenous mutant p53 protein.

In contrast, wild type *p53* expression was not detected in any clones arising after transfer of wild type *p53* expression vectors. Vectors encoding either a *p53* cDNA under the transcriptional control of the SV40 early gene promoter/enhancer or a gene copy of *p53* were used. Southern blot analysis showed that the frequency of integration of the exogenous wild type *p53* sequences was low compared with exogenous mutant *p53* DNA (Table 1). Of 29 clones examined, only 3 had integrated the exogenous wild type *p53* DNA, and none of these expressed p53 protein. RNA was available from two of these clones, and northern analysis revealed that one clone expressed a truncated *p53* related transcript, whereas the other expressed no *p53* mRNA (Johnson *et al*, 1991). Thus, DP16-1 Friend cells supported long term expression of mutant *p53* but not wild type *p53*. Surprisingly, electroporation of the wild type *p53* sequence together with the drug resistance plasmid did not cause a significant reduction in the number of drug resistant colonies compared with the drug resistance plasmid alone. DP16-1 cells may therefore be able to eliminate genes detrimental to their growth.

Similar studies were performed using different *p53* negative tumour cell lines as recipients. When SKOV-3 (human ovarian adenocarcinoma) (Johnson *et al*, 1991) or Saos-2 (human osteosarcoma) (Diller *et al*, 1990) cells were cotransfected with wild type *p53* cDNA and a drug resistance plasmid, there was a marked reduction in the number of colonies compared with controls transfected with mutant *p53* DNA or with the drug resistance plasmid alone. Thus, constitutive overexpression of wild type *p53* inhibited the clonogenic growth of *p53* negative cells. This may be a reflection of the high copy number of exogenous plasmids that commonly integrate as tandem repeats in cells transfected by calcium phosphate coprecipitation. To address this concern, Chen *et al* (1990) used recombinant retroviruses to introduce a single copy of mutant or wild type *p53* into Saos-2 cells. Integration of a single copy of wild type *p53* cDNA led to stable expression of wild type *p53* in the resulting clones, with no apparent reduction in the number of colonies compared with controls infected with a retroviral vector encoding mutant *p53*. Cells expressing wild type *p53* became larger, flatter and less refractile and had prolonged doubling times in culture. These cells also lost their ability to grow in soft agar and to form tumours in nude mice.

Dominance of Wild Type Over Mutant *p53* Alleles

To explain the transforming activity of mutant *p53* alleles in REF transformation assays, it has been proposed that mutant p53 protein may act in *trans* to render the endogenous rat wild type *p53* functionally inactive either through the formation of mutant/wild type *p53* heteroligomers or by competitive inhibition of the normal interactions between wild type p53 protein and its targets in the cell (Sturzbecher *et al*, 1988; Baker *et al*, 1989; Benchimol *et al*, 1989a; Eliyahu *et al*, 1989; Finlay *et al*, 1989; Lavigueur *et al*, 1989). We examined whether the expression of endogenous mutant *p53* in FCLs might confer tolerance to wild type *p53* expression. Two FCLs were used as recipients for transfer of wild type *p53*. DP16-1 1.7 cells were derived from DP16-1 cells after transfer of a mutated *p53* allele in pMR53; these cells express high levels of mutant p53 protein. DP15-1 cells express an endogenous, aberrant p53 polypeptide suspected of being the product of a mutated *p53* allele (Munroe *et al*, 1990). The results summarized in Table 1 indicate that wild type *p53* expression was not detected in either cell line. The inability of DP16-1 1.7 and DP15-1 cells to support long term expression of a wild type *p53* gene in the presence of a mutated *p53* allele indicates that wild type *p53* alleles are dominant over mutated *p53* alleles and reflects the situation that arises during Friend cell transformation. In all FCLs that have sustained a mutation in the *p53* coding sequence and consequently express an aberrant *p53* polypeptide, there is loss of the corresponding normal allele.

The dominant, growth suppressing phenotype of wild type *p53* has also been observed in other studies. Human colorectal carcinoma cell lines SW837 and SW480 (Baker *et al*, 1990) and the osteosarcoma cell lines KHOS-240S (Diller *et al*, 1990), which express endogenous mutant p53 protein, were unable to support long term expression of wild type p53 protein. Overexpression of wild type p53 protein relative to mutant protein may have accounted for this effect. However, Saos-2 cells, containing one integrated copy of wild type *p53* and one integrated copy of mutant *p53* after recombinant retrovirus infection, had a suppressed tumorigenic phenotype indistinguishable from clones expressing only wild type p53. The increased stability of the mutant p53 protein in these cells resulted in steady state levels that were about tenfold higher than those of wild type p53 (Chen *et al*, 1990). Taken together, these gene transfer experiments demonstrate the potency of the wild type p53 protein, even in the presence of mutant p53 polypeptides, in suppressing the growth and tumorigenic phenotype of transformed cells.

Several studies reported that overexpression of a transfected wild type *p53* gene in transformed cells induced growth arrest through a block in cell cycle progression at the G_1/S boundary (Baker *et al*, 1990; Diller *et al*, 1990; Mercer *et al*, 1990a,b; Michalovitz *et al*, 1990; Martinez *et al*, 1991). Studies with REFs transformed by *ras* and a temperature sensitive mutant *p53* allele supported this conclusion (Michalovitz *et al*, 1990; Martinez *et al*, 1991). At the non-permissive temperature of 32.5°C, the mutant p53 protein underwent a conformational change and behaved as wild type, inducing growth arrest in G_1. The overexpression of wild type p53 protein in all of these experiments needs to be critically considered. It is important to note that low level expression of wild type p53 resulting from the introduction of a single copy of *p53* cDNA into Saos-2 cells did not restrict growth (Chen *et al*, 1990). It is also possible that different transformed cell lines respond differently to p53 expression; some cells may be more sensitive to the growth suppressing effect of wild type p53.

Gain of Function: *p53* as a Dominant Oncogene?

The transforming activity of mutant *p53* alleles differs widely for the different mutants. One explanation is that only a subset of all mutations are dominant negatives and hence transforming in rat embryo fibroblasts. However, it is also possible that highly transforming mutant *p53* alleles contribute to transformation through a mechanism that is more elaborate than the removal or inactivation of endogenous wild type p53 protein. There is accumulating experimental evidence that some mutant alleles of *p53* contain "gain of function" mutations that have a positive role in transformation. Although these alleles may have suffered mutations that abrogate the tumour suppressor function of *p53*, the encoded, aberrant p53 proteins may have acquired novel, growth promoting activity. For example, expression of mutant *p53* in a *p53* negative cell line, L12, increased the tumorigenicity of these cells (Wolf *et al*, 1984; Shaulsky *et al*, 1990). Chen *et al* (1990) demonstrated that Saos-2 cells expressing a mutant human cDNA grew to higher saturation densities than the *p53* negative parental cell line. Recently, two groups have found a high proportion of in vivo mutations in the human *p53* locus at codon 249 of hepatocellular carcinoma patients from southern Africa and China. The specificity of this mutation, transversion from G to T/C, resulting in a putative change from arginine to serine, strongly suggests that inactivation of *p53* is insufficient and that the mutant protein resulting from this mutation may contribute to the development of malignancy (Bressac *et al*, 1991; Hsu *et al*, 1991). In addition, several studies have shown that transfection of certain mutant *p53* alleles increased the plating efficiencies of early passage rat embryo cells (Finlay *et al*, 1989) and of some transformed cell lines (Eliyahu *et al*, 1985; Finlay *et al*, 1989; Johnson *et al*, 1991). Since REFs express endogenous p53 protein, however, these experiments do not distinguish between dominant negative mutations and gain of function mutations.

We wished to examine the possibility that the mutant p53 protein encoded by pMR53 might possess growth promoting activity that was independent of any putative dominant negative activity. The mutant *p53* allele was introduced and expressed, together with a drug resistance plasmid, in a *p53* negative FCL, DP16-1. In such a system, where there is no endogenous wild type p53 protein, the dominant negative properties of the exogenous mutant *p53* are irrelevant. Five independent clones expressing mutant *p53* and five clones electroporated with the drug resistance plasmid alone were compared for their plating efficiency in methylcellulose and tumorigenicity in syngeneic animals. The *p53* positive and *p53* negative clones had similar plating efficiencies under different growth conditions. There appeared to be no growth advantage in methylcellulose for clones that were expressing the mutant *p53* allele (Table

2). The tumorigenicity of different clones varied considerably and was not correlated with mutant *p53* expression (Fig. 2). This finding is in contrast to the previously described work (Wolf *et al*, 1984; Shaulsky *et al*, 1990) demonstrating a *p53* mediated enhancement of tumorigenicity in L12 cells. This difference may arise from differences in the cell lines or *p53* alleles used in the various experiments.

SUMMARY

The development of Friend virus induced murine erythroleukaemia is associated with specific genetic events. One of these events is loss of wild type *p53* expression, which can occur by internal deletion or proviral insertion in the *p53* gene and by single point mutations in the coding sequence. In all cases, the corresponding wild type allele is absent. The high frequency of observed *p53* mutations strongly suggests that inactivation of *p53* may be an obligatory step in the development of Friend disease. Further evidence that abrogation of normal *p53* expression contributes to the development of malignant clones was provided by in vitro reconstitution experiments in Friend cell lines: whereas exogenous mutant *p53* was stably expressed in *p53* negative FCLs, long term wild type *p53* expression was not detected.

Friend erythroleukaemia arises as a late consequence of infection of susceptible mice with Friend virus. In addition to *p53* gene mutations, proviral insertions occur frequently adjacent to one of two cellular genes, *Spi-1/PU.1* or *Fli-1*. Aberrant expression of these genes may therefore be involved in virus induced erythroleukaemia. Interaction of SFFV *env* gp55 with the EPO-R also

TABLE 2. Plating efficiency of *p53* negative and *p53* positive clones of DP16-1

Clone	p53 protein	Plating efficiency (%)		
		αMEM +10% FCS[b]	Opti[c] +5% FCS	Opti +2% FCS
1	−	6.7	3.7	2.8
2	−	10.7	12.9	7.3
3	−	7.2	11.2	8.6
4	−	12.0	nd	nd
5	−	10.7	8.7	11.5
6	+	10.4	6.0	4.8
7	+	23.7	14.5	6.6
8	+	9.9	10.1	4.8
9	+	12.6	11.3	11.0
10	+	5.4	nd	nd

nd - not done
[a]Average of two dishes
[b]FCS, fetal calf serum
[c]GIBCO, Inc.

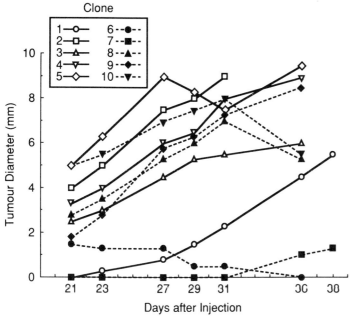

Fig. 2. Tumorigenic growth of DP16-1 derived clones expressing resistance to G418 only (clones 1–5; solid lines, open symbols) or expressing mutant *p53* encoded on pMR53 and resistance to G418 (clones 6–10; dashed lines, closed symbols)

appears to be important in providing a mitogenic signal to infected cells. The order in which these events occur and whether the order is relevant to the progression of the disease are not known. Investigation of the stepwise appearance of these events could provide information on the possible interactions of the gene products involved.

Abrogation of normal *p53* expression is not restricted to Friend erythroleukaemia: the observation of *p53* mutations and allele loss in human breast, lung, colon and hepatocellular carcinomas and in leukaemia suggests that mutation of *p53* may be the most common genetic abnormality detected in human cancer (reviewed in this issue).

Studies of *p53* expression in FCLs provided an early indication that *p53* was a tumour suppressor gene. Further studies of the mechanisms by which wild type and mutant *p53* affect the growth of *p53* negative FCLs may reveal important biochemical properties of *p53* in relation to cell cycle control and differentiation of erythroid cells.

Acknowledgements

This work was supported by grants from the Medical Research Council of Canada and the National Cancer Institute of Canada. We thank Bob Kuba for help with the tumorigenicity studies and Irene Ng for help with preparation of the manuscript.

References

Aizawa S, Suda Y, Furuta Y et al (1990) Env-derived gp55 gene of Friend spleen focus-forming virus specifically induces neoplastic proliferation of erythroid progenitor cells. EMBO Journal 9 2107–2116

Baker SJ, Fearon ER, Nigro JM et al (1989) Chromosome 17 deletions and p53 gene mutations in colorectal carcinomas. Science 244 217–221

Baker SJ, Markowitz S, Fearon ER, Willson JKV and Vogelstein B (1990) Suppression of human colorectal carcinoma cell growth by wild-type p53. Science 249 912–915

Benchimol S, Munroe DG, Peacock J, Gray D and Smith LJ (1989a) Abnormalities in structure and expression of the p53 gene in leukemia. Cancer Cells 7 121–125

Benchimol S, Munroe DG, Rovinski B, Ben-David Y and Bernstein A (1989b) Inactivation of the cellular p53 gene in Friend virus-transformed erythroleukemia cell lines, In: Lother H, Dernick R and Ostertag W (eds). Vectors as Tools for the Study of Normal and Abnormal Growth and Differentiation, pp 409–417, NATO ASI Series, Vol. H34, Springer-Verlag, Berlin

Ben-David Y, Prideaux VR, Chow V, Benchimol S and Bernstein A (1988) Inactivation of the p53 oncogene by internal deletion or retroviral integration in erythroleukemic cell lines induced by Friend leukemia virus. Oncogene 3 179–185

Ben-David Y, Giddens EB and Bernstein A (1990a) Identification and mapping of a common proviral integration site Fli-1 in erythroleukemia cells induced by Friend murine leukemia virus. Proceedings of the National Academy of Sciences of the USA 87 1332–1336

Ben-David Y, Lavigueur A, Cheong GY and Bernstein A (1990b) Insertional inactivation of the p53 gene during Friend leukemia: a new strategy for identifying tumor suppressor genes. New Biologist 2 1015–1023

Bienz B, Zakut-Houri R, Givol D and Oren M (1984) Analysis of the gene coding for the murine cellular tumour antigen p53. EMBO Journal 3 2179–2183

Bressac B, Kew M, Wands J and Ozturk M (1991) Selective G to T mutations of p53 gene in hepatocellular carcinoma from southern Africa. Nature 350 429–431

Chen P-L, Chen Y, Bookstein R and Lee W-H (1990) Genetic mechanisms of tumor suppression by the human p53 gene. Science 250 1576–1580

Chow V, Ben-David Y, Bernstein A, Benchimol S and Mowat M (1987) Multistage friend erythroleukemia: independent origin of tumor clones with normal or rearranged p53 cellular oncogenes. Journal of Virology 61 2777–2781

Clark SP and Mak TW (1983) Complete nucleotide sequence of an infectious clone of Friend spleen focus-forming provirus: gp55 is an envelope fusion glycoprotein. Proceedings of the National Academy of Sciences of the USA 80 5037–5041

Diller L, Kassel J, Nelson CE et al (1990) p53 functions as a cell cycle control protein in osteosarcomas. Molecular and Cellular Biology 10 5772–5781

Dreyfus F, Sola B, Fichelson S et al (1990) Rearrangements of the Pim-1, c-myc, and p53 genes in Friend helper virus-induced mouse erythroleukemias. Leukemia 4 590–594

Eliyahu D, Michalovitz D and Oren M (1985) Overproduction of p53 antigen makes established cells highly tumorigenic. Nature 316 158–160

Eliyahu D, Michalovitz D, Eliyahu S, Pinhasi-Kimhi O and Oren M (1989) Wild-type p53 can inhibit oncogene-mediated focus formation. Proceedings of the National Academy of Sciences of the USA 86 8763–8767

Finlay CA, Hinds PW and Levine AJ (1989) The p53 proto-oncogene can act as a suppressor of transformation. Cell 57 1083–1093

Friend C (1957) Cell-free transmission in adult Swiss mice of a disease having the character of a leukemia. Journal of Experimental Medicine 105 307–318

Friend C and Pogo BGT (1985) The molecular pathology of Friend erythroleukemia virus strains: an overview. Biochimica et Biophysica Acta 780 181–195

Goebl MG (1990) The PU.1 transcription factor is the product of the putative oncogene Spi-1. Cell 61 1165–1166

Hicks G and Mowat M (1988) Integration of Friend murine leukemia virus into both alleles of the p53 oncogene in an erythroleukemic cell line. *Journal of Virology* **62** 4752–4755

Hoatlin ME, Kozak SL, Lilly F, Chakraborti A, Kozak CA and Kabat D (1990) Activation of erythropoietin receptors by Friend viral gp55 and by erythropoietin and down-modulation by the murine Fv-2r resistance gene. *Proceedings of the National Academy of Sciences of the USA* **87** 9985–9989

Hsu IC, Metcalf RA, Sun T, Welsh JA, Wang NJ and Harris CC (1991) Mutational hotspot in the p53 gene in human hepatocellular carcinomas. *Nature* **350** 427–428

Johnson P, Gray D, Mowat M and Benchimol S (1991) Expression of wild-type p53 is not compatible with continued growth of p53-negative tumor cells. *Molecular and Cellular Biology* **11** 1–11

Khochbin S, Chabanas A and Lawrence JJ (1988) Early events in murine erythroleukemia cells induced to differentiate: variation of the cell cycle parameters in relation to p53 accumulation. *Experimental Cell Research* **179** 565–574

Klemsz MJ, McKercher SR, Celada A, Van Beveren C and Maki RA (1990) The macrophage and B cell-specific transcription factor PU.1 is related to the ets oncogene. *Cell* **61** 113–124

Lavigueur A, Maltby V, Mock D, Rossant J, Pawson T and Bernstein A (1989) High incidence of lung, bone, and lymphoid tumors in transgenic mice overexpressing mutant alleles of the p53 oncogene. *Molecular and Cellular Biology* **9** 3982–3991

Li JP, D'Andrea AD, Lodish HF and Baltimore D (1990) Activation of cell growth by binding of Friend spleen focus-forming virus gp55 glycoprotein to the erythropoietin receptor. *Nature* **343** 762–764

Mager D, Mak TW and Bernstein A (1980) Friend leukemia virus-transformed cells, unlike normal stem cells, form spleen colonies in Sl/Sld mice. *Nature* **288** 592–594

Mager DL, Mak TW and Bernstein A (1981a) Quantitative colony method for tumorigenic cells transformed by two distinct strains of Friend leukemia virus. *Proceedings of the National Academy of Sciences of the USA* **78** 1703–1707

Mager D, MacDonald ME, Robson IB, Mak TW and Bernstein A (1981b) Clonal analysis of the late stages of erythroleukemia induced by two distinct strains of Friend leukemia virus. *Molecular and Cellular Biology* **1** 721–730

Martinez J, Georgoff I, Martinez J and Levine AJ (1991) Cellular localization and cell cycle regulation by a temperature-sensitive p53 protein. *Genes and Development* **5** 151–159

Mercer WE, Shields MT, Amin M *et al* (1990a) Negative growth regulation in a glioblastoma tumor cell line that conditionally expresses human wild-type p53. *Proceedings of the National Academy of Sciences of the USA* **87** 6166–6170

Mercer WE, Amin M, Sauve GJ, Appella E, Ullrich SJ and Romano JW (1990b) Wild type human p53 is antiproliferative in SV40-transformed hamster cells. *Oncogene* **5** 973–980

Michalovitz D, Halevy O and Oren M (1990) Conditional inhibition of transformation and of cell proliferation by a temperature-sensitive mutant of p53. *Cell* **62** 671–680

Milner J and Cook A (1986) The cellular tumour antigen p53: evidence for transformation-related, immunological variants of p53. *Virology* **154** 21–30

Moreau-Gachelin F, Tavitian A and Tambourin P (1988) *Spi-1* is a putative oncogene in virally induced murine erythroleukaemias. *Nature* **331** 277–280

Moreau-Gachelin F, Ray D, Mattei MG, Tambourin P and Tavitian A (1989) The putative oncogene *Spi-1*: murine chromosomal localization and transcriptional activation in murine acute erythroleukemias. *Oncogene* **4** 1449–1456

Moreau-Gachelin F, Ray D, Tambourin P *et al* (1990) The PU.1 transcription factor is the product of the putative oncogene *Spi-1*. *Cell* **61** 1166

Mowat M, Cheng A, Kimura N, Bernstein A and Benchimol S (1985) Rearrangements of the cellular p53 gene in erythroleukemic cells transformed by Friend virus. *Nature* **314** 633–636

Munroe DG, Rovinski B, Bernstein A and Benchimol S (1988) Loss of a highly conserved domain on p53 as a result of gene deletion during Friend virus- induced erythroleukemia.

Oncogene **2** 621–624

Munroe DG, Peacock JW and Benchimol S (1990) Inactivation of the cellular p53 gene is a common feature of Friend virus-induced erythroleukemia: relationship of inactivation to dominant transforming alleles. *Molecular and Cellular Biology* **10** 3307–3313

Paul R, Schuetze S, Kozak SL and Kabat D (1989) A common site for immortalizing proviral integrations in Friend erythroleukemia: molecular cloning and characterization. *Journal of Virology* **63** 4958–4961

Paul R, Schuetze S, Kozak SL, Kozak CA and Kabat D (1991) The Sfpi-1 proviral integration site of Friend erythroleukemia encodes the ets-related transcription factor Pu1. *Journal of Virology* **65** 464–467

Rovinski B and Benchimol S (1988) Immortalization of rat embryo fibroblasts by the cellular p53 oncogene. *Oncogene* **2** 445–452

Rovinski B, Munroe D, Peacock J, Mowat M, Bernstein A and Benchimol S (1987) Deletion of 5′-coding sequences of the cellular p53 gene in mouse erythroleukemia: a novel mechanism of oncogene regulation. *Molecular and Cellular Biology* **7** 847–853

Ruscetti SK and Scolnick EM (1983) Expression of a transformation-related protein (p53) in the malignant stage of Friend virus-induced diseases. *Journal of Virology* **46** 1022–1026

Ruscetti S and Wolff L (1984) Spleen focus-forming virus: relationship of an altered envelope gene to the development of a rapid erythroleukemia. *Current Topics in Microbiology and Immunology* **112** 21–44

Ruscetti S and Wolff L (1985) Biological and biochemical differences between variants of spleen focus-forming virus can be localized to a region containing the 3′ end of the envelope gene. *Journal of Virology* **56** 717–722

Ruscetti SK, Janesch NJ, Chakraborti A, Sawyer ST and Hankins WD (1990) Friend spleen focus-forming virus induces factor independence in an erythropoietin-dependent erythroleukemia cell line. *Journal of Virology* **63** 1057–1062

Shaulsky G, Goldfinger N, Ben-Ze'ev A and Rotter V (1990) Nuclear accumulation of p53 protein is mediated by several nuclear localization signals and plays a role in tumorigenesis. *Molecular and Cellular Biology* **10** 6565–6577

Shen D-W, Real FX, DeLeo AB, Old LJ, Marks PA and Rifkind RA (1983) Protein p53 and inducer-mediated erythroleukemia cell commitment to terminal cell division. *Proceedings of the National Academy of Sciences, USA* **80** 5919–5922

Soussi T, de Fromentel CC and May P (1990) Structural aspects of the p53 protein in relation to gene evolution. *Oncogene* **5** 945–952

Sturzbecher HW, Addison C and Jenkins JR (1988) Characterization of mutant p53-hsp72/73 protein-protein complexes by transient expression in monkey COS cells. *Molecular and Cellular Biology* **8** 3740–3747

Tambourin PE, Wendling F, Jasmin C and Smadja-Joffe F (1979) The physiopathology of Friend leukemia. *Leukemia Research* **3** 117–129

Tan T-H, Wallis J and Levine AJ (1986) Identification of the p53 protein domain involved in formation of the simian virus 40 large T-antigen-p53 protein complex. *Journal of Virology* **59** 574–583

Troxler DH and Scolnick EM (1978) Rapid leukemia induced by cloned strain of replicating murine type-C virus: association with induction of xenotropic-related RNA sequences contained in spleen focus-forming virus. *Virology* **85** 17–27

Wolf D, Harris N and Rotter V (1984) Reconstitution of p53 expression in a nonproducer Ab-MuLV-transformed cell line by transfection of a functional p53 gene. *Cell* **38** 119–126

Wolff L and Ruscetti S (1988) The spleen focus-forming virus (SFFV) envelope gene, when introduced into mice in the absence of other SFFV genes, induces acute erythroleukemia. *Journal of Virology* **62** 2158–2163

Wolff L, Kaminchik J, Hankins WD and Ruscetti SK (1985) Sequence comparisons of the anemia- and polycythemia-inducing strains of Friend spleen focus-forming virus. *Journal of Virology* **53** 570–578

Yewdell JW, Gannon JV and Lane DP (1986) Monoclonal antibody analysis of p53 expression in normal and transformed cells. *Journal of Virology* **59** 444–452

Yoshimura A, D'Andrea AD and Lodish HF (1990) Friend spleen focus-forming virus glycoprotein gp55 interacts with the erythropoietin receptor in the endoplastic reticulum and affects receptor metabolism. *Proceedings of the National Academy of Sciences of the USA* **87** 4139–4143

The authors are responsible for the accuracy of the references.

Functional Analysis of the Retinoblastoma Gene Product and of RB-SV40 T Antigen Complexes

DAVID M LIVINGSTON

Dana-Farber Cancer Institute and Harvard Medical School, Boston, Massachusetts 02115

Introduction
SV40 T antigen, a multifunctional protein, binds to RB
T binds selectively to un(der)phosphorylated RB
RB phosphorylation is cell cycle dependent
RB structure-function relationships
Summary

INTRODUCTION

Three different DNA tumour viral oncoproteins are now known to form stable complexes with the product of the retinoblastoma (RB) susceptibility locus (DeCaprio *et al*, 1988; Whyte *et al*, 1988; Dyson *et al*, 1989), a molecule endowed with the ability to contribute to cellular growth control. They are: papovavirus T antigen (T), adenovirus E1A and the E7 product of the transforming strains of human papillomavirus. Although these three polypeptides are, in large part, wholly different molecules, they do share at least one small, colinear segment of high homology, and this segment is in significant measure responsible for RB complex formation. Moreover, this is a critical region in all three proteins for executing certain steps necessary for cellular transformation (Hu *et al*, 1990; Huang *et al*, 1990; Kaelin *et al*, 1990, 1991). Indeed, an analysis of the effects of mutants in this region shows a strong positive correlation between the ability of these three proteins to serve their transforming function and to bind to RB, suggesting in each case that the viral protein probably suppresses one or more aspects of the growth suppression function(s) of RB. From this set of clues, new insights have arisen into how RB functions, at least generically. In this chapter, I will try to review the evidence that now links viral protein RB binding to a possible cell cycle control function for RB and, where possible, attempt to look beyond the existing data to a view of how RB functions biochemically.

Cancer Surveys Volume 12: *Tumour Suppressor Genes, the Cell Cycle and Cancer*
© 1992 Imperial Cancer Research Fund. 0-87969-369-X/92. $3.00 + .00

SV40 T ANTIGEN, A MULTIFUNCTIONAL PROTEIN, BINDS TO RB

Following the observation by E Harlow that E1A forms a complex with RB (Whyte *et al*, 1988), a protein then strongly suspected of having growth suppression properties in mammalian cells, we asked a similar question of SV40 T antigen. This 708 aminoacid protein can perform all of the acts needed to bring a primary or untransformed immortal cell to a transformed state in tissue culture. Moreover, it shares a region of approximately ten aminoacids (aa 105–114) of clear homology with an E1A region of similar size, devoted both to the maintenance of tranforming function and to RB binding (Figge *et al*, 1988). Knowing these facts, we asked whether complexes could be detected by coimmunoprecipitation and detected them in a variety of cell species—both stably transformed and acutely transfected by T encoding plasmids (DeCaprio *et al*, 1988). Study of mutants of the 105–114 region, most of which were non-transforming, showed that the non-transforming mutants were uniformly noted to be defective in RB binding, whereas mutants that were non-defective or partially defective in transformation were non-defective or partially defective in RB binding. These data strongly suggested that a strong correlation existed between RB binding and the ability of T to serve its transforming function. This, in turn, clearly implied that at least one contribution of T to the viral transforming function was to modulate (? suppress) one or more aspects of the growth suppression function of RB. In short, T, like E1A, could be viewed as a mobile governor of the function of an element that (as seen from the genetics of the human RB syndrome) helps to protect a variety of cells against the acquisition of neoplastic characteristics. How might this be accomplished?

T BINDS SELECTIVELY TO UN(DER)PHOSPHORYLATED RB

Lee *et al* (1987) first noted that RB exists as a phosphorylated nuclear protein with a non-specific DNA binding function. Extensive gel electrophoretic analysis strongly suggested to us that RB migrated as a complex set of products, and from ^{32}P labelling and in vitro phosphatase treatment experiments, it became clear that the fastest migrating member of the family did not readily label, whereas the other members did (Ludlow *et al*, 1989). Indeed, from examining the effects of treatment of this set of bands with alkaline phosphatase, it became clear that the various slowly migrating members of this set were all phosphorylated and owed their abnormally slow gel migration to their being phosphorylated. Indeed, we now know that they are differentially phosphorylated. Thus, it was possible to separate, generically, phosphorylated from unphosphorylated or underphosphorylated RB.

With the ability to separate underphosphorylated and overtly phosphorylated RB species from one another, we then asked whether the state of RB phosphorylation affects T binding in any obvious way. It became clear, through a number of approaches, that T bound selectively to the un(der)phosphorylated member(s) of the family, showing no readily detectable affinity for the phosphorylated species (Ludlow *et al*, 1989). Moreover, it was clear that whether or not T was present in a given cell type, the absolute abundance of RB and the relative abundances of pRB (the unphosphorylated species) and pRB^{phos} (the phosphorylated species) were the same. Moreover, with the presence of enough T in a given cell, it was possible to show that in crude extracts of those cells, more than 95% of the ambient pRB was complexed to T, whereas no detectable pRB^{phos} was so bound. From these data, it was possible to hypothesize that the major role for T in the "life" of RB was to serve as a titrant of pRB and that it did not alter its phosphorylation or dephosphorylation.

We argued further that it was pRB and not pRB^{phos} that performed those elements of RB growth suppression that T could perturb and that phosphorylation of this species should be linked to the cancellation of those particular functions. This did not mean that pRB^{phos} was inert. Rather, it remains possible that this collection of differentially phosphorylated species performs one or more aspects of the overall RB growth suppression function that T does not perturb.

RB PHOSPHORYLATION IS CELL CYCLE DEPENDENT

Given the hypothesis that the state of RB phosphorylation determines, at least in part, which functions RB will and will not perform and the suggestion that certain RB species lack functions that others maintain, we asked whether a cell contains phosphorylated and unphosphorylated RB at the same time. Or are the two species mutually exclusive? To answer this question, cells were synchronized in multiple ways, and the result was always the same. In G_1 only pRB was present, whereas in S and G_2, only pRB^{phos} was present. The same results were obtained with primary and established cells, and similar data were noted with monkey, mink and human cells (DeCapio *et al*, 1989; Laiho *et al*, 1990). Moreover, when the first evidence of pRB phosphorylation was timed in cycling cells, we found it to occur at or near the G_1/S boundary. Thus, pRB is phosphorylated just before a cell begins to replicate its DNA.

In keeping with the lack of affinity of T for pRB^{phos}, we also noted, in an established T transformant, that pRB-T complexes exist in G_1 and disappear at G_1/S (Ludlow *et al*, 1990).

These observations can be integrated with the reasoning derived from the studies on T binding to the various RB subspecies noted above. In particular, the cell cycle findings could be interpreted to mean that a major species of RB loses one or more elements of its growth suppression function as a cell enters S. If certain aspects of RB function are lost at G_1/S, one might then argue that, since pRB is a growth suppressing element, at least part of its function is to help block exit from G_1. The model further proposes that in cells which cannot phosphorylate pRB at the end of G_1, T binding can cancel the G_1 exit blocking function of pRB. In cells that can phosphorylate pRB at G_1/S, the act of phosphorylation should have a similar effect.

The data are thus consistent with a picture of RB as a growth regulating element, operating at a key cell cycle gate in a growth suppressing manner. They also point to T as a mobile inhibitor of this function, in keeping with the long established fact that T is a potent G_1/S mitogen.

New findings support this cyclical regulation model of RB. Work carried out together with Y Furukawa and J Griffin (Furukawa *et al*, 1990) showed that certain primary human haematopoietic cells (neutrophils and monocytes), which cannot replicate under any circumstances but can be activated by growth factors to perform certain specialized functions, contain only pRB, even after activation. Moreover, they remain pure populations of G_1 arrested cells even after stimulation. By contrast, primary T cells, which represent a pure G_0 population before stimulation and can be driven into cycle by exposure to phytohaemagglutinin, contain only pRB before stimulation and accumulate pRB^{phos} after stimulation and entry into S.

More direct evidence for the aforementioned model comes from work done together with M Laiho and J Massagué (Laiho *et al*, 1990). Transforming growth factor-β (TGF-β), a known inhibitor of epithelial replication, was found to block exit of mink lung epithelial cells from G_1 late in this period of the cycle. Moreover, the block was specific to cells containing intact TGF-β receptors. In addition, cells that were in cycle before TGF-β exposure ceased cycling at a point late in G_1 and simultaneously underwent a transition from a state in which pRB^{phos} was present to one in which only unphosphorylated RB could be detected. In short, it appeared as if activation of the late G_1 RB kinase was being inhibited by action of the factor.

To determine whether the apparent inhibition of the RB kinase was merely a byproduct of cessation of replication under the influence of the hormone, several clones of mink cells transformed by T were analysed. Clones transformed, in parallel, by a plasmid encoding a transformation defective, non-RB binding T mutant were also studied. In both cases, the RB kinase was inhibited by the hormone, but only in the mutant cells was there overt inhibition of replication. Therefore, one could argue that RB might have a role in TGF-β mediated G_1 blockade. In addition, it appeared that the hormone blocked activation of the RB kinase by a route that did not depend on cessation of cell growth before the time that the kinase was normally activated. These data, then, support the hypothesis that there are at least two potential ways around the pRB mediated block at G_1/S-pRB phosphorylation and T binding.

Further analysis of the kinetics of kinase activation in the naive and the T containing cells showed that the enzyme was inhibited with the same kinetics and to the same extent (approximately 40–50%) in both lines over the first 9 hours of the experiment. Thereafter, however, in the T containing clones, no further inhibition was noted. By contrast, in the mutant clones, inhibition rose to about 90% over the next 12 hours. These data suggest that there may be at least one more RB kinase, different from that sensitive to TGF-β, which operates after the point of inactivation of the former by TGF-β. Experiments aimed at testing this possibility are in progress. If successful, one would be required to consider the phosphorylation of RB a multistep process. One might speculate from such a conclusion that different phosphorylation events have different functional effects on RB.

RB STRUCTURE-FUNCTION RELATIONSHIPS

Although the results noted above point to a cell cycle regulatory role for RB, they fail to speak to any other effects, if any, that RB might bring to bear upon mammalian cells. Moreover, they imply that RB has certain generic functions but say little about how this protein operates biochemically. In an effort to approach the question of how RB works, we began experiments aimed at determining how it binds to T/E1A/E7.

Specifically, the *RB* cDNA was subjected to deletion mutagenesis to determine whether its product contains an independent domain responsible for T and E1A binding. If such a segment exists, we wanted to know how large it was and what sequences were involved. To summarize the relevant experiments, which used in vitro transcription and translation coupled with coimmunoprecipitation as an assay, we found, as did two other laboratories (Hu *et al*, 1990; Huang *et al*, 1990), that the segment extending from residues 379 to 793 could operate as a discrete, independent unit in the binding of both viral proteins and that peptide replicas of the minimal T sequence needed to bind to RB (residues 105–114) competed effectively and specifically with T and E1A for binding to both intact RB and this subsegment. These data demonstrated that RB contains a colinear domain devoted to viral protein binding. Moreover, they indicated that T contains a short, colinear domain that can operate as an independent unit in binding to RB (Hu *et al*, 1990; Huang *et al*, 1990; Kaelin *et al*, 1990).

In vitro recombination experiments showed that this approximately 400 aminoacid domain could be fused to a foreign polypeptide and retain T/E1A binding function (Kaelin *et al*, 1991). Furthermore, they led to the development of an affinity binding method, which was used to "pan" for cellular proteins that could bind to this domain (Kaelin *et al*, 1991). We have termed this domain the RB "pocket" or simply "pocket".

There are two major reasons for searching for cellular RB binding proteins. Firstly, this domain is large and displays strong, independent binding of three viral proteins that are related primarily by their content of a homologous RB binding peptide sequence. The existence of such a sequence suggests, among various possibilities, that there are cellular proteins containing related sequences that normally bind to this RB domain. Secondly, there are now an increasing number of stable, naturally occurring, loss of function *RB* mutants that have sustained mutations in the "pocket" and cannot bind to T or

E1A (Kaelin *et al*, 1991). This further underscores the suspicion that cells contain one or more proteins that normally bind to the "pocket".

The affinity binding system alluded to above was used to search for such putative proteins (Kaelin *et al*, 1991). Specifically, the wild type RB "pocket" and various mutant derivatives were fused to *Schistosoma japonicum* glutathione transferase. The fusion proteins were purified from *Escherichia coli* transformants and bound to glutathione Sepharose beads. The complexes were then used to pan for labelled binding proteins present in various human cell extracts. The first question was whether cells produce proteins that can bind to a wild type "pocket" but not to any of a series of non-binding mutant "pockets." Secondly, do such proteins also fail to bind to a wild type "pocket" that had been preloaded with a peptide replica of the 105–114 sequence of T? A set of proteins displaying these characteristics were detected, ranging in size from approximately 150 kDa down to 36 kDa. These elements were detected in a variety of RB –/– and RB +/+ human cell lines. All appear to cosediment with the nuclear fraction. One, p68–72, appeared only in extracts of S phase cells, raising the possibility that its binding is cell cycle regulated.

The detection of these bands indicates that cells do contain proteins that share at least one property with T and E1A. Moreover, since the specificity of their binding was indistinguishable from that of the viral proteins, it seems likely that the binding of one or more of them contributes to the expression of RB biochemical and biological function. In part, one might speculate that there is cell cycle regulatory value to the interactions of at least one (p68–72) and perhaps more of these proteins with RB.

The key questions now are: what is the identity of these proteins and does RB binding affect their function, or vice versa? Are any of these proteins able to recognize a specific canonical DNA sequence? If so, are any of them transcription regulation factors? Are any proteins specifically involved in DNA replication or mitosis or already known to be involved in the regulation of certain gates in the cell cycle? Ideally, from knowledge of the functions of these species, it may be possible to define areas of biochemical function that are regulated by or that regulate RB action.

One could imagine RB having one of two generic roles. In the first, it might be viewed as having an intrinsic biochemical function not yet discovered. In that case, binding of one or more of the "pocket" binding proteins might be seen to modulate that function and the modulation is played out differently depending on which proteins are bound. In another model, the main efferent function of RB might be to bind these proteins and to modulate their function.

In either case, the existing data are consistent with certain possibilities. Differential phosphorylation of RB might determine which proteins can bind in the pocket. Or it might determine not which proteins can bind but rather how they are bound and therefore how they will perform once complexed to RB. Or it might govern how their binding will affect an as yet undiscovered intrinsic function of RB.

How RB acts cyclically is not yet understood in biochemical detail. Clearly, one clue is its cyclical phosphorylation and dephosphorylation. Ideally, with further genetic and biochemical analyses of the "pocket" and its binding proteins, new clues that will lead to a more detailed appreciation of how RB functions will come to light.

SUMMARY

The *RB* gene product has properties of a cell cycle control element. Its function is, in part, controlled by its cyclical and specific phosphorylation and dephosphorylation and effected through specific interactions with certain cellular proteins.

References

DeCaprio JA, Ludlow JW, Figge J *et al* (1988) SV40 large tumor antigen forms a specific complex with the product of the retinoblastoma susceptibility gene. *Cell* **54** 275–283

DeCaprio JA, Ludlow JW, Lynch DC *et al* (1989) The product of the retinoblastoma susceptibility gene has properties of a cell cycle regulatory element. *Cell* **58** 1085–1095

Dyson N, Howley PM, Munger K and Harlow E (1989) The human papilloma virus-16 E7 oncoprotein is able to bind to the retinoblastoma gene product. *Science* **243** 934–937

Figge J, Webster T, Smith TF and Paucha E (1988) Prediction of similar transforming regions in simian virus 40 large T, adenovirus E1A, and *myc* oncoproteins. *Journal of Virology* **62** 1814–1818

Furukawa Y, DeCaprio JA, Freedman A *et al* (1990) Expression and state of phosphorylation of the retinoblastoma susceptibility gene product in cycling and noncycling human hematopoietic cells. *Proceedings of the National Academy of Sciences of the USA* **87** 2770–2774

Hu Q, Dyson N and Harlow E (1990) The regions of the retinoblastoma protein needed for binding to adenovirus E1A or SV40 large T antigen are common sites for mutations. *EMBO Journal* **9** 1147–1155

Huang H-J S, Wang N-P, Tseng BY, Lee W-H and Lee E Y-H (1990) Two distinct and frequently mutated regions of retinoblastoma protein are required for binding to SV40 T antigen. *EMBO Journal* **9** 1815–1822

Kaelin WG Jr, Ewen ME and Livingston DM (1990) Definition of the minimal simian virus 40 large T antigen- and adenovirus E1A-binding domain in the retinoblastoma gene product. *Molecular and Cellular Biology* **10** 3761–3769

Kaelin WG Jr, Pallas DC, DeCaprio JA, Kaye FJ and Livingston DM (1991) Identification of cellular proteins that can interact specifically with the T/E1A-binding region of the retinoblastoma gene product. *Cell* **64** 521–532

Laiho M, DeCaprio JA, Ludlow JW, Livingston DM and Massagué J (1990) Growth inhibition by TGF-β linked to suppression of retinoblastoma protein phosphorylation. *Cell* **62** 175–185

Lee W-H, Shew J-Y, Hong FD *et al* (1987) The retinoblastoma susceptibility gene encodes a nuclear phosphoprotein associated with DNA binding activity. *Nature* **329** 642–645

Ludlow JW, DeCaprio JA, Huang C-M, Lee W-H, Paucha E and Livingston DM (1989) SV40 large T antigen binds preferentially to an underphosphorylated member of the retinoblastoma susceptibility gene product family. *Cell* **56** 57–65

Ludlow JW, Shon J, Pipas JM, Livingston DM and DeCaprio JA (1990) The retinoblastoma susceptibility gene product undergoes cell cycle-dependent dephosphorylation and binding to and release from SV40 large T. *Cell* **60** 387–396

Whyte P, Buchkovich KJ, Horowitz JM *et al* (1988) Association between an oncogene and an antioncogene: the adenovirus E1A proteins bind to the retinoblastoma gene product. *Nature* **334** 124–129

The author is responsible for the accuracy of the references.

Adenovirus E1A Targets Key Regulators of Cell Proliferation

NICHOLAS DYSON • ED HARLOW

Massachusetts General Hospital Cancer Center, Building 149, 13th Street,
Charlestown, Massachusetts 02129

INTRODUCTION

Small DNA viruses rely heavily on their host cells for many of the steps needed for their own propagation. Since these viruses often use the same metabolic processes as the host cell but are easier to study, DNA viruses have become, somewhat paradoxically, powerful systems for analysing cellular metabolism. Many important developments in our knowledge of molecular biology have come first from the study of simple virus model systems. Our current understanding of many cellular events, such as eukaryotic DNA replication, transcriptional regulation, RNA processing, translational control and oncogenic transformation, relies heavily on observations of viral systems.

Cancer Surveys Volume 12: *Tumour Suppressor Genes, the Cell Cycle and Cancer*
© 1992 Imperial Cancer Research Fund. 0-87969-369-X/92. $3.00 + .00

Although viruses utilize many of the basic processes of cellular metabolism, they often perturb these routines, tailoring them to their own needs. Two types of changes that are commonly initiated by viruses are the inappropriate timing of normal cellular functions and the reprogramming of cellular metabolism to handle viral products at the expense of cellular ones. To induce these changes, viruses have evolved powerful systems to target key regulatory events. Presumably because viruses replicate frequently and are under intense evolutionary pressure, they have adapted to induce these changes efficiently.

Since viruses attack fundamental points of the cell's regulatory controls, the interface between the virus and host cell has become an important and fruitful field of study. Typically, studies of viral mutants are used to identify the viral products that are responsible for a particular change. The viral products, often proteins, then provide an entry into the study of their cellular targets. As these targets are often proteins that sit at key regulatory points in cellular metabolism, the viral proteins often provide an advantageous starting point to study cellular regulation.

One aspect of the life cycle of DNA viruses that is particularly crucial to their survival is the replication of the viral genome. Different viruses have developed diverse strategies to ensure the synthesis of their DNA. Larger viruses, such as the herpes simplex virus or the pox viruses, encode most of the enzymes needed to initiate and maintain replication of their DNA. For example, both of these viruses have their own DNA polymerase, thymidine kinase and ribonucleotide reductase (reviewed in Wittek, 1982; Moss, 1985; Knipe, 1989). These viruses have only a marginal need for host cell factors in replication. This is easily illustrated by considering the unusual subcellular location of poxvirus DNA synthesis. Poxvirus DNA is replicated in virus specific structures found only in the cytoplasm, and the nucleus is not required for viral DNA replication. As might be expected, these large DNA viruses are able to replicate their DNA irrespective of the cell cycle stage of the infected cell.

In contrast, the smallest of the DNA viruses, the parvoviruses, depend heavily on the host cell for the replication of their DNA. The only viral proteins needed for replication of the parvoviral genome bind to the termini of the viral DNA molecules. The functions of these proteins appear to be twofold: firstly, to ensure that viral DNA is recognized by the cellular replication machinery, and secondly, to release viral length genomes by an endonuclease action. Because the parvovirus contributes so little to the synthesis of viral DNA, these viruses depend heavily on their hosts for the machinery of DNA replication. This is illustrated by the observation that parvoviral DNA synthesis occurs only when host DNA is replicated. The strategy of these viruses is simply to wait for cellular DNA synthesis to begin, then to ensure that their DNA is replicated along with the cell's.

Other DNA viruses, notably the adenoviruses, papillomaviruses and polyomaviruses that are intermediate in size between the smaller parvoviruses and the larger pox virus or herpesviruses, have adopted a strategy for DNA synthesis between the two extremes discussed above. These viruses rely on the host cell to provide most of the enzymes for DNA synthesis, and they encode proteins which ensure that the DNA synthesis machinery efficiently replicates the viral genome. What distinguishes these viruses from other groups of viruses is that they also synthesize proteins that compel infected cells to replicate their own DNA. This strategy provides a unique relationship with the host cell. These viruses provide a strong stimulatory force that induces infected cells to assemble all of the machinery needed for DNA synthesis. Once assembled, special viral proteins ensure that the cellular enzymes process the virus genome with high priority.

The induction of cellular DNA synthesis by products of adenoviruses, polyomaviruses and papillomaviruses provides an excellent system for the study of virus/host cell interactions. These viruses synthesize proteins that are potent inducers of cellular DNA synthesis and thus act as strong deregulators of cell cycle control. For polyomaviruses, the induction of DNA synthesis is carried out primarily by proteins known as the large T antigens, for papillomaviruses, the E7 proteins are the major inducers of cell cycle regulation and for adenoviruses, the E1A gene products are the major mitogens. Studies of these viral products have provided important insights into the control of cell proliferation. As discussed below, these three proteins have a number of common properties, including the way in which they interact with the host cell. The common cellular targets for these viral proteins appear to be key points of regulation in cell cycle control and have become important points of research over the last several years.

Analyses of all three groups of viruses, the polyomaviruses, papillomaviruses and adenoviruses, have been part of an integrated effort from a number of laboratories to study the loss of controlled cell growth. This chapter will concentrate primarily on the study of the adenovirus E1A proteins.

E1A MEDIATED ONCOGENESIS

The E1A proteins are the first virus specific polypeptides synthesized following adenovirus infection (Lewis and Mathews, 1980; Nevins, 1981). One of major roles for these proteins is to initiate changes in the host cell that produce an environment suitable for viral propagation. To do this, the E1A proteins perform a number of different functions. E1A appears to be an authentic example of a multifunctional protein with different activities being carried out by separate protein domains. The data for the multifunctional nature of E1A are discussed in more detail below, but for convenience in this presentation, they will be divided into two groups, those of transcriptional *trans*-activation and cell cycle deregulation. It is not clear that these are the only changes induced by E1A, only that these are the best studied and understood.

As early products of adenovirus infection, one of the functions of the E1A polypeptides is to reorder the priorities of the cellular transcriptional machinery to recognize the viral promoters preferentially. In fact, the E1A proteins are among the most potent *trans*-activators that have been identified. The molecular mechanism of E1A mediated *trans*-activation is just beginning to be understood and appears to involve the specific activation of particular cellular transcription factors. Although the exact mechanism of alteration is not well understood at present, recent evidence suggests that it may involve direct physical interaction with transcription factors, such as ATF (Liu and Green, 1990), TFIID (Lee *et al*, 1991) and Oct 4 (Schöler *et al*, 1991). Although more work will be needed to determine whether physical interaction is the sole mechanism of *trans*-activation, it is interesting that this same strategy is also important for initiating changes in control of cell proliferation. For more information on *trans*-activation, see Lillie and Green (1989) and reviews by Berk (1986) and Flint and Shenk (1989).

The second class of E1A mediated changes can be generally grouped as cell cycle deregulation. These activities are most often studied by testing for the ability of E1A to immortalize primary cells in tissue culture, to cooperate with other oncogenes to transform cells or to induce host cell DNA synthesis in quiescent cells. These assays are somewhat artificial, as they measure gross phenotypic changes that are induced by E1A but may not reflect an immediate biochemical change induced by E1A. However, they have provided a reliable and reproducible set of criteria to compare various E1A mutations. Although the assays may seem different, they appear to depend on similar functions of E1A. As a group, all of these assays relate to the ability of E1A to act as an oncogene.

Adenoviruses were first shown to be oncogenic in newborn hamsters (Trentin *et al*, 1962) and were later shown to transform primary rodent cells (Freeman *et al*, 1967). Work from several laboratories showed that cells transformed by adenovirus always contained the left end of the adenovirus genome (Gallimore, 1974; Graham *et al*, 1974; Flint *et al*, 1976). Genetic analysis of adenovirus mutants and transfection experiments showed that two early genes of adenovirus, E1A and E1B, were both capable and sufficient for adenovirus transformation (Van der Eb *et al*, 1979; Houweling *et al*, 1980; Land *et al*, 1983; Ruley, 1983).

Although the focus of this review is on the mechanism of E1A's oncogenic activities, two points that are sometimes overlooked in this context should be considered. Firstly, at least as far as one can tell at present, adenoviruses do not cause tumours in their natural hosts. Although many serotypes of adenoviruses have been isolated from various human sources, no link has been demonstrated between adenovirus infection and any human cancer. E1A's oncogenic activities are apparent when it is assayed in the absence of the remainder of the viral genome or in cells, such as rodent cells, that do not support an efficient lytic infection. Thus, it appears that it is the continued expression of E1A in the absence of its viral context that leads to continued cell proliferation. Secondly, E1A is among the most potent of the nuclear oncogenes that have been identified. This feature probably reflects E1A's viral origin. Since

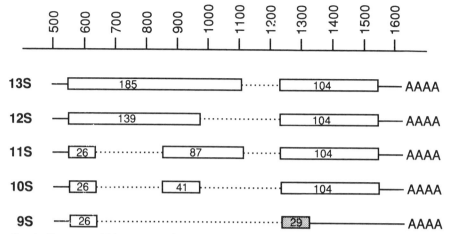

Fig. 1. Structure of E1A mRNAs. The structures of the five E1A mRNAs that were synthesized by alternative splicing of a primary transcript are shown by the relative positions of their coding sequences in the viral genome (numbered). Boxes indicate open reading frames, and dotted lines represent sequences that are removed during RNA maturation. The carboxyterminal 29 aminoacids of the 9S mRNA are shaded to indicate that they are encoded by a reading frame that is different from the reading frame encoding the carboxyterminus of the other mRNAs

adenovirus replication normally leads to the lysis of infected cells, the continued survival of the host cell is not necessary. Consequently, viral functions are able to evolve to be somewhat more harsh than their cellular counterparts and may be insusceptible to cellular regulation. Likewise, the survival of the virus depends at least in part on how effective the virus is at redirecting the host activities to those that are advantageous to the virus. Therefore, viral proteins that specialize in these changes can be expected to be potent, properties that are consistent with the oncogenic functions of E1A.

Structural Organization of the E1A Proteins

The E1A gene products are a heterogeneous family of polypeptides that contain a large number of polypeptide species when detected on high resolution two dimensional gel electrophoresis (Stephens *et al*, 1986). This remarkable heterogeneity arises from both alternative splicing of the primary transcript and extensive posttranslational modification of the primary products. For adenovirus types 2 and 5, five different messenger RNA (mRNA) transcripts from the E1A gene have been identified. They have sizes of 9S, 10S, 11S, 12S and 13S (Berk and Sharp, 1978; Chow *et al*, 1979; Perricaudet *et al*, 1979; Kitchingman and Westphal, 1980; Stephens and Harlow, 1987; Ulfendahl *et al*, 1987). The four largest mRNAs represent differentially processed mRNAs that encode different portions of a single open reading frame as illustrated in Fig. 1. The most abundant of these are the 12S and 13S transcripts, which are synthesized early in infection and encode proteins of 243 and 289 aminoacids,

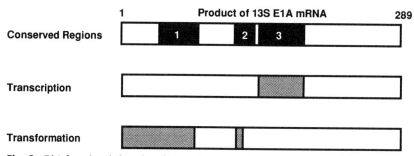

Fig. 2. E1A functional domains. Comparison of E1A sequences from different viral serotypes reveals three regions that are highly conserved. Conserved region 3 corresponds to a domain of E1A that has potent *trans*-activation activity. Two regions of E1A are required for its oncogenic properties. These two domains of E1A contain part of conserved regions 1 and 2

respectively (Perricaudet *et al*, 1979). Later in infection after the initiation of viral DNA synthesis, the 9S, 10S and 11S transcripts are detectable. The 10S and 11S transcripts produce proteins of 171 and 217 aminoacids, respectively (Stephens and Harlow, 1987; Ulfendahl *et al*, 1987). The product of the 9S transcript has not yet been found in infected cells (Virtanen and Pettersson, 1983).

Much of the heterogeneity of the E1A proteins is produced by posttranslational modifications. The primary translation products from all of the E1A mRNAs are rapidly phosphorylated, primarily on serine residues (Yee *et al*, 1983; Harlow *et al*, 1985; Stephens *et al*, 1986). Surprisingly, mutagenesis of several of the sites of phosphorylation has failed to show any major role for these modifications in transformation or *trans*-activation functions of E1A (Tsukamoto *et al*, 1986; Tremblay *et al*, 1988). Little is yet known about the significance of these modifications.

The first clues to the structural organization of E1A came from comparisons of the aminoacid sequences of E1A found in various serotypes of adenovirus (van Ormondt *et al*, 1980; Kimelman *et al*, 1985). These revealed three blocks of aminoacids that were highly conserved between the various adenovirus serotypes (Fig. 2). These regions are aminoacids 40–80 (conserved region 1), 121–139 (conserved region 2) and 140–188 (conserved region 3) (Moran and Mathews, 1987). Since these regions were conserved, it seemed likely that they represented important functional domains in E1A. In general, this view has been found to be accurate.

Mutagenesis studies have shown that the regions of E1A needed to perform individual tasks could be localized to certain domains of the primary structure. Discrete portions of E1A have been identified that provide the major *trans*-activation or transformation activities. *Trans*-activation of early viral promoters was found to be an activity of E1A proteins encoded by the 13S mRNA but not by the 12S mRNA (Graham *et al*, 1978; Esche *et al*, 1980; Carlock and Jones, 1981; Ricciardi *et al*, 1981; Montell *et al*, 1982; Glenn and Ricciardi, 1985; Lillie *et al*, 1986). The 12S mRNA encodes proteins that contain conserved regions 1 and 2 but lacks the coding region for conserved region 3. Conserved region 3 is encoded by the 13S mRNA. This was the first indication that conserved region 3 might specify the functions needed for *trans*-activation. Furthermore, mutations within conserved region 3 abolished *trans*-activation, whereas mutations elsewhere in E1A had little effect (Glenn and Ricciardi, 1985; Lillie *et al*, 1986; Moran *et al*, 1986a,b; Moran and Mathews, 1987). Compelling evidence that conserved region 3 contains E1A's potent *trans*-activation activity came from Lillie *et al* (1987), who demonstrated that the microinjection of a peptide which corresponds to this region was sufficient to *trans*-activate the E2A promoter in HeLa cells.

In contrast to *trans*-activation, the transformation functions of E1A require sequences in both conserved regions 1 and 2, but conserved region 3 is completely dispensable (Haley *et al*, 1984; Lillie *et al*, 1986; Moran *et al*, 1986a,b; Zerler *et al*, 1986; Lillie *et al*, 1987; Schneider *et al*, 1987; Stephens and Harlow, 1987; Moran and Zerler, 1988; Smith and Ziff, 1988; Subramanian *et al*, 1988; Whyte *et al*, 1988b; Jelsma *et al*, 1989). Further analysis of the transforming regions showed that E1A mutants lacking conserved region 1 will complement E1A mutants lacking region 2. This suggests that these regions contain discrete activities that can function in *trans* (Moran and Zerler, 1988). Thus, the data support a general view of E1A as a collection of independently acting domains. The structure and properties of the domains that comprise the transforming regions of E1A are discussed in more detail below.

Immortalization of Primary Cells by the Adenovirus E1A Proteins

The transfection of E1A into primary cells converts these cells into established cell lines (Van der Eb *et al*, 1979; Houweling *et al*, 1980). These cells have the characteristics of immortalized cells and arise at a frequency which suggests that E1A expression alone or E1A expression in combination with one or a very small number of cellular gene mutations is sufficient to produce an established cell line (see eg Cone *et al*, 1988). However, these immortalized, E1A expressing cells are not fully transformed. To gain a transformed phenotype, other oncogenes need to be activated, which can be demonstrated experimentally by transfecting oncogenes into the previously immortalized cells or by performing the original transfections with additional cooperating oncogenes. E1A has been shown to cooperate with several oncogenes to achieve full transformation. These include the *ras*, polyomavirus middle T and adenovirus E1B oncogenes (van den Elsen *et al*, 1982, 1983; Ruley, 1983). Like the immortalization assays, these transformation events occur with a frequency which suggests either that the expression of these two exogenous oncogenes is sufficient for transformation or that only one or a small number of cellular mutations are needed to produce fully transformed cells.

During the last few years, the analysis of E1A mediated transformation has provided the first clues about the possible biochemical mechanism of E1A's role in transformation. It appears that E1A mediated changes are induced by physical interactions with cellular proteins. In adenovirus infected or transformed cells, the E1A proteins associate with a large number of cellular proteins. These proteins were first detected by immunochemical methods (Yee and Branton, 1985; Harlow et al, 1986). Antibodies specific for E1A were used to immunoprecipitate E1A and its associated proteins from these cells. In the earliest studies, ten proteins were found to be associated with E1A (Harlow et al, 1986). Originally, these were known by their relative molecular masses of 300, 130, 107, 105, 90, 80, 60, 50, 40, and 28 kDa. Recently, one additional protein of 33 kDa found to be associated with E1A has been identified (Giordano et al, 1991; Tsai et al, in press; Faha B, unpublished). Four of these proteins have now been identified. The first to be identified was p105, now known to be the product of the retinoblastoma tumour suppressor gene (Whyte et al, 1988a). The p107 protein has recently been cloned by Ewen et al (1991) and shown to be structurally related to pRB. The p60 protein was shown to interact with human cdc2 like kinase (Giordano et al, 1989) and then was identified as human cyclin A (Pines and Hunter, 1990). The 33 kDa protein has been shown to be a kinase that is closely related to cdc2 (Giordano et al, 1989, 1991a; Tsai et al, 1991; Faha B, unpublished). Recent cloning of this gene has identified it as $p33^{cdk2}$ (Tsai et al, 1991), the human homologue of Xenopus Eg-1 (Paris et al, 1991). The other proteins that are found in the E1A immunoprecipitations are still known only by their relative molecular weights.

The biochemical consequences of E1A's interactions with cellular proteins are still largely unknown. However, mutational studies of E1A suggest that these interactions are essential for transformation. The regions of E1A that are needed to bind to the cellular proteins are the same regions that are needed for transformation (Egan et al, 1988, 1989; Jelsma et al, 1989; Whyte et al, 1989; Howe et al, 1990; Giordano et al, 1991b). Similarly, mutations that destroy the ability of E1A to interact with these cellular proteins also abolish the ability of E1A to act as an oncogene. The binding sites of these cellular proteins have been mapped to the aminoterminal 127 residues of E1A (Whyte et al, 1989). These same sequences will cooperate with an activated ras oncogene to convert primary baby rat kidney cells to fully transformed cells (Whyte et al, 1988b). In this case, the frequency of transformation is reduced but the transformed cells that arise from cotransfection with E1A aminoacids 1 to 127 appear to have all of the phenotypes of transformed cells prepared using full length wild type E1A.

The analysis of mutations in E1A that destroy binding to the cellular proteins provided two interesting findings. Firstly, any mutation that significantly diminishes binding to any of the cellular proteins also significantly diminishes transforming ability. For example, removing two more aminoacids from the carboxyterminal 127 residue fragment of E1A yields a protein that fails to bind to many of the cellular proteins and fails to transform (Whyte et al, 1988b, 1989). Similar correlations are seen in all of the binding regions. Some of the mutations are very dramatic, correlating total loss of binding with total loss of transforming activity. Other mutations are less dramatic, but equally consistent, and show concomitant decreases in levels of binding and transformation efficiencies. No mutants have yet been characterized that break this correlation. If E1A fails to bind, transforming activity is destroyed. This observation has led to a simple hypothesis that the interactions have identified the cellular targets for E1A mediated transformation. As a first estimate, this appears to be correct. The interacting domains correspond remarkably well to the regions needed for transformation, and the binding proteins themselves have activities that suggest important roles in control of cell propagation.

The second striking finding is that the binding sites for these host proteins on E1A often overlap with one another. Some of the cellular proteins appear to have identical sequence requirements for interaction, some appear to overlap but have unique regions and some appear to have unique interaction sites. These observations have led to several problems. Firstly, these patterns of overlapping binding have made it difficult to assign functional domains to individual associations. If more than one protein binds to the same regions of E1A, then assigning a function to either protein interaction is difficult to do using viral mutagenesis. Secondly, the demonstration of overlapping binding sites also brings into question what the binding assays are actually measuring. Our strategy to determine the binding sites of the associated proteins has been to make successive deletions in the E1A coding region and test the resulting mutants for stable interactions with cellular proteins. This approach has been particularly successful in identifying small regions of E1A that sustain stable protein-protein interactions. The regions that remain using this strategy must then contain residues that contact the cellular proteins. However, this strategy also has its limitations. It may eliminate other contact sites that are not necessary for binding but contribute to the overall stability of the interaction. Therefore, although the correlations derived from these mapping studies are interpretable in a general sense, one should not consider them to be the sole determinants of the total contact sites. Similarly, this approach will include regions of E1A that contribute to stable folding of binding domains and may not only detect actual contact sites.

The most extensively studied of the interactions between E1A and the cellular proteins is the association with pRB. Two segments of E1A were shown to be important for binding to pRB using the deletion mutant strategy outlined above. These included aminoacids 30–60 and 120–127 (Whyte *et al*, 1989). Deletion of either region destroyed the interactions with pRB seen in vivo. Smaller deletions into each region likewise prevented detection of an in vivo complex. More detailed in vitro studies showed that both regions of E1A were able to interact directly with pRB. This was first demonstrated by using the same mutants used for in vivo studies in the in vitro binding experiments. These binding assays relied on the ability of pRB and various mutant E1As to bind in vitro. They showed that mutations in the 30–60 region were able to bind to pRB in vitro, although with a lower binding affinity than any E1A

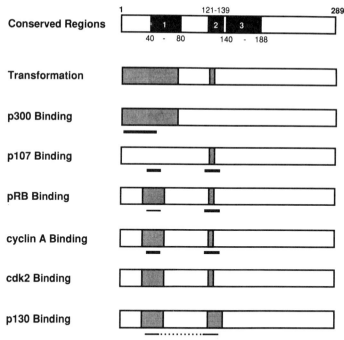

Fig. 3. Regions of E1A required for association with cellular proteins. The shaded boxes represent regions of E1A that have been identified by analysis of E1A mutants to be important for E1A mediated transformation or for protein binding. The unshaded areas show regions of E1A that could be deleted without loss of binding activity. The black bars represent synthetic peptides or bacterially produced polypeptides that were sufficient for stable association with the cellular proteins. The different thicknesses of the bars representing pRB binding peptides indicate that the peptides bind to pRB with considerably different affinities. Proteins p107, pRB and cyclin A bound more strongly to a peptide that combines both regions, but interaction with p130 was detected only with this combined peptide as indicated by the broken line

protein that had both regions. These results were underscored by assays using synthetic peptides (Dyson N, Guida P, McCall C and Harlow E, unpublished). Two peptides were prepared that represented each region individually, and these were compared with one that linked the two regions as a single unit. These peptides were used in two types of experiments. In one set, the peptides were used to block the binding of E1A and pRB in vitro, and in the other, the peptides were covalently linked to agarose beads, which then were used as adsorbents to bind to pRB in vitro. In both assays, all three of the E1A derived peptides were able to bind to pRB. The peptide from region 1 bound weakly, the region 2 peptides bound more avidly and the peptide containing both sequences was the strongest binder. These results suggested that each site could bind independently to pRB.

The use of synthetic peptides also allowed an important combined experiment. Using E1A peptides coupled to beads as an adsorbent for pRB, peptides representing one binding region of E1A were tested for the ability to block the interaction of pRB with the other region of E1A. This tested whether the peptides had independent sites of interaction. In both cases, peptides were able only to block the interaction of pRB with their cognate peptide bead and showed no activity when tested against peptides from the other region. Therefore, both regions of E1A make discrete contacts with pRB.

Less is known about the physical characteristics of the interactions with the other E1A associated proteins. Peptide experiments similar to those described for pRB suggest that at least two regions of E1A are involved in association with p107. These experiments reinforce the conclusion that these small regions of E1A provide stable association with multiple cellular proteins (Dyson N, Guida P, Munger K, Howley PM and Harlow E, unpublished). This is illustrated in Fig. 3, which shows the combination of data from studies of E1A mutants and synthetic peptides.

p105 IS THE RETINOBLASTOMA GENE PRODUCT

The 105 kDa protein was the first E1A associated polypeptide to be identified. Whyte *et al* (1988a) noted the similarity in size between the E1A associated 105 kDa protein and the product of the human retinoblastoma susceptibility gene *RB* (Lee *et al*, 1987). On the basis of their potential roles in cell transformation, these two proteins were compared and by several criteria were found to be indistinguishable. These nuclear phosphoproteins co-migrated on SDS polyacrylamide gel electrophoresis and yielded identical proteolytic fragments when cleaved by *Staphylococcus aureus* V8 protease and N chlorosuccinimide under several different digestion conditions. Monoclonal antibodies to the E1A associated 105 kDa protein recognized the products of in vitro transcription and translation of the *RB* human cDNA clone. Conversely, anti-peptide antibodies raised against the predicted sequence deduced from the *RB* cDNA sequences recognized the E1A associated protein. Although the 105 kDa E1A associated protein was found in a wide variety of cell lines, it was missing from retinoblastoma cells, cells that contained homozygous deletions of both alleles of the *RB* gene. These criteria made it clear that the E1A associated 105 kDa protein was the product of the retinoblastoma tumour suppressor gene. DeCaprio *et al* (1988) quickly expanded these observations to show that another viral transforming protein, the simian virus 40 (SV40) large T antigen, could also form stable protein-protein complexes with pRB. From subsequent experiments, pRB is now known to bind to the early products of several small DNA tumour viruses, including the E7 oncoproteins of human papillomaviruses (Dyson *et al*, 1989b; Munger *et al*, 1989) as well as the large T antigens of other polyomaviruses (Dyson *et al*, 1990).

pRB Is One of the Key Tumour Suppressor Gene Products

The study of the retinoblastoma gene and its product has laid the foundation for much of our understanding about tumour suppressor genes. The retinoblastoma gene was the first member of this family to be identified and is probably one of the simplest to comprehend. A number of other tumour suppressor genes have now been cloned and characterized, and the current list includes *p53* (Finlay *et al*, 1989), Wilms' tumour (*WT1*) (Haber *et al*, 1990), deleted in colon carcinoma (*DCC*) (Fearon *et al*, 1990), neurofibromatosis 1 (*NF1*) (Cawthon *et al*, 1990; Wallace *et al*, 1990) and adenomatous polyposis coli (*APC*) (Groden *et al*, 1991; Joslyn *et al*, 1991; Kinzler *et al*, 1991; Nishisho *et al*, 1991).

Retinoblastomas are childhood tumours of the developing retina, which arise in both sporadic and inherited forms. These tumours are probably the simplest of all the human tumours, because they appear to arise after the fewest number of mutations. Their genesis is controlled by two rate limiting steps, in contrast to the many adult tumours that show evidence of five or more steps. The two rate limiting steps for retinoblastoma development are mutations of the two alleles of the *RB* gene (Knudson, 1971, 1987). Both copies of the *RB* gene are mutated or deleted in all retinoblastoma tumour cells that have been characterized to date. In the sporadic form of retinoblastoma, both *RB* mutations arise during somatic development of the retina, and the low incidence of retinoblastoma (1 in 23 000 births) reflects the low probability of the two mutations occurring in a single cell during retinal development. Once full terminal differentiation of the retina has taken place, the chance of developing a retinoblastoma drops to near zero.

Familial predisposition to retinoblastoma accounts for only 10% of patients (Vogel, 1979) and is caused by the inheritance of a mutated *RB* allele. The appearance of the retinoblastoma tumour in these cases follows the mutation of the remaining normal allele in the developing retina. In most of the children who inherit a mutated *RB* allele, this second mutation occurs at least once in each eye. Consequently, retinoblastomas appear as an autosomal dominant trait with a very high level of penetrance (approximately 90%) (Knudson, 1975; Francois *et al*, 1976; Matsunaga, 1976).

The loss of an active pRB protein in every retinoblastoma tumour suggests that one key function of pRB is as a negative regulator of cell proliferation. Thus, the loss of pRB would remove an inhibitory control and consequently promote cell growth, although the molecular mechanism by which pRB would impart this regulation is unknown. It appears that this function of pRB is important in a wide variety of cells, since pRB has been found to be ubiquitously expressed in most tissues and developmental stages that have been examined to date. Furthermore, it is believed that pRB must be active in a wide variety of cells, because *RB* mutations have been found in tumours and cell lines isolated from many sources. These include osteosarcoma, bladder carcinoma, prostate carcinoma, breast carcinoma, small cell lung carcinomas, leukaemia and cervical carcinoma (Friend *et al*, 1986, 1987; Fung *et al*, 1987; Dunn *et al*, 1988, 1989; Harbour *et al*, 1988; Lee *et al*, 1988; T'Ang *et al*, 1988; Yokota *et al*, 1988; Horowitz *et al*, 1989a,b, 1990; Toguchida *et al*, 1989; Chen *et al*, 1990; Cheng *et al*, 1990; Hensel *et al*, 1990; Scholz *et al*, 1990; Shew *et al*, 1990). Thus, the current model for the action of pRB is that it performs a negative regulatory role in a wide variety of cells and tissues.

The frequency of the *RB* mutation, however, varies considerably between different types of tumours. Although not all tumours have been studied in detail, *RB* mutations have been found in all retinoblastomas and most small cell lung carcinomas, suggesting that inactivation of the *RB* gene function is an obligatory step in the development of these types of tumours. In bladder carcinoma, prostate carcinoma and osteosarcomas, the *RB* mutation occurs with lower frequencies, showing that although the *RB* mutation may be a contributing event in the development of these tumours, it is clearly not essential for tumorigenesis. In cervical carcinomas, an interesting combination of these findings has been observed. Examples of cells containing either wild type or mutant pRB proteins have been identified, but in all of the cases with wild type pRB, these cells also contain the human papillomavirus E7 oncoprotein (Scheffner *et al*, 1991). Since, as discussed below, E7 association is thought to inactivate the pRB protein, pRB function must be overcome in these cells during tumour formation. However, inactivation of pRB can be accomplished by more than one method.

Not all tumour sources that have been examined show mutations in pRB. For example, some tumours, such as colon carcinoma, have shown no *RB* mutations. This indicates that inactivation of *RB* function probably has no selective advantage for these cells, and therefore pRB function appears to have varying importance, depending on the type of cell affected. Presumably other pathways provide the key growth suppressor functions in these cells.

Similar conclusions are drawn from studies of individuals with an inherited mutation in one of the *RB* alleles (see eg Abramson *et al*, 1976; Cullen, 1991). These children must have a mutated *RB* allele in all of their cells, yet the primary tumour that arises after mutation of the other *RB* alleles is a retinoblastoma. Presumably mutations in the second *RB* allele occur throughout the body, but childhood tumours are not commonly seen in other tissues. Likewise, after removal of the retinoblastoma, these individuals do not develop tumours in all tissues. Many continue to lead normal lives for years but then suffer from second malignancies in a few selected sites, most frequently osteosarcomas.

All of these data lead to several characteristics of the retinoblastoma tumour suppressor gene. pRB appears to exert negative control over some aspect of cell proliferation, and functional inactivation of pRB leads to a change in growth potential. The importance of this change appears to be tissue specific, as different cells display different sensitivities to the loss of pRB. For reasons that are still not completely clear, developing retinal cells appear to be the most sensitive to these changes.

The pRB/E1A Complex

The discovery that the E1A associated 105 kDa protein was pRB provided the first clue to the potential function of the E1A's strong physical association with cellular proteins. Given the ability of E1A to act as a dominant oncogene and pRB's apparent function as a negative regulator of growth in normal cells, a simple hypothesis was suggested by Whyte *et al* (1988a). These authors suggested that E1A binds to pRB to inactivate it, thus mimicking the loss of *RB* in tumour cell lines. Although the biochemical proof for this hypothesis is still missing, a number of observations support this model. Firstly, the regions of pRB that are needed for interaction with E1A and large T are also required for the correct function of this protein. Secondly, pRB undergoes cell cycle dependent modifications that appear to change its potential to act as a negative regulator, and the association with large T antigen, E7 and to a lesser extent E1A is sensitive to these changes. Thirdly, E1A is capable of overcoming the ability of pRB to interact with its natural targets in the cell. These observations are discussed in more detail below, but collectively they argue quite strongly that viral oncoproteins, such as E1A, large T and E7, have evolved to target key regulatory proteins like pRB and have done so in ways that disrupt its normal function within the cell.

The Regions of pRB Needed for Interaction with E1A Are Key Functional Domains

The regions of pRB that are required for association with the viral proteins are also important functional sites for pRB function. Two regions of pRB, 393–572 and 646–772, are required for high affinity binding with E1A and large T antigen (Hu *et al*, 1990; Huang *et al*, 1990; Kaelin *et al*, 1990). A comparison of the regions of pRB that are required for association with E1A or large T antigen and the regions of pRB that are mutated in tumour cells provides two pieces of information (Hu *et al*, 1990; Huang *et al*, 1990; Kaelin *et al*, 1990). The first is that the regions targeted by the viral proteins are essential for normal pRB function, since small mutations within these regions are apparently sufficient to render it inactive. Where known, these same mutations also destroy the ability of pRB to interact with E1A or large T. The second is that although the E1A/T binding domains are hot spots for mutation, mutants do exist that lie outside these regions, suggesting that pRB may contain several domains that are essential for normal growth control.

pRB Exists in Different Forms That May Be Functionally Distinct

During the search for *RB* mutations in various tumours, it became clear that most cells contain wild type *RB* genes and produce pRB that is apparently normal. In addition, pRB was found throughout the cell cycle in normal cells that were actively dividing. Given the proposed role of pRB as a negative regulator of cell growth, these results seemed to be somewhat paradoxical at first glance. How does a cell divide when expressing a known negative regulator of cell proliferation? A solution to this paradox is suggested by the observation that pRB is phosphorylated in a cell cycle dependent manner

(Buchkovich *et al*, 1989; Chen *et al*, 1989; DeCaprio *et al*, 1989; Mihara *et al*, 1989). pRB is un- or underphosphorylated during the G_0 and G_1 phases of the cell cycle but becomes heavily phosphorylated near the G_1-S boundary and remains in this hyperphosphorylated state until it is dephosphorylated near the end of mitosis (Ludlow *et al*, 1990). It seems reasonable to hypothesize that this posttranslational modification acts to regulate pRB function such that the cell is temporarily relieved from pRB's negative control. The suggestion that pRB is functionally modulated by phosphorylation is supported by the observation that SV40 large T antigen binds preferentially to underphosphorylated pRB (Ludlow *et al*, 1989). Since large T, like E1A, is thought to inactivate pRB by protein association, it follows that the activity of pRB that is targeted by large T must be provided in G_1 by unphosphorylated pRB. This activity is therefore either missing from the phosphorylated forms of pRB or irrelevant to large T antigen.

Since it appears that pRB is functionally regulated by phosphorylation, it is important to determine the kinase(s) and phosphatases responsible for this control. There is now strong evidence that pRB is phosphorylated by cdc2 or a closely related kinase. This conclusion comes from two complementary sets of data, one study showing that sites on pRB that are phosphorylated in vivo are consensus cdc2 phosphorylation sites (Lees *et al*, 1991), and the second demonstrating a physical association in vivo between pRB and a cdc2 kinase (Hu *et al*, in press). In these experiments, immunological reagents to cdc2 and cyclin A detected the predominant pRB associated kinase activity. pRB associated kinase activity is regulated in a cell cycle dependent manner, being largely absent from G_1 phase cells, appearing in S phase and extending through to M phase (Hu *et al*, in press). However, it is possible that this kinase may not be the only one to phosphorylate pRB. It is clear that there exists a large family of kinases that are closely related to cdc2 (Meyerson *et al*, 1991; Pines and Hunter, 1991), and each may be regulated by association with an equally large family of cyclins (reviewed in Hunter and Pines, 1991). Thus, determining the kinase that is responsible for *RB* phosphorylation at the G_1-S transition, which is presumably the key site of regulation, may not be simple. In addition, pRB is phosphorylated on multiple sites (Lees *et al*, 1991; Lin, 1991). Within the degree of synchrony afforded by cell cycle experiments, most of these occur simultaneously (Lees *et al*, 1991). Thus, at present, it is unclear how many kinases are involved and which site, if any, is the key regulatory modification.

Cellular Partners for pRB

Given the considerable amount of research into the *RB* gene and its products, the biochemical basis for its tumour suppressor function has remained surprisingly obscure. The sequence of this gene reveals no easily recognizable motifs and provides no clues to its function. The attempt to determine its function has turned to pRB associated proteins in the hope that these might offer some insight into its mechanism of action. Initial attempts to identify RB associated proteins using conventional immunological approaches have proven un-successful. However, using large amounts of bacterially produced wild type pRB or fragments of pRB to drive the binding to proteins from radioactively labelled cells, Huang *et al* (1991) and Kaelin *et al* (1991) have identified several cellular proteins that can bind to pRB. Many of these proteins interact with the same binding domains, or pocket, of pRB that provides its association with viral proteins. Therefore, these represent candidates for cellular interac-tions that are targeted by the viruses. Fragments of genes encoding two such candidates have been recently cloned from expression libraries by screening procedures using bacterially produced pRB (Defeo-Jones *et al*, 1991). These genes, termed *RBP1* and *RBP2*, contain motifs that are homologous to the pRB binding sequences of E1A/E7/T, and these motifs mediate binding of the cellular proteins to pRB. To date, these interactions have only been shown for in vitro assays, and it is still unclear at present whether analogous interactions occur in vivo. Unfortunately, the remaining sequences of *RBP1* and *RBP2* con-tain no significant homology with other known genes and give no clue to their biochemical activities (Defeo-Jones *et al*, 1991; Fattaey A, unpublished).

Recent observations suggest that pRB may play a direct role in regulation of cellular transcription. This suggestion comes from the discovery that pRB is physically associated with two closely related transcription factors E2F (Chel-lappan *et al*, 1991; Mudryj *et al*, 1991) and DRTF1 (Bandara and La Thangue, 1991; Bandara *et al*, 1991), and also from the observations that pRB binds in vitro to members of the *myc* family of oncogenes (Rustgi *et al*, 1991).

E2F and DRTF1 are multisubunit factors that bind to elements in the adenovirus E2 promoter and mediate *trans*-activation of the E2 promoter by E1A (Kovesdi *et al*, 1986; Yee *et al*, 1989). Sequences that are similar to the E2F binding site in the E2 promoter have been found upstream of several cel-lular genes, and these may also be involved in transcriptional regulation. Ac-tivation of E2 transcription by E1A is correlated with an increase in E2F DNA binding affinity (Raychaudhuri *et al*, 1990) and the release of cellular proteins from the multimeric complex (Bagchi *et al*, 1990). Chellepan *et al* (1991) and Bandara and La Thangue (1991) have shown that pRB is one of the com-ponents of E2F/DRTF1 and is dissociated from the DNA binding factors by incubation with E1A. This activity requires the regions of E1A that are essen-tial both for binding to pRB and for transforming activity (Bandara *et al*, 1991; Chellappan *et al*, 1991; Raychaudhuri *et al*, 1991). Together, these results sug-gest that the regulation of E2F activity is a function of pRB that is targeted by the viral oncoproteins. At least three additional lines of evidence support this model. Firstly, Bagchi *et al* (1991) isolated an inhibitor of E2F, E2F-I, that in-hibits E2F from binding to DNA. Analysis of E2F-I reveals that it contains pRB. Removal of pRB either with E1A sequences or with antibodies to pRB inactivated the inhibitory function of E2F-I. Secondly, in a different approach, Chittenden *et al* (1991) used polymerase chain reaction amplification to select DNA sequences that bound specifically to pRB associated proteins from a pool of random oligonucleotides. Analysis of the enriched sequences revealed that the cellular proteins that bind to pRB included a factor that binds strongly to sequences closely related to E2F. Third is the observation that E2F appears to bind only to unphosphorylated pRB (Chellappan *et al*, 1991), suggesting that the pRB/E2F interaction is regulated by phosphorylation. Since unphosphorylated pRB is thought to provide the anti-proliferative function that is targeted by SV40 large T antigen, this observation is consistent with the model that pRB regulation of E2F is at least one of the processes targeted. As would be expected in this model, E2F activity has been shown to be cell cycle regulated and activated at points in the cell cycle when pRB is known to be phosphorylated (Mudryj *et al*, 1990, 1991).

Results from Rustgi *et al* (1991) suggest that pRB may regulate other transcription factors in addition to E2F. A variety of in vitro binding assays were used to show that pRB is able to interact with the c-*myc* and N-*myc* oncogenes (Rustgi *et al*, 1991). Like the associations between pRB and RBP1, RBP2, or E2F/DRTF1, the pRB/c-*myc* interaction could be competed by viral proteins containing pRB binding sequences. c-*myc* and N-*myc* contain structural motifs that are conserved among many families of transcription factors, and it is likely that these oncogenes also function at the level of transcriptional regulation, although precise functions of these proteins are not known. By analogy with the E2F/pRB interaction, it is tempting to speculate that pRB is a negative regulator of c-*myc* mediated transcriptional activation. However, the interpretation of this interaction, like those with RBP1 and RBP2, depends on the demonstration and functional analysis of these protein complexes in vivo.

THE E1A ASSOCIATED PROTEIN, p107

Studies of the E1A associated 107 kDa protein (p107) have shown that it has many properties in common with pRB. Initial experiments showed that both pRB and p107 were nuclear phosphoproteins that appeared to be expressed in many cell types and species. More recent work has continued to emphasize the similarities between these proteins. The recent cloning of the p107 gene (Ewen *et al*, 1991) confirms the idea that pRB and p107 are related and lends support to the idea that they share similar biochemical activities. However, as is the case for pRB, the precise definition of these activities is unclear, and the targets for p107 action are not known.

Like pRB, p107 is a potential target for E1A's role in transformation based on the mapping of its binding sites on E1A (Whyte *et al*, 1989). As with pRB, mutants that fail to bind to p107 also fail to transform. Detailed genetic analysis showed that aminoacids 120–127 of E1A are required for it to associate with p107 (Whyte *et al*, 1989). Furthermore, a synthetic peptide containing E1A aminoacids 117–132 is sufficient for binding to p107 (Dyson N, Guida P, and Harlow E, unpublished). Whereas these studies mapped the binding of E1A to p107 to a small region, it appears likely that additional sequences in E1A also contribute to this interaction. This is best illustrated by experiments which demonstrate that small synthetic peptides from other regions of E1A can bind to p107 directly and that E1A fusion proteins that lack the 120–127 region also bind to p107, although with a reduced affinity (Zhu L, Dyson N and Harlow E, unpublished). These data suggest that the 120–127 region of E1A represents a high affinity binding site for p107 and that the region between residues 30 and 60 also provides a second binding site with lower affinity for p107. Although the relative affinity of these regions for p107 appears to be different, these are the same regions that E1A uses for interaction with pRB.

The ability to bind to p107 is also conserved in the oncoproteins of other DNA tumour viruses that bind to pRB. p107 forms stable protein complexes with the large T antigens of SV40 and JC polyomaviruses (Dyson *et al*, 1989a; Ewen *et al*, 1989). As with E1A, the genetic analysis of SV40 large T antigen shows that mutants of large T that fail to bind to p107 have lost transforming activity (Ewen *et al*, 1989). It is highly likely that p107 is also targeted by the E7 protein of human papillomavirus type 16 (HPV-16), since synthetic peptides containing aminoacids 2–32 or 16–32 of the E7 sequence bind to p107 with affinity equivalent to the homologous E1A and SV40 large T antigen sequences (Dyson N, Guida P, Munger K, Howley PM and Harlow E, unpublished). Curiously, the p107 protein that associates with E1A is a phosphoprotein, whereas the p107 that is associated with SV40 large T antigen is un- or underphosphorylated (Dyson *et al*, 1989a; Ewen *et al*, 1989). This is highly reminiscent of the observation that SV40 large T antigen binds only to unphosphorylated pRB. By analogy, this may suggest that p107 exists in differentially phosphorylated forms that are functionally distinct. To date, only one study of phosphorylation of p107 through the cell cycle has been carried out. Herrmann *et al* (1991) showed that in an E1A containing derivative of HeLa cells, E1A associated p107 was phosphorylated at all phases of the cell cycle but was most heavily modified during S phase. Since E1A associated p107 may represent only a subset of the total pool of this protein, and p107 phosphorylation may be altered in these cells by the presence of viral oncoproteins, the overall pattern of p107 phosphorylation in normal cells may be quite different. Hopefully, the preparation of immunological reagents to p107 will give a more complete picture.

Although pRB and p107 have similar features, these proteins are clearly the products of different genes. WERI-1 cells that carry a homozygous deletion of the *RB* gene express p107 protein that is apparently wild type and binds to E1A and SV40 T antigen (Dyson *et al*, 1989a; Ewen *et al*, 1989). Nevertheless, the observation that p107 and pRB bind to overlapping sites on E1A raised the possibility that they might contain similar structures in their binding regions. This idea was supported by the isolation of a monoclonal antibody to pRB that cross reacted to p107 (Hu *et al*, in press). This antibody, XZ37, was prepared after immunizing mice with a fragment of pRB that contained the E1A binding regions. Since most monoclonal antibodies to pRB fail to recognize p107, the isolation of XZ37 suggests that these proteins contain a limited amount of structural homology. The recent cloning of the human gene for p107 confirms that this is indeed the case (Ewen *et al*, 1991). These genes share aminoacid homology of approximately 30% within the regions that mediate binding to E1A but show little similarity outside these domains. More information on the similarities of pRB and p107 can be found in Livingston (this issue).

One feature of p107 that appears to distinguish it from pRB is that it forms a relatively stable and readily detectable complex with cyclin A in either the presence or absence of E1A (Ewen *et al*, in press; Faha *et al*, in press). p107, like pRB, contains two regions that are required for association with viral proteins. These regions are separated by a stretch of aminoacids termed the spacer region. In pRB, the length but not the sequence of the spacer region is important for association with viral proteins. The spacer region of p107 shows virtually no sequence homology with the pRB spacer and is considerably longer. The binding site for cyclin A on p107 maps to this spacer region and is genetically distinct from association with E1A or T antigen. This interaction provides a clear link between p107 and the machinery that regulates the cell cycle (see below), but until more is known about what other proteins are present, the functional implications of this observation are not clear.

The degree of similarity between pRB and p107 may indicate that their biochemical activities are related. These similarities have led to the speculation that p107 may also be a tumour suppressor gene. To test this suggestion, we have analysed cell lines isolated from a number of human tumours for changes in the pattern of p107 expression; however, we have been unable to find any type of tumour cell that consistently shows abnormalities in p107. Even though p107 and pRB may have similar activities, the consequences of these activities may be quite different. It is important to note that in retinoblastoma cell lines that lack pRB but contain apparently normal p107, the presence of p107 is unable to compensate for lack of pRB function. Nevertheless, one compelling observation, which continues to force one to consider a role for p107 in cell proliferation, is that it is targeted by several viral oncoproteins.

CELL CYCLE CONNECTIONS: CYCLIN A AND p33[cdk2]

Studies of the E1A associated p60 have led to the first discovery of direct link between cancer genes and cell cycle control. The p60 protein, known originally only by its molecular weight, was characterized more fully by Giordano *et al* (1989). These authors noted that in the absence of E1A, p60 could be found bound to an approximately 33 000 dalton protein (p33) that had many properties of the cell cycle regulated kinase p34[cdc2]. This complex had kinase activity that was temporally regulated during the cell cycle. At the time it appeared that the p33 protein was likely to be p34[cdc2]. As described below, this now appears to be incorrect, as the cDNA for p33 has been cloned and it encodes another kinase closely related to p34^{cdc2}. However, the discovery of a kinase associated with p60 laid the groundwork for its investigation.

p60 Is Human Cyclin A

The identity of p60 was determined by Pines and Hunter (1990), after cloning the human cyclin A cDNA. The product of this cDNA was shown to be the E1A associated p60 protein. Cyclins are a large class of proteins that participate in cell cycle regulation. It is thought that cyclins are regulatory subunits that bind to kinases and help control the timing of the activation of the kinase activity. Although the molecular basis for activation of the kinases following cyclin association is not clear, these interactions appear to be required to turn the inactive catalytic subunit into an active one. At present, there are six classes of cyclins, designated A, B, C, D, E and CLN (recently reviewed in Hunter and Pines, 1991). The A, C, D and E cyclins have been found only in vertebrates, whereas the CLN cyclins have only been found in the budding yeast *Saccharomyces cerevisiae* and the fission yeast *Schizosaccharomyces pombe* (puc 1). Cyclins from the B class have been identified in all eukaryotes studied to date. In addition to their interaction with kinases, most cyclins have been shown to oscillate in their levels throughout the cell cycle.

The best characterized of the cyclins are those of the A and B classes. These cyclins interact with the major cell cycle regulating kinase p34^{cdc2}. The cyclin A/p34^{cdc2} kinase is activated first in the cell cycle, and it continues to be active until metaphase of mitosis, where degradation of the cyclin leads to downregulation of the kinase activity. The kinase activity of the cyclin B/p34^{cdc2} complex appears later in the cell cycle, being the major regulator of the entry into and progression through mitosis. Like the cyclin A/p34^{cdc2} complex, the cyclin B/p34^{cdc2} complex is inactivated by degradation of the cyclin subunit, but with the cyclin B complex, this occurs at the end of mitosis.

The demonstration that the E1A associated p60 was cyclin A provided the first direct link between known cell cycle regulatory proteins and oncoproteins. The connection relies on physical interaction, although, as discussed below, the exact architecture of these interactions is still not fully understood. In the initial characterization of human cyclin A, Pines and Hunter (1990) reported that cyclin A bound to a 33 000 dalton protein (p33) that appeared to be related to but different from the p34^{cdc2} kinase. Giordano *et al* (1991a) also characterized an approximately 33 000 dalton protein that they showed was found in E1A immunoprecipitations. At this time, the exact origin of p33 was not clear. Work by Faha *et al* (unpublished) gave the first detailed characterization of this protein and its association with cyclin A. Using monoclonal antibodies specific for cyclin A, they were able to show that cyclin A immunoprecipitations contained both authentic p34^{cdc2} and p33. p33 was shown to be structurally related to p34^{cdc2}, but these proteins were clearly distinct. As demonstrated originally by Giordano *et al* (1991a), the p33 protein was found in E1A complexes; however, no evidence for p34^{cdc2} binding to E1A has been established.

To characterize p33 further, we set about to clone its cDNA. Using a polymerase chain reaction protocol (Lehner and O'Farrell, 1990), a number of human cdc2 related clones have been isolated (Meyerson *et al*, 1991; Pines and Hunter, 1991; Tsai *et al*, 1991). Eight novel genes encoding members of this family of kinases have been isolated to date. One of these genes, the human cyclin dependent kinase 2 (*cdk2*) gene, encodes p33. The *cdk2* gene is the human homologue of a previously isolated *Xenopus* clone, Eg-1 (Paris *et al*, 1991), that has been implicated in the regulation of entry into S phase of the cell cycle in *Xenopus* (Fang and Newport, 1991). The cloning of this gene confirms that cyclin A binds to more than one kinase subunit. As p34^{cdc2} and p33^{cdk2} share extensive sequence homology (approximately 65% identity), it is often assumed that both of these kinases have related roles in the cell. The demonstration that one cyclin can bind to more than one kinase suggests strongly that combinatorial regulation is important in controlling cell cycle progression. Vertebrates have multiple cyclins and multiple kinases that appear to be able to form a variety of complexes in cells. Presumably, the different complexes are used to respond to different environmental stimuli and to dictate cell cycle progression. Although the mere discovery of different complexes does not demand that these complexes have different functions, the observation that E1A binds only to one of the cyclin A/kinase complexes suggests strongly that these kinases will have different roles in the cell.

Cyclin A Binds to Other Cellular Proteins, Including p107

During the analysis of the cyclin A associated kinases, we found that cyclin A also associated with other proteins, one of which has now been identified as p107 (Ewen *et al*, in press; Faha *et al*, in press). This complex was observed in cells that do not contain E1A, so it appears that cyclin A associates with p107 without the need of E1A as an intermediate. This independence was confirmed by mapping studies that showed that cyclin A binds to a different region of p107 than E1A and T antigen (Ewen *et al*, in press). These findings have important repercussions on the mechanism of cyclin A's association with E1A. Now, it is not necessary to postulate that E1A binds directly to cyclin A; instead, cyclin A may be found in E1A complexes only through its interaction with p107. If these suggestions prove to be true, these observations present a confusing question. What is the physiological significance of the p107/cyclin A association? Will a kinase also be found in this complex and the association just represents a stable enzyme-substrate interaction? Or is this an example of how a cyclin targets a key substrate? An alternative possibility is that the association is a novel function of cyclin A that is independent of its role as a regulator of kinases. As a first step, we need to learn in more precise detail how this complex is formed in vivo, how many proteins are present, and the identities of the individual components.

OTHER E1A ASSOCIATED PROTEINS

Considerably less is known about the other polypeptides that associate with E1A. The binding sites of p300 and p130 have been mapped and are located in or overlap with the transforming regions of E1A. These proteins therefore represent excellent candidates for cellular targets of E1A action. The remaining polypeptides, p90, p80, p50 and p28, are difficult to detect by immunoprecipitation and are apparently minor components of the E1A complexes, at least as judged by signal intensity using metabolically labelled cells. In the absence of any reagents to these proteins, it has been impossible to gauge the significance of the interactions of p90, p80, p50, p40 and p28 with E1A.

p300

The binding site of p300 maps to the extreme aminoterminus of E1A (Egan *et al*, 1988; Howe *et al*, 1990; Whyte *et al*, 1989), but the minimal sequences required for binding vary depending on the experimental procedures used. Using bacterially expressed E1A fusion proteins, aminoacids 1–49 are sufficient for association (Lee M-H, unpublished). Genetic studies have shown that this region of E1A is important for several of its activities, including stimulation of cellular DNA synthesis in quiescent cells (Lillie *et al*, 1987; Zerler *et al*, 1987; Moran and Zerler, 1988; Howe *et al*, 1990; Stein *et al*, 1990), immortalization (Quinlan *et al*, 1988; Subramanian *et al*, 1988), transformation (Lillie *et al*, 1986; Moran *et al*, 1986; Schneider *et al*, 1987; Smith and Ziff, 1988; Subramanian *et al*, 1988; Whyte *et al*, 1988b; Jelsma *et al*, 1989) and transcriptional repression of several cellular and viral genes (Schneider *et al*, 1987; Subramanian *et al*, 1988; Velcich and Ziff, 1988; Jelsma *et al*, 1989; Stein *et al*, 1990). Where tested with mutants of E1A, many of these activities have been found to correspond with the ability of the E1A to bind to p300. Hence, p300 has become a good candidate for a cellular protein that is instrumental in at least some stage of these E1A induced changes.

p300 is a nuclear phosphoprotein that is ubiquitously expressed in all types of human cells tested to date. Homologues of p300 probably exist in many species, since similarly sized E1A associated proteins are detected in experiments using mouse, rat, cow and frog cells (Hu Q, Lee M-H and Harlow E, unpublished). Low percentage polyacrylamide gels resolve p300 into at least two distinct forms. In addition to their mobility differences, these forms yield different, but related patterns after cleavage with *S aureus* V8 protease (Dyson N and Harlow E, unpublished). These two forms show slightly different binding properties when tested with a panel of E1A deletion mutants (Dyson N and Harlow E, unpublished). It is unclear whether these different forms of p300 are differentially modified proteins synthesized from a single gene or whether these are the products of a family of related genes. Similarly, it is unclear whether the polypeptides are functionally distinct.

In addition to binding to E1A, p300 also associates with SV40 large T antigen (Morgan J, Ludlow JW, Modjtahedi N, Livingston DM, Harlow E and

Dyson N, unpublished). A variety of experimental approaches have been used to locate the region of T antigen that is involved in binding. These experiments have shown that the small domain of SV40 large T that provides contact with pRB and p107 is essential for large T transforming activity. This segment also contributes to p300 binding. This result was surprising since the sequences of E1A that are homologous to this portion of SV40 T are dispensable for the association of E1A with p300. As p300 shares overlapping binding sites on E1A with pRB and on SV40 T with pRB and p107, it seems possible that these proteins might contain elements of structural similarity at least within their E1A binding regions. Consistent with this idea, Hu *et al* (1991) have characterized an anti-pRB monoclonal antibody, XZ77, which cross reacts with p300.

Although the studies of p300 are in the earliest stages, these investigations promise to provide important new information about the function of E1A. Mutants of E1A that fail to interact with p300 have a much reduced or absent ability to act as oncogenes, as well as having lost the ability to repress transcription from various test promoters. Therefore, the identity of p300 will likely tell us important information about the function of E1A, as well as provide new insights into key cellular controls.

p130

The E1A associated p130 possesses several features that are similar to those of pRB and p107. As shown by binding to E1A mutants (Giordano *et al*, 1991b) and by peptide binding or competition (Dyson N and Harlow E, unpublished), the regions of E1A that provide association with pRB closely map to the binding regions of p130. Synthetic peptides containing these regions of E1A or homologous sequences of SV40 large T or HPV-16 E7 also block E1A-p130 binding, suggesting that association with p130 may also be conserved between these viral oncoproteins.

p130 is one of the E1A associated proteins which are less easily detected in immunoprecipitations and as a result, p130 has been poorly studied. Low percentage gels resolve p130 into two forms, one of which is heavily phosphorylated. It is unclear whether this modification is cell cycle regulated. Like p107, p130 is an excellent substrate for a kinase present in immunoprecipitations of E1A-protein complexes (Herrmann *et al*, 1991), but it is not known whether p130 also associates with cyclin A.

CURRENT (AND FUTURE) AFFAIRS

Although the analysis of the adenovirus E1A proteins and their interactions with cellular proteins is rapidly advancing, it is clear that major questions still exist. To discuss these questions, we have divided these concerns into two groups: a consideration of the physical structure of the complexes and of models that might explain their functions.

The Architecture of the E1A Complexes

Missing in our knowledge of the E1A complexes is a detailed understanding of the architecture of these interactions. Although for some protein-protein interactions, this information would be important primarily for the mechanics of the physical associations, for the E1A complexes, identifying the directly interacting proteins is essential to determine how E1A perturbs these systems. Only by knowing how E1A interacts with these complicated multicomponent systems can we understand how E1A mediates change.

When the E1A complexes were first identified, it was unclear whether the associated proteins bound independently or in multimeric complexes. In the absence of any experimental data, the simplest way of thinking of the associated proteins was as molecules that were individually targeted by E1A. However, information from studies of E1A associated proteins shows that several of these proteins interact with one another while executing their normal functions. Protein complexes between pRB and $p34^{cdc2}$, p107 and cyclin A, and cyclin A and $p33^{cdk2}$ are readily apparent in immunoprecipitations of labelled cell lysates, even in the absence of E1A. A weaker or less prevalent interaction between pRB and cyclin A has also been detected. Therefore, to understand how E1A effects its changes, we need to know how E1A interacts with the targets and how the targets interact with one another.

It appears likely that E1A affects the function of its targets by physical interaction. The discovery of additional interactions between E1A associated proteins highlights the importance of discriminating between cellular proteins that are directly targeted by E1A and those that are indirectly associated. The proteins that are bound indirectly may be important in determining the purpose of the association, but characterization of the function of the direct targets will be of primary importance.

At present, it is still unclear how many of the E1A associated proteins are direct targets. Many of the proteins are not yet available in the required purity and abundance to test for direct interaction. However, a number of arguments allow good guesses to be made about authentic E1A targets. The earliest evidence came from analysis of the binding properties of various E1A mutants. One of the easiest proteins to study in this way is p107, since most of E1A is not required for p107 association. E1A mutants that can synthesize only the carboxyterminal residues beginning at residue 120 are able to bind to p107. These mutants do not bind to any of the other E1A associated proteins and also establish the aminoterminal boundary of the minimal p107 binding region (see above). Since no other proteins are found in these immunoprecipitations, it is fair to assume that p107 interacts directly with E1A. Similar arguments can be made for p300. Here, sequences at the extreme aminoterminus are all that is needed for interaction with p300. None of the other E1A associated proteins require the same sequences for interaction, and mutations in the aminoterminal sequence do not change the interactions with the other cellular proteins yet no longer bind to p300. Since no other proteins have similar binding sequences nor respond in similar ways to certain mutations, it appears that p300 must bind directly. The conclusion that p107 and p300 bind directly to E1A is supported by experiments with bifunctional cross linkers which show that 107 kDa and 300 kDa proteins can be cross linked to E1A (Galvin K, unpublished). However, although it seems likely that p300 and p107 bind directly to E1A, we cannot exclude the possibilities that there are low molecular weight molecules or molecules without methionine residues that mediate or stabilize their association with E1A.

Although pRB uses sequences for interaction that are similar to those used by other E1A associated proteins, the availability of a good panel of antibodies for pRB first indicated that it is directly bound by E1A. These antibodies immunoprecipitate pRB and its associated E1A molecules, but none of the other E1A associated proteins were detected in the immune complexes. These immunoprecipitations remove all of the pRB from these lysates, and there is no evidence for forms or complexes of pRB that are sterically hindered from precipitation. More recently, it has been shown that synthetic E7 and E1A peptides bind to purified fragments of pRB expressed in bacteria (Jones *et al*, 1990). Since p107 and pRB show sequence homology in their domains that interact with E1A and large T interaction, it is consistent that both proteins are targeted directly by the viral proteins. A general conclusion that pRB, p107 and p300 all bind directly to E1A is supported by the observations that they share elements of structural homology that are revealed either by sequence comparisons or by the characterization of cross reacting antibodies (Ewen *et al*, 1991; Hu *et al*, 1991.

There is no evidence to date to show that E1A binds directly to cyclin A. For example, an E1A-cyclin A complex could not be detected after mixing cell lysates from insect cells after infection with baculovirus constructs expressing cyclin A and E1A, even though both proteins were shown to be active in other assays (Tsai LT and Faha B, unpublished). Conversely, results from several different approaches provide a considerable quantity of circumstantial data to suggest that the association is indirect. As has been described, p107 and cyclin A form stable complexes in the absence of E1A, raising the possibility that cyclin A does not bind directly to E1A. In addition, the binding sites for cyclin A on E1A overlap with the regions needed for pRB and p107 to bind. Mutants of E1A have been described that bind to p107 but fail to associate with cyclin A, but all of the mutants that were shown to bind to cyclin A also bind to p107 (Whyte *et al*, 1989; Giordano *et al*, 1991b). Ewen *et al* (in press) mapped the regions of p107 that are needed for interaction with E1A and cyclin A, and found that they were different, suggesting that E1A and cyclin A could bind to the same molecule of p107. Comparison of the aminoacid sequences of pRB and p107 reveals strong sequence similarities between the domains of pRB and p107 that bind directly to E1A (Ewen *et al*, in press, a), but these regions have no significant homology with the domain of cyclin A that is necessary for E1A association (Lees E, unpublished). At present, it seems more likely that cyclin A is associated with E1A through p107 and/or p130.

There are several reasons for speculating that p33^{cdk2} is also only indirectly associated with E1A. p33^{cdk2} is stably associated with cyclin A in the presence or absence of E1A. Analysis of E1A mutants reveals a perfect correlation between association of E1A with p33 (Giordano *et al*, 1991a), with histone kinase activity (Herrmann *et al*, 1991), and association with cyclin A (Giordano *et al*, 1991b). Furthermore, the sequence of p33^{cdk2} has no significant homology with the domains of pRB or p107 that bind to E1A. Neither does E1A appear to be a substrate for p33^{cdk2} . In in vitro kinase reactions performed on E1A immune complexes, two E1A associated proteins, p107 and p130, are excellent substrates for an E1A associated kinase, whereas E1A is only weakly phosphorylated. Little is known about the architecture of E1A's interaction with the less easily detected proteins that are found in E1A immunoprecipitations.

Models and Questions

The available information about the E1A associated proteins and their functions has allowed the establishment of the first models to explain E1A's action in cells. The clues to these early models come from the analysis of pRB. pRB is thought to regulate negatively some aspect of cell proliferation, since loss of pRB function leads to deregulated cell growth in a number of cell types. The simplest model to explain E1A's direct association with pRB is that physical association with E1A causes an inhibition of pRB's normal function. How might this inhibition occur? To understand this, we need to know how pRB normally effects its control of cell growth. What are the downstream targets of pRB? In the past year, several candidates have been suggested. The clearest picture of how pRB may act comes from the suggestion that pRB functions in normal cells to regulate the action of the transcription factor E2F. E2F associates with pRB in high molecular weight complexes in the absence of E1A. When E1A is present, either added to in vitro preparations or expressed in vivo, the pRB/E2F complex is disrupted, releasing free E2F. In the recently proposed model (Bandara and La Thangue, 1991; Chellappan *et al*, 1991), E1A causes the release of E2F by binding directly to pRB. The negative regulation of pRB is thus overcome, and "activated" E2F is then be able to stimulate the transcription of a set of genes that promote cell division.

What then are the normal controls that regulate the pRB/E2F complex? Since only unphosphorylated pRB appears able to bind to E2F (Chellappan *et al*, 1991), it seems likely that phosphorylation of pRB is a key element in the activation of E2F. Un- or underphosphorylated pRB is found only during the G_0 and G_1 phases of the cell cycle, and this is the same time for the appearance of the pRB/E2F complex. These observations then provide the first clear suggestion of a function for pRB. pRB appears to act in the negative regulation of E2F, and phosphorylation by the cell cycle regulated kinases acts to tie this regulation to the general status of the cell cycle. Although this model is appealing, it raises several new questions. Is pRB's role limited to the regulation of E2F or to transcription factors in general? And does the pRB regulate one factor at one time or are there multiple points of regulation that vary by the type of interacting protein or the particular promoter that is targeted?

At present, it is unclear whether E2F represents the sole target for pRB function. Several additional proteins have been shown to bind to pRB. These include two members of the *myc* family of oncogenes (Rustgi *et al*, 1991), several proteins known only by their molecular weight (Huang *et al*, 1991; Kaelin *et al*, 1991), and two proteins, RBP1 and RBP2, that have been cloned by their ability to bind to pRB (Defeo-Jones *et al*, 1991). Of these, only c-*myc* and N-*myc* have been studied extensively. Since c-*myc* and N-*myc* are believed to function at the level of transcriptional regulation, it is possible that pRB may function more generally to control the activities of several transcription factors. However, since so little is known about these interactions in general, it is not clear whether these proteins are authentic targets for pRB. Answering this question will go a long way to understanding whether pRB helps to regulate more than one pathway. It may be important to remember that other pathways that are regulated by pRB need not be restricted to transcriptional control, but might include any cellular process that would need to be under strict temporal control.

Whether there are one or many targets for pRB, there is still no way of determining whether all of the activities targeted by pRB occur at the same time. The interaction of pRB and E2F appears to be tightly controlled to one stage near the G_1/S boundary, but other events, either with other DNA binding proteins or with various E2F preparations, might be controlled by different timing events. Thus, although the original E2F/pRB interaction suggests one specific change that may be regulated at one time in the cell cycle, other possible regulatory schedules must be still considered.

By analogy with pRB, can we expect all of the proteins that are targeted by the transforming regions of E1A to be regulators of transcription factors, and the mode of E1A's action to be sequestration? Two major problems hinder answering this question. Firstly, very little is known about several of these targets, and as all models are still possible, it may be a mistake to categorize these targets into models based on information about pRB. Secondly, the analogy to pRB seems less likely for proteins that are indirectly associated with E1A. Here, the effects of E1A association may be subtle and important or may be irrelevant.

Of all the E1A associated proteins, the most likely to follow the pRB paradigm is p107. The striking sequence similarity between pRB and p107 argues strongly that their biochemical activities may be related. Recent evidence indicates that p107 like pRB is associated with E2F in an E2F complex that also contains cyclin A (Cao L, Faha B, Dembski M, Tsai L-H, Harlow E and Dyson N, unpublished) and is dissociated by E1A (Chellappan *et al*, 1991; Mudryj *et al*, 1991). However, a number of observations suggest that the functions of pRB and p107 may be quite distinct. pRB and p107 are associated with E2F complexes that appear to arise at different stages of the cell cycle (Chellappan *et al*, 1991; Mudryj *et al*, 1991). Furthermore, the p107/E2F complex contains cyclin A (Cao L, Faha B, Dembski M, Tsai L-H, Harlow E and Dyson N, unpublished), and although the significance of this association is not known, the fact that cyclin A is not detected in pRB/E2F may be an important difference between these complexes.

SUMMARY

Studies of E1A support the notion that small DNA tumour viruses target cellular pathways at key points that are amenable to regulation. In the case of E1A, these targets appear to be points of control of cellular proliferation and, in particular, proteins that regulate the progression of cells from G_0 and G_1 phases of the cell cycle into the S phase. In several cases, recent studies have identified complexes between the viral targets and other cellular proteins. These interactions may provide insight not only into the mechanism of E1A mediated transformation but also into the control of proliferation in normal cells.

Acknowledgements

We thank our colleagues at the Massachusetts General Hospital Cancer Center for vigorous discussions. In particular, we thank Liang Cao, Barbara Faha, Katherine Galvin, Ali Fattaey, Kristian Helin, Myung Ho Lee, Emma Lees, Jacqueline Lees, Matthew Meyerson, Steven Schiff, Li Huei Tsai, Chin Lee Wu and Liang Zhu for permission to quote unpublished work and for critical reading of the manuscript. This work was funded by the Massachusetts General Hospital Cancer Center and grants from the National Institutes of Health.

References

Abramson DH, Ellsworth RM and Zimmerman LE (1976) Nonocular cancer in retinoblastoma survivors. *Transactions of the American Academy of Ophthalmology* **81** 454–457

Bagchi S, Raychaudhuri P and Nevins J (1990) Adenovirus E1A proteins can dissociate heteromeric complexes involving the E2F transcription factor: a novel mechanism for E1A trans-activation. *Cell* **62** 659–669

Bagchi S, Weinmann R and Raychaudhuri P (1991) The retinoblastoma protein copurifies with E2F-I, an E1A-regulated inhibitor of the transcription factor E2F. *Cell* **65** 1063–1072

Bandara LR and La Thangue NB (1991) Adenovirus E1a prevents the retinoblastoma gene product from complexing with a cellular transcription factor. *Nature* **351** 494–497

Bandara L, Adamczewski J, Hunt T and La Thangue N (1991) Cyclin A and the retinoblastoma gene product complex with a common transcription factor. *Nature* **352** 249–251

Berk AJ (1986) Adenovirus promoters and E1A transactivation. *Annual Review of Genetics* **20** 45–79

Berk AJ and Sharp PA (1978) Structure of the adenovirus 2 early mRNAs. *Cell* **14** 695–711

Buchkovich K, Duffy LA and Harlow E (1989) The retinoblastoma protein is phosphorylated during specific phases of the cell cycle. *Cell* **58** 1097–1105

Carlock LR and Jones NC (1981) Transformation-defective mutant of adenovirus type 5 containing single altered E1a mRNA species. *Journal of Virology* **40** 657–664

Cawthon RM, Weiss R, Xu G *et al* (1990) A major segment of the neurofibromatosis type 1 gene: cDNA sequence, genomic structure, and point nutations. *Cell* **62** 192–201

Chellappan S, Hiebert S, Mudryj M, Horowitz J and Nevins J (1991) The E2F transcription factor is a cellular target for the RB protein. *Cell* **65** 1053–1061

Chen P-L, Scully P, Shew J-Y, Wang J and Lee W-H (1989) Phosphorylation of the retinoblastoma gene product is modulated during the cell cycle and cellular differentiation. *Cell* **58** 1193–1198

Chen YC, Chen PJ, Yeh SH *et al* (1990) Deletion of the human retinoblastoma gene in primary leukemias. *Blood* **76** 2060–2064

Cheng J, Scully P, Shew JY, Lee WH, Vila V and Haas M (1990) Homozygous deletion of the retinoblastoma gene in an acute lymphoblastic leukemia (T) cell line. *Blood* **75** 730–735

Chittenden T, Livingston D and Kaelin W (1991) The T/E1A-binding domain of the retinoblastoma product can interact selectively with a sequence-specific DNA-binding protein. *Cell* **65** 1073–1082

Chow LT, Broker TR and Lewis JB (1979) Complex splicing patterns of RNAs from the early regions of adenovirus-2. *Journal of Molecular Biology* **134** 265–303

Cone RD, Grodzicker T and Jaramillo M (1988) A retrovirus expressing the 12S adenoviral E1A gene product can immortalize epithelial cells from a broad range of rat tissues. *Molecular and Cellular Biology* **8** 1036–1044

Cullen JW (1991) Second malignant neoplasms in survivors of childhood cancer. *Pediatrician* **18** 82–89

DeCaprio JA, Ludlow JW, Figge J *et al* (1988) SV40 large tumor antigen forms a specific complex with the product of the retinoblastoma susceptibility gene. *Cell* **54** 275–283

DeCaprio JA, Ludlow JW, Lynch D *et al* (1989) The product of the retinoblastoma susceptibility gene has properties of a cell cycle regulatory element. *Cell* **58** 1085–1095

Defeo-Jones D, Huang PS, Jones RE *et al* (1991) Cloning of cDNAs for cellular proteins that bind to the retinoblastoma gene product. *Nature* **352** 251–254

Dunn JM, Phillips RA, Becker AJ and Gallie BL (1988) Identification of germline and somatic mutations affecting the retinoblastoma gene. *Science* **241** 1797–1800

Dunn JM, Phillips RA, Zhu X, Becker A and Gallie BL (1989) Mutations in the RB1 gene and their effects on transcription. *Molecular and Cellular Biology* **9** 4596–4604

Dyson N, Buchkovich K, Whyte P and Harlow E (1989a) The cellular 107K protein that binds to adenovirus E1A also associates with the large T antigens of SV40 and JC virus. *Cell* **58** 249–255

Dyson N, Howley PM, Munger K and Harlow E (1989b) The human papilloma virus-16 E7 oncoprotein is able to bind to the retinoblastoma gene product. *Science* **243** 934–937

Dyson N, Bernards R, Friend SH *et al* (1990) Large T antigens of many polyomaviruses are able to form complexes with the retinoblastoma protein. *Journal of Virology* **64** 1353–1356

Egan C, Jelsma TN, Howe JA, Bayley ST, Ferguson B and Branton PE (1988) Mapping of cellular protein-binding sites on the products of early-region 1A of human adenovirus type 5. *Molecular and Cellular Biology* **8** 3955–3959

Egan C, Bayley ST and Branton PE (1989) Binding of the Rb1 protein to E1A products is required for adenovirus transformation. *Oncogene* **4** 383–388

Esche H, Mathews MB and Lewis JB (1980) Proteins and messenger RNAs of the transforming region of wild-type and mutant adenoviruses. *Journal of Molecular Biology* **142** 399–417

Ewen ME, Ludlow JW, Marsilio E *et al* (1989) An N-terminal transformation-governing sequence of SV40 large T antigen contributes to the binding of both p110Rb and a second cellular protein, p120. *Cell* **58** 257–267

Ewen M, Xing Y, J L and Livingston D (1991) Molecular cloning, chromosonal mapping, and expression of the cDNA for p107, a retinoblastome gene product-related protein. *Cell* **66** 1155–1164

Ewen M, Faha B, Harlow E and Livingston D p107 interacts with cyclin A independent of complex formation with SV40 T antigen and adenovirus E1A. *Science* (in press)

Faha B, Ewen M, Tsai L-H, Livingston D and Harlow E Association between human cyclin A and adenovirus E1A-associated p107 protein. *Science* (in press)

Fang F and Newport JW (1991) Evidence that the G1-S and G2-M transitions are controlled by different cdc2 proteins in higher eukaryotes. *Cell* **66** 731–742

Fearon ER, Cho KR, Nigro JM *et al* (1990) Identification of a chromosome 18q gene that is altered in colorectal cancers. *Science* **247** 47–56

Finlay CA, Hinds PW and Levine AJ (1989) The p53 proto-oncogene can act as a suppressor of transformation. *Cell* **57** 1083–1093

Flint J and Shenk T (1989) Adenovirus E1A protein paradigm viral transactivator. *Annual Review of Genetics* **23** 141–161

Flint SJ, Sambrook J, Williams JF and Sharp PA (1976) Viral nucleic acid sequences in transformed cells IV A study of the sequences of adenovirus 5 DNA and RNA in four lines of adenovirus 5-transformed rodent cells using specific fragments of the viral genome. *Virology* **72** 456–470

Francois J, Matton MT, DeBic J, Tanaka Y and Vandenbulker D (1976). Genesis and genetics of retinoblastoma. *Ophthalmologica* **70** 405–425

Freeman AE, Black PH, Vanderpool EA, Henry PH, Austin JB and Huebner RJ (1967) Transformation of primary rat embryo cells by adenovirus type 2. *Proceedings of the National Academy of Sciences of the USA* **58** 1205–1212

Friend SH, Bernards R, Rogelj S *et al* (1986) A human DNA segment with properties of the gene that predisposes to retinoblastoma and osteosarcoma. *Nature* **323** 643–646

Friend SH, Horowitz JM, Gerber MR *et al* (1987) Deletions of a DNA sequence in retinoblastomas and mesenchymal tumors: organization of the sequence and its encoded protein. *Proceedings of the National Academy of Sciences of the USA* **84** 9059–63 (erratum appears in *Proceedings of the National Academy of Sciences of the USA* 1988 **85** 2234

Fung YK, Murphree AL, T'Ang A, Qian J, Hinrichs SH and Benedict WF (1987) Structural evidence for the authenticity of the human retinoblastoma gene. *Science* **236** 1657–1661

Gallimore PH (1974) Viral DNA in transformed cells II A study of the sequences of adenovirus 2 DNA in nine lines of transformed rat cells using specific fragments of the viral genome. *Journal of Molecular Biology* **89** 49–72

Giordano A, Whyte P, Harlow E, Franza BR, Beach D and Draetta G (1989) A 60 kd cdc2-associated polypeptide complexes with the E1A proteins in adenovirus-infected cells. *Cell* **58** 981–990

Giordano A, Lee JH, Scheppler JA *et al* (1991a) Cell cycle regulation of histone H1 kinase activity associated with the adenoviral protein E1A. *Science* **253** 1271–1275

Giordano A, McCall C, Whyte P and Franza Jr BR (1991b) Human cyclin A and the retinoblastoma protein interact with similiar but distinguishable sequences in the adenovirus E1A gene product. *Oncogene* **6** 481–486

Glenn GM and Ricciardi RP (1985) Adenovirus 5 early region 1A host range mutants hr3, hr4, and hr5 contain point mutations which generate single amino acid substitutions. *Journal of Virology* **56** 66–74

Graham FL, Harrison T and Williams J (1978) Defective transforming capacity of adenovirus type 5 host-range mutants. *Virology* **86** 10–21

Graham FL, van der Eb AJ and Heijneker HL (1974) Size and location of the transforming region in human adenovirus type 5 DNA. *Nature* **251** 687–691

Groden J, Thliveris A, Samowitz W *et al* (1991) Identification and characterization of the familial adenomatous polyposis coli gene. *Cell* **66** 589–600

Haber DA, Buckler AJ, Glaser T *et al* (1990) An internal deletion within an 11p13 zinc finger gene contributes to the development of Wilms' tumor. *Cell* **61** 1257–1269

Haley KP, Overhauser J, Babiss LE, Ginsberg HS and Jones NC (1984) Transformation properties of type 5 adenovirus mutants that differentially express the E1A gene products. *Proceedings of the National Academy of Sciences of the USA* **81** 5734–5738

Harbour JW, Lai SL, Whang PJ, Gazdar AF, Minna JD and Kaye FJ (1988) Abnormalities in structure and expression of the human retinoblastoma gene in SCLC. *Science* **241** 353–357

Harlow E, Franza BR and Schley C (1985) Monoclonal antibodies specific for adenovirus early region 1A proteins: extensive heterogeneity in early region 1A products. *Journal of Virology* **55** 533–546

Harlow E, Whyte P, Franza BR and Schley C (1986) Association of adenovirus early-region 1A proteins with cellular polypeptides. *Molecular and Cellular Biology* **6** 1579–1589

Hensel CH, Hsieh CL, Gazdar AF *et al* (1990) Altered structure and expression of the human retinoblastoma susceptibility gene in small cell lung cancer. *Cancer Research* **50** 3067–3072

Herrmann C, Su L-K and Harlow E (1991) Adenovirus E1A is associated with a serine/threonine protein kinase. *Journal of Virology* **65** 5848–5859

Horowitz Park S-H, Yandell DW and Weinberg R (1989a) Involvement of the retinoblastoma gene in the genesis of various human tumors In: Cavenee W, Hastie N and Stanbridge E (eds). *Current Communications in Molecular Biology, Recessive Oncogenes and Tumor Suppression*, Cold Spring Harbor Laboratory Press, New York

Horowitz JM, Yandell DW, Park SH *et al* (1989b) Point mutational inactivation of the retinoblastoma antioncogene. *Science* **243** 937–940

Horowitz JM, Park SH, Bogenmann E *et al* (1990) Frequent inactivation of the retinoblastoma anti-oncogene is restricted to a subset of human tumor cells. *Proceedings of the National Academy of Sciences of the USA* **87** 2775–2779

Houweling A, van den Elsen P and van der Eb AJ (1980) Partial transformation of primary rat cells by the leftmost 4.5% fragment of adenovirus 5 DNA. *Virology* **105** 537–550

Howe JA, Mymryk JS, Egan C, Branton PE and Bayley ST (1990) Retinoblastoma growth suppressor and a 300-kDa protein appear to regulate cellular DNA synthesis. *Proceedings of the National Academy of Sciences of the USA* **87** 5883–5887

Hu QJ, Dyson N and Harlow E (1990) The regions of the retinoblastoma protein needed for binding to adenovirus E1A or SV40 large T antigen are common sites for mutations. *EMBO Journal* **9** 1147–1155

Hu Q, Bautista C, Edwards G, Defeo-Jones D, Jones R and Harlow E (1991) Antibodies specific for the human retinoblastoma protein identify a family of related polypepides. *Molecular and Cellular Biology* **11** 5792–5799

Hu Q, Lees J, Buchkovich K and Harlow E The retinoblastoma protein physically associates with the human cdc2 kinase. *Molecular and Cellular Biology* (in press)

Huang S, Wang NP, Tseng BY, Lee WH and Lee EH (1990) Two distinct and frequently mutated regions of retinoblastoma protein are required for binding to SV40 T antigen. *EMBO Journal* **9** 1815–1822

Huang S, Lee W-H and Lee EY-H (1991) A cellular protein that competes with SV40 T antigen for binding to the retinoblastoma gene product. *Nature* **350** 160–162

Hunter T and Pines J (1991) Cyclins and cancer. *Cell* **66** 1071–1074

Jelsma TN, Howe JA, Mymryk JS, Evelegh CM, Cunniff NF and Bayley ST (1989) Sequences in E1A proteins of human adenovirus 5 required for cell transformation, repression of a transcriptional enhancer, and induction of proliferating cell nuclear antigen. *Virology* **171** 120–130

Jones RE, Wegrzyn RJ, Patrick DR *et al* (1990) Identification of HPV-16 E7 peptides that are potent antagonists of E7 binding to the retinoblastoma suppressor protein. *Journal of Biological Chemistry* **265** 12782–12785

Joslyn G, Carlson M, Thliveris A *et al* (1991) Identification of deletion mutations and three new genes at the familial polyposis locus. *Cell* **66** 601–613

Kaelin WJ, Ewen ME and Livingston DM (1990) Definition of the minimal simian virus 40 large T antigen- and adenovirus E1A-binding domain in the retinoblastoma gene product. *Molecular and Cellular Biology* **10** 3761–3769

Kaelin WG, Pallas DC, DeCaprio JA, Kaye FJ and Livingstone DM (1991) Identification of cellular proteins that can interact specifically with the T/E1A-binding region of the retinoblastoma gene product. *Cell* **64** 521–532

Kimelman D, Miller JS, Porter D and Roberts BE (1985) E1a regions of the human adenoviruses and of the highly oncogenic simian adenovirus 7 are closely related. *Journal of Virology* **53** 399–409

Kinzler KW, Nilbert MC, Su L-K *et al* (1991) Identification of FAP locus genes from chromosome 5q21. *Science* **253** 661–665

Kitchingman GR and Westphal H (1980) The structure of adenovirus 2 early nuclear and cytoplasmic RNAs. *Journal of Molecular Biology* **137** 23–48

Knipe DM (1989) The role of viral and cellular nuclear proteins in herpes simplex virus replication. *Advances in Virus Research* **37** 85–123

Knudson AG (1971) Mutation and cancer: statistical study of retinoblastoma. *Proceedings of the National Academy of Sciences of the USA* **68** 820–823

Knudson A (1975) The genetics of childhood cancer. *Cancer* **35** 1022–1026

Knudson AG (1987) A two-mutation model for human cancer. *Advances in Viral Oncology* **7** 1–17

Kovesdi I, Reichel R and Nevins JR (1986) Identification of a cellular transcription factor involved in E1A trans-activation. *Cell* **45** 219–228

Land H, Parada LF and Weinberg RA (1983) Tumorigenic conversion of primary embryo fibroblasts requires at least two cooperating oncogenes. *Nature* **304** 596–602

Lee EY, To H, Shew JY, Bookstein R, Scully P and Lee WH (1988) Inactivation of the retinoblastoma susceptibility gene in human breast cancers. *Science* **241** 218–221

Lee WH, Shew JY, Hong FD *et al* (1987) The retinoblastoma susceptibility gene encodes a nuclear phosphoprotein associated with DNA binding activity. *Nature* **329** 642–645

Lee WS, Kao CC, Byrant GO, Liu X and Berk AJ (1991) Adenovirus E1A activation domain binds the basic repeat in the TATA box transcription factor. *Cell* **67** 365–376

Lees JA, Buchkovich KJ, Marshak DR, Anderson CW and Harlow E (1991) The retinoblastoma protein is phosphorylated on multiple sites by human cdc2. *EMBO Journal* **10** 4279–4289

Lehner CF and O'Farrell PH (1990) The roles of Drosophila cyclins A and B in mitotic control. *Cell* **61** 535–547

Lewis JB and Mathews MB (1980) Control of adenovirus early gene expression: a class of immediate early products. *Cell* **21** 303–313

Lillie JW and Green MR (1989) Transcription activation by the adenovirus E1A protein. *Nature* **338** 39–44

Lillie JW, Green M and Green MR (1986) An adenovirus E1a protein region required for transformation and transcriptional repression. *Cell* **46** 1043–1051

Lillie JW, Loewenstein PM, Green MR and Green M (1987) Functional domains of adenovirus type 5 E1a proteins. *Cell* **50** 1091–1100

Lin BT-Y, Gruenwald S, Morla AO, Lee W-H and Wang JYJ (1991) Retinoblastoma cancer suppressor gene product is a substrate of the cell cycle regulator cdc2 kinase. *EMBO Journal* **10** 857–864

Liu F and Green MR (1990) A specific member of the ATF transcription factor family can mediate transcription activation by the adenovirus E1a protein. *Cell* **61** 1217–1224

Ludlow JW, DeCaprio JA, Huang CM, Lee WH, Paucha E and Livingston DM (1989) SV40 large T antigen binds preferentially to an underphosphorylated member of the retinoblastoma susceptibility gene product family. *Cell* **56** 57–65

Ludlow JW, Shon J, Pipas JM, Livingston DM and DeCaprio JA (1990) The retinoblastoma susceptibility gene product undergoes cell cycle-dependent dephosphorylation and binding to and release from SV40 large T. *Cell* **60** 387–396

Matsunaga E (1976) Hereditary retinoblastoma; penetrance, expressivity and age of onset. *Human Genetics* **33** 1–15

Mihara K, Cao XR, Yen A *et al* (1989) Cell cycle-dependent regulation of phosphorylation of the human retinoblastoma gene product. *Science* **246** 1300–1303

Montell C, Fisher EF, Caruthers MH and Berk AJ (1982) Resolving the functions of overlapping viral genes by site-specific mutagenesis at a mRNA splice site. *Nature* **295** 380–384

Moran E and Mathews MB (1987) Multiple functional domains in the adenovirus E1A gene. *Cell* **48** 177–178

Moran E and Zerler B (1988) Interactions between cell growth-regulating domains in the products of the adenovirus E1A oncogene. *Molecular and Cellular Biology* **8** 1756–1764

Moran E, Grodzicker T, Roberts RJ, Mathews MB and Zerler B (1986a) Lytic and transforming functions of individual products of the adenovirus E1A gene. *Journal of Virology* **57** 765–775

Moran E, Zerler B, Harrison TM and Mathews MB (1986b) Identification of separate domains in the adenovirus E1A gene for immortalization activity and the activation of virus early genes. *Molecular and Cellular Biology* **6** 3470–3480

Moss B (1985) Replication of the poxviruses. 68–703

Mudryj M, Hiebert SW and Nevins JR (1990) A role for the adenovirus inducible E2F transcription factor in a proliferation dependent signal transduction pathway. *EMBO Journal* **9** 2179–2184

Mudryj M, Devoto S, Hiebert S, Hunter T, Pines J and Nevins J (1991) Cell cycle regulation of the E2F transcription factor involves an interaction with cyclin A. *Cell* **65** 1243–1253

Munger K, Werness BA, Dyson N, Phelps WC, Harlow E and Howley PM (1989) Complex formation of human papillomavirus E7 proteins with the retinoblastoma tumor suppressor gene product. *EMBO Journal* **8** 4099–4105

Nevins JR (1981) Mechanism of activation of early viral transcription by the adenovirus E1A gene product. *Cell*

Nishisho I, Nakamura Y, Miyoshi Y *et al* (1991) Mutations of chromosome 5q21 genes in FAP and colorectal cancer patients. *Science* **253** 665–669

Paris J, Guellec R, Couturier A *et al* (1991) Cloning by differential screening of a Xenopus cDNA coding for a protein highly homologous to cdc2. *Proceedings National Academy of Sciences of the USA* **88** 1039–1043

Perricaudet M, Akusjarvi G, Virtanen A and Pettersson U (1979) Structure of two spliced mRNAs from the transforming region of human subgroup C adenoviruses. *Nature* **281** 694–696

Pines J and Hunter T (1990) Human cyclin A is adenovirus E1A-associated protein p60 and behaves differently from cyclin B. *Nature* **346** 760–763

Pines J and Hunter T (1991) The Cell Cycle. *Cold Spring Harbor Symposia on Quantitative Biology* **56** 449–463

Quinlan MP, Whyte P and Grosdzicker T (1988) Growth factor induction by the adenovirus type 5 E1A 12S protein is required for immortalization of primary epithelial cells. *Molecular and Cellular Biology*

Raychaudhuri P, Bagchi S, Neill S and Nevins JR (1990) Activation of the E2F transcription factor in adenovirus infected cells involves an E1A-dependent stimulation of DNA binding activity and induction of cooperative binding mediated by an E4 gene product. *Journal of Virology* **64** 2702–2710

Raychaudhuri P, Bagchi S, Devoto SH, Kraus VB, Moran E and Nevins JR (1991) Domains of the adenovirus E1A protein that are required for oncogenic activity are also required for dissociation of E2F transcription factor complexes. *Genes and Development* **5** 1200–1211

Ricciardi RP, Jones RL, Cepko CL, Sharp PA and Roberts BE (1981) Expression of early adenovirus genes requires a viral encoded acidic polypeptide. *Proceedings of the National Academy of Sciences of the USA* **78** 6121–6125

Ruley HE (1983) Adenovirus early region 1A enables viral and cellular transforming genes to transform primary cells in culture. *Nature* **304** 602–606

Rustgi AK, Dyson NJ and Bernards R (1991) Amino-terminal domains of c-*myc* and N-*myc* proteins mediate binding to the retinoblastoma gene product. *Nature* **352** 541–544

Scheffner M, Munger K, Byrne JC and Howley PM (1991) The state of the p53 and retinoblastoma genes in human cervical carcinoma cell lines. *Proceedings of the National*

Academy of Sciences of the USA **88** 5523–5527

Schneider JF, Fisher F, Goding CR and Jones NC (1987) Mutational analysis of the adenovirus E1a gene: the role of transcriptional regulation in transformation. *EMBO Journal* **6** 2053–2060

Schöler HR, Ciesiolka T and Fruss P (1991) A nexus between Oct-4 and E1A: implications for gene regulation in embryonic stem cells. *Cell* **66** 291–304

Scholz RB, Kabisch H, Delling G and Winkler K (1990) Homozygous deletion within the retinoblastoma gene in a native osteosarcoma specimen of a patient cured of a retinoblastoma of both eyes. *Pediatric Hematology and Oncology* **7** 265–273

Shew JY, Lin BT, Chen PL, Tseng BY, Yang FT and Lee WH (1990) C-terminal truncation of the retinoblastoma gene product leads to functional inactivation. *Proceedings National Academy of Sciences of the USA* **87** 6–10

Smith DH and Ziff EB (1988) The amino-terminal region of the adenovirus serotype 5 E1a protein performs two separate functions when expressed in primary baby rat kidney cells. *Molecular and Cellular Biology* **8** 3882–3890

Stein RW, Corrigan M, Yaciuk P, Whelan J and Moran E (1990) Analysis of E1A mediated growth regulation functions: binding of the 300kDa cellular product correlates with E1A enhancer repression function and DNA systhesis inducing activity. *Journal of Virology* **64** 4421–4427

Stephens C and Harlow E (1987) Differential splicing yealds novel adenovirus 5 E1A mRNAs that encode 30 kd and 35 kd proteins. *EMBO Journal* **6** 2027–2035

Stephens C, Franza BR, Schley C and Harlow E (1986) Heterogeneity of adenovirus E1a proteins is due to post-translational modification of the primary translation products of the 12s and 13s mRNAs. *Cancer Cells* **4** 429–434

Subramanian T, Kuppuswamy M, Nasr RJ and Chinnadurai G (1988) An N-terminal region of adenovirus E1a essential for cell transformation and induction of an epithelial cell growth factor. *Oncogene* **2** 105–112

T'Ang A, Varley JM, Chakraborty S, Murphree AL and Fung YK (1988) Structural rearrangement of the retinoblastoma gene in human breast carcinoma. *Science* **242** 263–266

Toguchida J, Ishizaki K, Sasaki MS *et al* (1989) Preferential mutation of paternally derived RB gene as the initial event in sporadic osteosarcoma. *Nature* **338** 156–158

Tremblay ML, McGlade CJ, Gerber GE and Branton PE (1988) Identification of the phosphorylation sites in early region 1A proteins of adenovirus type 5 by amino acid sequencing of peptide fragments. *Journal of Biological Chemistry* **263** 6375–6383

Trentin JJ, Yabe Y and Taylor G (1962) The quest for human cancer viruses. *Science* **137** 835–841

Tsai L, Harlow E and Meyerson M (1991) Isolation of the human cdk2 gene that encodes the cyclin A- and adenovirus E1A-associated p33 kinase. *Nature* **353** 174–177

Tsukamoto AS, Ponticelli A, Berk AJ and Gaynor RB (1986) Genetic mapping of a major site of phosphorylation in adenovirus type 2 E1A proteins. *Journal of Virology* **59** 14–22

Ulfendahl PJ, Linder S, Kreivi JP *et al* (1987) A novel adenovirus-2 E1A mRNA encoding a protein with transcription activation properties. *EMBO Journal* **6** 2037–2044

van den Elsen P, de Pater S, Houweling A, van der Veer J van der Eb AJ (1982) The relationship between region E1a and E1b of human adenoviruses in cell transformation. *Gene* **18** 175–85

van den Elsen P, Houweling A and van der Eb AJ (1983) Expression of region E1b of human adenoviruses in the absence of region E1a is not sufficient for complete transformation. *Virology* **128** 377–390

van der Eb AJ, van Ormondt H, Schrier PI *et al* (1979) Structure and function of the transforming genes of human adenoviruses and SV40. *Cold Spring Harbor Symposia on Quantitative Biology* **44** 383–399

van Ormondt H, Maat J and Dijkema R (1980) Comparison of nucleotide sequences of the early E1a regions for subgroups A, B and C of human adenoviruses. *Gene* **12** 63–76

Velcich A and Ziff E (1988) Adenovirus E1a ras cooperation activity is separate from its positive and negative transcription regulatory functions. *Molecular and Cellular Biology* **8** 2177–2183

Virtanen A and Pettersson U (1983) The molecular structure of the 9S mRNA from early region 1A of adenovirus serotype 2. *Journal of Molecular Biology* **165** 496

Vogel F (1979) Genetics of retinoblastoma. *Human Genetics* **52** 1–54

Wallace MR, Marchuk DA, Anderson LB *et al* (1990) Type 1 neurofibromatosis gene: identification of a large transcript disrupted in three NF1 patients. *Nature* **249** 181–186

Whyte P, Buchkovich KJ, Horowitz JM *et al* (1988a) Association between an oncogene and an anti-oncogene: the adenovirus E1A proteins bind to the retinoblastoma gene product. *Nature* **334** 124–129

Whyte P, Ruley HE and Harlow E (1988b) Two regions of the adenovirus early region 1A proteins are required for transformation. *Journal of Virology* **62** 257–65

Whyte P, Williamson NM and Harlow E (1989) Cellular targets for transformation by the adenovirus E1A proteins. *Cell* **56** 67–75

Wittek R (1982) Organization and expression of the poxvirus genome. *Experientia* **38** 285–310

Yee AS, Raychaudhuri P, Jakoi L and Nevins JR (1989) The adenovirus-inducible factor E2F stimulates transcription after specific DNA binding. *Molecular and Cellular Biology* **9** 578–585

Yee SP and Branton PE (1985) Detection of cellular proteins associated with human adenovirus type 5 early region 1A polypeptides *Virology* **147** 142 153

Yee SP, Rowe DT, Tremblay ML, McDermott M and Branton PE (1983) Identification of human adenovirus early region 1 products by using antisera against synthetic peptides corresponding to the predicted carboxy termini. *Journal of Virology* **46** 1003–1013

Yokota J, Akiyama T, Fung YK *et al* (1988) Altered expression of the retinoblastoma (RB) gene in small-cell carcinoma of the lung. *Oncogene* **3** 471–475

Zerler B, Moran E, Maruyama K, Moomaw J, Grodzicker T and Ruley HE (1986) Adenovirus E1A coding sequences that enable ras and pmt oncogenes to transform cultured primary cells. *Molecular and Cellular Biology* **6** 887–899

Zerler B, Roberts RJ, Mathews MB and Moran E (1987) Different functional domains of the adenovirus E1A gene are involved in regulation of host cell cycle products. *Molecular and Cellular Biology* **7** 821–829

The authors are responsible for the accuracy of the references.

Interactions of HPV E6 and E7 Oncoproteins with Tumour Suppressor Gene Products

KARL MÜNGER • MARTIN SCHEFFNER • JON M HUIBREGTSE
PETER M HOWLEY

Laboratory of Tumour Virus Biology, National Cancer Institute, Bethesda, Maryland 20892

INTRODUCTION

The papillomaviruses are a group of small DNA viruses that induce benign skin lesions, including squamous warts and papillomas. These viruses have been isolated and characterized from a variety of vertebrate species including humans. More than 65 different human papillomavirus types (HPVs) have been described thus far, and a subgroup of about 20 HPVs has been associated with lesions of the anogenital tract (reviewed in DeVilliers, 1989). These HPVs can be further divided into two groups: the "low risk" HPVs, including HPV-6 and HPV-11, which are associated with lesions such as condyloma acuminata which generally remain benign, and the "high risk" HPVs such as HPV-16 and HPV-18, which are associated with lesions that can progress to cancer (zur Hausen and Schneider, 1987). Cervical intraepithelial neoplasia (CIN) is recognized as a precursor to cervical carcinoma, and about 85% of cervical

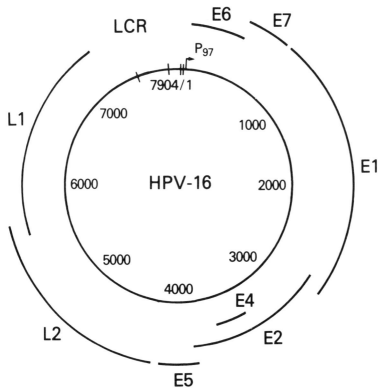

Fig. 1. Circular genomic organization of HPV-16. The early (E) and late (L) open reading frames (ORFs) are represented by the discontinuous outer arcs. The positions of the long control region (LCR) and the early viral promoter P_{97} are also indicated. Vertical marks in the LCR represent the locations of the E2 binding sites (ACCN₆GGT) in the genome

carcinomas contain HPV DNA sequences (Riou *et al*, 1990). Further evidence for an active role for HPV in the aetiology of cervical carcinogenesis is derived from studies demonstrating that the "high risk" HPVs can efficiently immortalize human squamous epithelial cells in vitro (Dürst *et al*, 1987b; Pirisi *et al*, 1987; Kaur and McDougall, 1988; Schlegel *et al*, 1988). The viral genomes are double stranded circular DNA molecules of about 8000 base pairs. All of the major open reading frames (ORFs) are located on one strand, and hybridization studies have shown that the viral mRNA species in productively infected cells correspond to that strand of the viral genome. In addition to the coding region, the papillomavirus genomes contain a 1 kbp region with no extensive coding potential. Since this region contains numerous *cis* elements that are important for the control of viral replication and gene expression, it is referred to as the long control region (LCR). A schematic diagram of the HPV-16 genome is shown in Fig. 1. The papillomaviruses have remained refractory to study with standard virological techniques because no tissue culture system that allows their replication has been devised. The failure to grow this virus can be explained at least partly by the intimate link between papillomavirus gene expression and the differentiation state of the host keratinocyte. Productive functions of the papillomaviruses are expressed only in fully differentiated squamous epithelial cells (reviewed in Baker, 1990). Tissue culture systems for epithelial cells that mimic these differentiation properties have not yet been developed, and many aspects of the papillomavirus life cycle are therefore poorly characterized.

ONCOGENIC FUNCTIONS ENCODED BY HPV

The precancerous CIN lesions contain extrachromosomal HPV sequences (Dürst *et al*, 1985). In the carcinomas, however, the HPV sequences are generally integrated, suggesting that integration may play a part in carcinogenic progression (Boshart *et al*, 1984; Dürst *et al*, 1985; Matsukura *et al*, 1989; Cullen *et al*, 1991). There do not appear to be specific sites of integration of the viral DNA into the host genome (Dürst *et al*, 1987a), but there is a characteristic pattern of integration with respect to the viral genome (Fig. 2). Integration of the viral DNA is probably a random event, but integration patterns that retain expression of the HPV E6 and E7 ORFs and disrupt and/or delete the E1 and E2 ORFs are regularly seen in the cancers, suggesting that they may provide a selective growth advantage to the cell (Schwarz *et al*, 1985; Matsukura *et al*, 1986; Baker *et al*, 1987). Molecular genetic studies have demonstrated that both the E6 and E7 ORFs encode oncoproteins, but the consequences of E1 and/or E2 disruption are less well understood. The E2 ORF encodes a DNA binding protein that interacts directly with its cognate binding sites located within the viral genome to regulate transcription from viral promoters (reviewed in McBride *et al*, 1989). The HPV-16 and HPV-18 E2 gene products have been shown to either activate or repress transcription, depending on the context of the E2 binding sites in the promoter (Phelps and Howley, 1987; Thierry and Yaniv, 1987; Bernard *et al*, 1989; Romanczuk *et al*, 1990; Thierry and Howley, 1991). In HPV-16 and HPV-18, the viral promoter that regulates E6 and E7 expression is repressed by E2. The functions of the HPV E1 ORF have not yet been extensively studied, but by analogy with bovine papillomavirus (BPV) E1, the encoded proteins are likely to be involved in viral replication (reviewed in Lambert, 1991). Recent studies have shown that disruption of either the E1 or the E2 ORF in the context of the full length cloned HPV-16 genome leads to enhanced transformation of primary human foreskin keratinocytes, suggesting that their encoded products directly or indirectly negatively regulate the expression of the viral E6 and E7 transforming functions (Romanczuk H and Howley PM, unpublished).

HPV E7 Oncoprotein

The E7 oncoprotein encoded by HPV-16 and HPV-18 is sufficient for transformation of established rodent fibroblast cell lines such as NIH3T3 cells

---

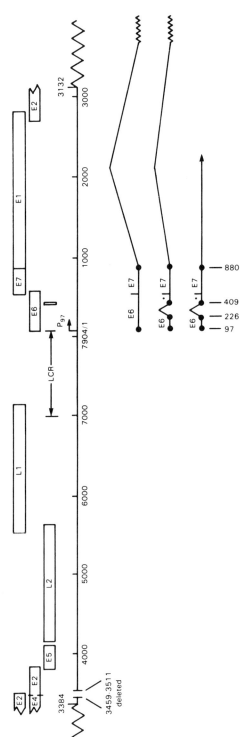

Fig. 2. Structure and expression of the single integrated copy of HPV-16 in the SiHa human cervical carcinoma cell line (Baker *et al*, 1987). Integration led to a disruption of the E2 ORF, and bases 3132 to 3384 and 3459 to 3511 have been deleted. The major viral mRNA species detected are expressed from the P_{97} promoter and are shown below. They all encode the full length E7 protein as well as the full length or internally spliced versions of E6, designated E6* (from Smotkin and Wettstein, 1986; Baker *et al*, 1987)

(Kanda *et al*, 1988; Phelps *et al*, 1988a; Vousden *et al*, 1988; Watanabe and Yoshiike, 1988; Bedell *et al*, 1989; Tanaka *et al*, 1989). Expression of the E7 gene induces focus formation in these cell lines and results in anchorage independence and tumorigenicity in nude mice. E7 has properties similar to adenovirus (Ad) E1A in that it can *trans*-activate the Ad E2 promoter and can cooperate with the activated *ras* oncogene to transform primary baby rat kidney cells (Matlashewski *et al*, 1987; Phelps *et al*, 1988a,b; Storey *et al*, 1988). Biochemical studies have revealed that HPV-16 E7 encodes a nuclear, zinc binding 98 aminoacid phosphoprotein (Smotkin and Wettstein, 1986; Sato *et al*, 1989a). The aminoterminal 38 aminoacids are strikingly similar to portions of conserved regions 1 and 2 of the Ad E1A proteins, as well as to the analogous regions of SV40 T antigen (Fig. 3) (Phelps *et al*, 1988a,b). Genetic studies of Ad E1A, SV40 T antigen and HPV E7 have shown that the conserved regions are required for cellular transformation (Kalderon and Smith, 1984; Lillie *et al*, 1987; Moran and Mathews, 1987; Cherington *et al*, 1988; Whyte *et al*, 1988a; Larose *et al*, 1991), as well as for the interaction with a number of host cellular proteins including the retinoblastoma tumour suppressor gene product pRB (DeCaprio *et al*, 1988; Münger *et al*, 1989a; Whyte *et al*, 1989). At the carboxyterminal boundary of the conserved aminoacid sequences are two serine residues, which can serve in vitro as substrates for phosphorylation by casein kinase (CK) II (Firzlaff *et al*, 1989; Barbosa *et al*, 1990). The carboxyterminal portion of E7 does not share any additional sequence similarity with Ad E1A or SV40 T antigen. It contains two copies of a Cys-X-X-Cys sequence motif, which are likely to be involved in the zinc binding property of E7 (Barbosa *et al*, 1989). The major properties of E7 are summarized in Table 1.

HPV E6 Oncoprotein

There are several species of viral mRNAs in cervical carcinomas and derived cell lines (Schwarz *et al*, 1985; Smotkin and Wettstein, 1986; Baker *et al*, 1987). One species has the capacity to encode the full length E6 protein, and several spliced versions of E6 (called E6*) are also produced (see Fig. 2). These internally spliced versions of E6 are unique to the "high risk" HPV types, and thus far, no biological activities have been described for the shortened E6* proteins potentially encoded by these spliced mRNAs. It is speculated that the E6* spliced mRNAs would be more efficiently translated into the E7 protein by bringing the initiation codon for E7 closer to the 5 ' end of the polycistronic mRNA (Smotkin *et al*, 1989). Moreover, this splicing event could constitute a mechanism for regulating the relative levels of E6 and E7. The full length E6 protein has transforming properties in that it is necessary for efficient transformation of primary human cells of both epithelial and fibroblastic origin (Hawley-Nelson *et al*, 1989; Münger *et al*, 1989b; Watanabe *et al*, 1989). The major properties of HPV-16 E6 are summarized in Table 2. It encodes a 151 aminoacid, basic, zinc binding protein (Androphy *et al*, 1987;

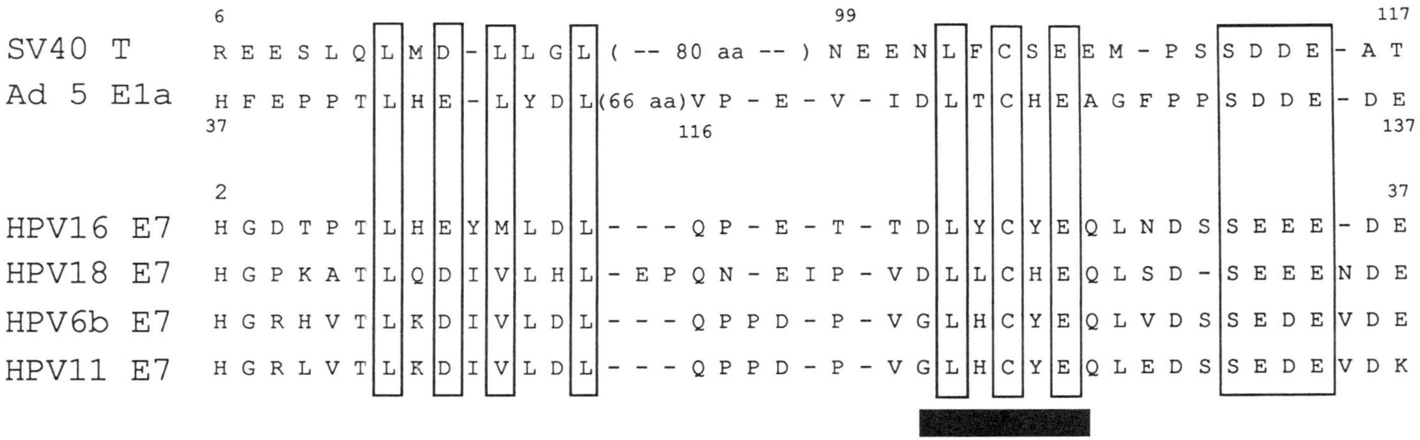

```
                          6                                                                                 117
SV40 T      R E E S L Q L M D - L L G L  ( -- 80 aa -- ) N E E N L F C S E E M - P S S D D E - A T
Ad 5 E1a    H F E P P T L H E - L Y D L (66 aa) V P - E - V - I D L T C H E A G F P P S D D E - D E
               37                                116                                                        137

               2                                                                                       37
HPV16 E7    H G D T P T L H E Y M L D L - - - Q P - E - T - T D L Y C Y E Q L N D S S E E E - D E
HPV18 E7    H G P K A T L Q D I V L H L - E P Q N - E I P - V D L L C H E Q L S D - S E E E N D E
HPV6b E7    H G R H V T L K D I V L D L - - - Q P P D - P - V G L H C Y E Q L V D S S E D E V D E
HPV11 E7    H G R L V T L K D I V L D L - - - Q P P D - P - V G L H C Y E Q L E D S S E D E V D K
```

Fig. 3. Aminoacid sequence comparison of regions of SV40 T antigen and portions of conserved regions 1 and 2 of the Ad E1A proteins with the aminoterminal portions of the E7 proteins of the anogenital associated HPVs. The standard one-letter code for aminoacids is used. Identical and isofunctional aminoacid residues are indicated by boxes. The E7 sequences which are necessary for pRB binding (Münger *et al*, 1989a) are indicated by the bar at the bottom of the figure

TABLE 1. Properties of the HPV-16 E7 oncoprotein[a]

Biochemical properties
  98 aminoacid, zinc binding, acidic nuclear phosphoprotein
  Phosphorylated at serine residue(s) by casein kinase II
  Apparent M_r: 19 kDa; predicted M_r: 11 kDa
  Aminoterminal region (aminoacid 1–39) structurally related to regions of adenovirus E1A and
    of large T antigens of the polyomaviruses
  Can complex with the retinoblastoma tumour suppressor gene product pRB
  Carboxyterminal region contains two Cys-X-X-Cys sequence motifs
  Can activate the cellular transcription factor E2F

Biological properties
  Sufficient for transformation of established rodent fibroblasts (eg NIH3T3 cells)
  Adenovirus E1A like transcriptional modulatory and transformation functions:
    Transactivates adenovirus E2 promoter
    Cooperates with *ras* to transform primary rodent cells
  Necessary together with E6 for the efficient immortalization of primary human squamous
    epithelial cells
  Abrogates TGF-β mediated repression of c-*myc* and G_1 growth arrest

[a]See text for references

Barbosa *et al*, 1989; Grossman and Laimins, 1989). It contains four repeats of a Cys-X-X-Cys sequence motif similar to the carboxyterminal region of E7. This led to the suggestion that E6 and E7 are evolutionarily related (Cole and Danos, 1987). Biochemical studies have shown that the E6 proteins derived from the "high risk" HPV types can associate with the tumour suppressor protein p53 (Werness *et al*, 1990). There are no significant aminoacid sequence similarities between HPV E6, Ad E1B and SV40 T antigen, which are all p53 binding proteins. Biochemical studies have indicated that the E6-p53 interaction can lead to the selective degradation of p53 in vitro (Scheffner *et al*, 1990). The E6 protein binds to double stranded DNA with high affinity (Mallon *et al*, 1987; Grossman *et al*, 1989; Imai *et al*, 1989), and there is some evidence that the E6 protein may be involved in transcriptional regulation (Lamberti *et al*, 1990).

TABLE 2. Properties of the HPV-16 E6 oncoprotein[a]

Biochemical properties
  151 aminoacid, zinc binding, basic protein (pI 9.9)
  Four copies of Cys-X-X-Cys sequence motif, which may serve as ligands for zinc binding
  Binds to double stranded DNA with high affinity
  Can form a complex with the p53 tumour suppressor protein and promote its in vitro
    degradation

Biological properties
  Cooperates with E7 for the efficient immortalization of primary human squamous epithelial
    cells
  May have transcriptional regulatory properties

[a]See text for references

Other Oncogenic Functions Encoded by HPVs

Although the E6/E7 region of the HPV genome is sufficient for cellular transformation in vitro, other HPV genes may also contribute to this phenomenon. In the context of the entire HPV-16 genome, disruption of E1 and E2 leads to increased transformation of primary human foreskin keratinocytes (Romanczuk H and Howley PM, unpublished). Although the exact mechanisms have not yet been delineated, it is presumed that disruption of E2 expression may lead to increased expression of the E6/E7 ORFs, resulting in enhanced transformation. Whether the effect of E1 disruption is mediated through the same transcriptional regulatory pathway is unknown, and other mechanisms involving the direct interaction of E1 and/or E2 with cellular factors cannot be excluded.

The E5 ORF of BPV encodes a small 44 aminoacid, membrane associated oncoprotein (reviewed in DiMaio and Neary, 1990). The BPV E5 protein is associated with a 16 kDa host cellular protein (Goldstein and Schlegel, 1990) and has been implicated in perturbing the growth factor responses of the virally infected host cells (Martin *et al*, 1989; Petti *et al*, 1991). Studies with the "high risk" HPVs have shown that they also have the capacity to encode E5 proteins (Bubb *et al*, 1988; Halbert and Galloway, 1988). Although they do not share extensive aminoacid sequence homology with BPV-1 E5, they have structural similarities to BPV-1 E5, with a very hydrophobic membrane anchor domain and a more hydrophilic domain. Additional studies are required to define further the biochemical and biological properties of the HPV E5 proteins. Owing to the integration of the HPV genome in the E1/E2 region, expression of E5 is generally not detected in cervical carcinomas and the derived cell lines. However, the possibility that expression of the HPV E5 genes could be important in participating in the HPV associated preneoplastic lesions cannot be excluded.

INTERACTION OF HPV E7 WITH CELLULAR PROTEINS

Interaction of HPV E7 with pRB

It was recognized some time ago that the Ad E1A proteins form specific complexes with several host cellular proteins in vivo (Yee and Branton, 1985; Harlow *et al*, 1986). Although some of these proteins interacted with sequences on the Ad E1A proteins which were recognized to be important for cellular transformation (ie conserved regions 1 and 2 of Ad E1A) (Whyte *et al*, 1988a), the biological importance of these interactions remained unclear. The hypothesis that the transforming functions of Ad E1A could, at least in part, be mediated through some of these protein/protein interactions received considerable support, however, when the 105 kDa Ad E1A associated protein was identified as the product of the retinoblastoma tumour suppressor gene, pRB (Whyte *et al*, 1988b). Given the functional and structural similarity between HPV-16 E7 and Ad E1A (Phelps *et al*, 1988a,b), the possibility of an interaction between the

E7 protein and pRB was investigated and confirmed (Dyson *et al*, 1989a). Coprecipitation experiments provided evidence for the complex in HPV-16 E7 expressing cells (Münger *et al*, 1989b). HPV-16 E7, much like SV40 T antigen (Ludlow *et al*, 1989), preferentially binds the underphosphorylated form of pRB (Münger K, unpublished). Cell cycle studies have shown that pRB has properties of a cell cycle regulatory factor in that its phosphorylation state varies through the cell cycle (Buchkovich *et al*, 1989; DeCaprio *et al*, 1989; Mihara *et al*, 1989). The underphosphorylated forms of pRB are present only during G_0 and G_1 of the cell cycle. Since pRB acts as a negative growth regulator at the G_1/S boundary, these underphosphorylated forms therefore must represent the forms of pRB that confer G_1 growth arrest. According to this model, G_1-S cell cycle progression is achieved by phosphorylation of pRB through the action of cell cycle specific serine/threonine protein kinase. Phosphorylated forms of pRB are present during S, G_2 and early M phases in the cell cycle and are dephosphorylated during M phase. These observations have led to the hypothesis that complex formation of the underphosphorylated forms of pRB with Ad E1A, SV40 T antigen or HPV E7 results, much like phosphorylation, in an "inactivation" of pRB and cell cycle progression (Fig. 4) (reviewed in Green, 1989). Ad E1A, SV40 T antigen and HPV E7 each has mitogenic activity and can induce DNA synthesis in quiescent cells (Mueller *et al*, 1978; Moran and Zerler, 1988; Sato *et al*, 1989b). This property of the DNA tumour viruses is thought to be essential in placing the infected host cells in a replicative state to permit viral DNA replication.

Quantitative mixing experiments with *in vitro* synthesized E7 proteins derived from "high risk" and "low risk" HPVs have shown that the E7 proteins of the "high risk" HPVs bind to pRB with higher affinity than the E7 proteins of the "low risk" HPVs (Münger *et al*, 1989a). Whereas the pRB binding affinities of HPV-16 and HPV-18 E7 were comparable, the HPV-11 and HPV-6 E7 proteins bound to pRB with significantly decreased affinities.

The pRB binding site on HPV-16 E7 was mapped using a series of mutant E7 proteins. It is confined to a portion of the region of sequence similarity of the E7 protein with the Ad E1A conserved region 2. The CK II phosphorylation site, which is also in this part of the E7 molecule, does not seem to be required for pRB binding (see Fig. 3) (Münger *et al*, 1989a; Barbosa *et al*, 1990; Firzlaff *et al*, 1991). Competition studies with a series of HPV-16 E7 specific synthetic peptides have confirmed the importance of this domain in binding pRB (Jones *et al*, 1990).

Mutant E7 proteins with a decreased affinity for pRB or unable to bind pRB were also transformation defective in NIH3T3 and in baby rat kidney cell *ras* cooperation assays. In contrast, some mutations in the portion of the E7 protein, which is similar to conserved region 1 of Ad E1A, were transformation defective, although they had wild type affinity for pRB in *in vitro* binding assays. This led to the conclusion that complex formation with pRB may be necessary but not sufficient for cellular transformation (Banks *et al*, 1990; Phelps WC, Münger K, Yee CL and Howley PM, unpublished).

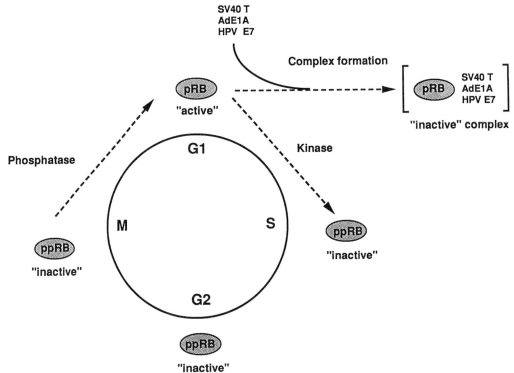

Fig. 4. "Inactivation" of pRB by complex formation with the oncogenes of different DNA tumour viruses. The retinoblastoma tumour suppressor protein is differentially phosphorylated during the cell cycle. The underphosphorylated form (pRB) is only detected during the G_0/G_1 phase of the cell cycle. Since the retinoblastoma protein is thought to act as a negative regulator of cell growth, pRB is regarded as the "active" form. Phosphorylation at serine and threonine residues at the G_1/S boundary is thought to result in an "inactivation" of the retinoblastoma protein and trigger cell cycle progression and entry into S phase. Complex formation of pRB with Ad E1A, SV40 T antigen or HPV E7 may also result in the "inactivation" of the negative growth regulatory functions of pRB and lead to cell cycle progression. Since the regulatory functions of the pRB kinase and phosphatase are annulled by complex formation with the viral oncoproteins, this may result in uncontrolled cell growth and differentiation

Interaction of HPV E7 with Other Host Cellular Proteins

Coprecipitation experiments have shown additional cellular proteins in complex with E7. Some of these E7 associated cellular proteins have electrophoretic mobilities similar to those of Ad E1A and SV40 T antigen associated proteins (Münger K, unpublished). The low levels of E7 present in HPV transformed cell lines have not yet permitted a full characterization of these host cellular proteins. Of particular interest is a protein designated p107, which seems to interact with the identical sequences on Ad E1A and SV40 T antigen as pRB (Dyson *et al*, 1989b; Ewen *et al*, 1989; Whyte *et al*, 1989). In vitro mixing experiments with purified E7 protein or coprecipitation experiments with E7 specific antibodies led to the detection of a protein with the same electrophoretic mobility as p107. HPV-16 E7 peptides compete with the Ad E1A bound p107. In addition, p107 can be detected in complex with HPV-16 E7 peptides immobilized on Sepharose beads (Dyson N, Münger K, Howley PM and Harlow E, unpublished).

Since mutations in the aminoacid sequence of HPV-16 E7 analogous to conserved region 1 of Ad E1A result in transformation defective proteins despite their ability to bind pRB in vitro with wild type affinity, other cellular proteins that interact with this aminoterminal domain of E7 must also be important for the transformed phenotype. A possible candidate is p300, which interacts with the Ad E1A proteins in conserved region 1 (Whyte *et al*, 1989). To date, there is no direct experimental evidence for an interaction of p300 with the E7 protein.

The E7 proteins encoded by the "high risk" HPVs differ from the "low risk" HPV E7 proteins in their CK II phosphorylation site. The "high risk" HPV E7 proteins are more rapidly phosphorylated by CK II in vitro than the "low risk" HPV E7 proteins (Barbosa *et al*, 1990). Mutations in the E7 phosphorylation site lead to a decrease in transformation without markedly affecting pRB binding (Barbosa *et al*, 1990; Firzlaff *et al*, 1991). The biological consequences of these findings are still unclear.

Ad E2 *Trans*-Activation Function of HPV E7

Since E7 does not share any significant aminoacid sequence similarity with conserved region 3 of Ad E1A, the portion of Ad E1A that has been shown to be important for its strong *trans*-activation function, it was clear that E7 must function differently from the 13S E1A product. The 12S form of Ad E1A, which lacks conserved region 3, is a weak *trans*-activator and functions on a subset of the 13S Ad E1A targets (reviewed in Nevins, 1989). Recent biochemical studies have shown that one of the targeted cellular transcription factors, E2F, is activated by Ad E1A through dissociation of a heteromeric macromolecular complex. This Ad E1A mediated dissociation is dependent on Ad E1A sequences in conserved region 2 and may be mediated by protein/protein interactions (Bagchi *et al*, 1990). Genetic and biochemical studies have shown that HPV E7 *trans*-activates a similar subset of 12S Ad E1A responsive promoters, and it can release E2F from the macromolecular complex. Although the sequences on the E7 protein required for this activity have not been mapped in detail, it is clear that the portion of E7 similar to conserved sequence 2 of Ad E1A is necessary for this activity (Phelps WC *et al*, in press). This is in agreement with previous findings with mutant E7 proteins, which showed that the sequences required for *trans*-activation were not clearly separable from those required for transformation (Edmonds and Vousden 1989; Phelps *et al*, 1990; Watanabe *et al*, 1990). The "low risk" HPV E7 proteins, although impaired for cellular transformation and pRB binding, can *trans*-activate the Ad E2 promoter with an efficiency similar to that of the "high risk" HPVs (Storey *et al*, 1990; Münger *et al*, 1991). This suggests that cellular transformation and transcriptional *trans*-activation may not be mediated through interactions with an identical set of host cellular proteins.

Abrogation of TGF-β Mediated Repression of c-*myc* Expression

Transforming growth factor-β (TGF-β) acts as a potent negative growth regulator of many epithelial cells and induces G_1 growth arrest (reviewed in Moses *et al*, 1990). TGF-β treatment of keratinocytes results in the rapid transcriptional repression of c-*myc* expression (Coffey *et al*, 1988). Studies with c-*myc* antisense oligodeoxynucleotides have suggested that the observed G_1 growth arrest may be a consequence of this transcriptional repression of c-*myc* expression (Pietenpol *et al*, 1990a). Many squamous epithelial derived tumour cell lines have lost their responsiveness to TGF-β. Moreover, human keratinocyte cell lines transformed by the HPV-16 E6/E7 region expressed from the human β-actin promoter, by HPV-18 or by SV40, are also resistant to growth inhibition by TGF-β (Pietenpol *et al*, 1990b). HPV-16 E7, SV40 T antigen and Ad E1A can each abrogate the TGF-β mediated transcriptional repression of c-*myc* expression in a transient transfection assay. This property is dependent on the integrity of the pRB binding site of each of these viral oncoproteins. This suggests that one of the cellular proteins that can form a complex with these viral oncoproteins through the pRB binding domain such as pRB or p107 may be involved in the transcriptional regulatory pathway of c-*myc* expression (Pietenpol *et al*, 1990b).

INTERACTION OF HPV E6 WITH THE p53 TUMOUR SUPPRESSOR PROTEIN

Like SV40 T antigen and the Ad5 E1B 55 kDa oncoprotein, the E6 proteins encoded by the "high risk" HPVs can form a complex with the tumour suppressor protein p53 (Lane and Crawford, 1979; Linzer and Levine, 1979; Sarnow *et al*, 1982; Werness *et al*, 1990). For the "low risk" HPV E6 proteins, no complex formation with p53 was detected. The aminoacid sequences of E6 that are necessary for this interaction have not yet been defined, but preliminary studies show that rather than a short linear aminoacid sequence, a specific conformational structure of the E6 protein may be required for the E6/p53 interaction (Huibregtse JM, unpublished). The truncated, internally spliced forms of E6, E6° do not interact with p53 (Werness BA, unpublished). Interaction of SV40 T antigen and Ad5 E1B with p53 leads to an extended half life and increased steady state levels of p53 in SV40 and adenovirus transformed cell lines (Oren *et al*, 1981; Reich *et al*, 1983). The levels of p53 in HPV positive cervical carcinoma cell lines and in HPV transformed keratinocyte cell lines are quite low (Scheffner *et al*, 1991). Indeed, it was previously reported that HeLa cells that contain HPV-18 contain no detectable p53 protein despite the presence of translatable *p53* mRNA (Matlashewski *et al*, 1986). Biochemical studies have revealed that binding of E6 promotes the degradation of p53 in an in vitro system. The E6 induced degradation of p53 is ATP dependent and involves the ubiquitin dependent proteolysis system (Scheffner *et al*, 1990). This property of E6 may account for the low levels of p53 detected in cervical carcinoma cell lines and in HPV transformed human keratinocyte cell lines.

Cotransfection studies with HPV-16 E7 and wild type and mutant forms of *p53* have shown that mutant *p53* can potentiate the ability of E7 and *ras* to transform baby rat kidney cells and confer growth factor independence on the transformed cell lines. The results with wild type *p53* were somewhat less conclusive. Using an anchorage independence assay in NIH3T3 cells, a decrease in transformation was observed. Whether this was due to a specific transformation inhibiting effect of wild type *p53* or a non-specific toxicity effect of overexpressing wild type *p53* in these cells is unknown (Crook *et al*, 1991a).

IS THE FUNCTIONAL INACTIVATION OF THE RB AND p53 GENE PRODUCTS IMPORTANT IN CERVICAL CARCINOGENESIS?

Although the biochemical nature of the interactions of the viral oncoproteins with p53 and pRB is well documented, the biological consequences of these interactions can still be viewed as speculative. Since the "high risk" HPVs are associated with cervical carcinomas, they provide a unique system to test the hypothesis that the complex formation of the HPV E6 and E7 oncoproteins with the p53 and pRB tumour suppressor proteins may be of significance for cervical carcinogenesis.

Approximately 85% of the human cervical cancers contain HPV sequences (Riou *et al*, 1990), and one can predict that if p53 and pRB are relevant and essential targets of E6 and E7, respectively, then there might be no selective advantage to a tumour for further mutations in their *p53* and *RB* genes, since the functions of the encoded tumour suppressor proteins would presumably be annulled through interactions with HPV E6 and E7 oncoproteins. Furthermore, in the HPV negative cervical carcinomas, one would expect p53 and pRB functions also to be abrogated through a different mechanism, most likely mutation. These predictions were tested on a panel of HPV positive and HPV negative cervical carcinoma cell lines. All the HPV positive cell lines had wild type p53 and normal pRB, whereas both HPV negative cervical carcinoma cell lines contained mutated *p53* and *RB* genes (Crook *et al*, 1991b; Scheffner *et al*, 1991) (Table 3). These experiments not only indicate that the *RB* and *p53* genes are frequently inactivated during cervical carcinogenesis but also strongly suggest that p53 and pRB may be physiologically relevant targets of the HPV E6 and E7 oncoproteins. The interactions of the viral oncoproteins and cellular tumour suppressor proteins detected in coprecipitation assays may

TABLE 3. Status of p53 and pRB in human cervical carcinoma cell lines[a]

Cell line	HPV	p53	pRB
HeLa	HPV-18	wt	wt
C4-II	HPV-18	wt	wt
SiHa	HPV-16	wt	wt
CaSki	HPV-16	wt	wt
Me180	HPV-39 related	wt	wt
C33-A	Negative	Mutated, R_{273} to C	Mutated (exon 20)
HT-3	Negative	Mutated, G_{245} to V	Mutated (exon 13)

wt = wild type
[a]See Scheffner *et al*, 1991, for details

therefore reflect an "inactivation" of some of the important regulatory functions encoded by these tumour suppressor gene products.

Some mutations of the *p53* gene are believed to result in a dominant gain, rather than merely a loss of function. Therefore, it is possible that the E6/p53 interaction may not have the exact same consequences as a p53 mutation but rather result in a "null" phenotype. In this context, it is interesting to note that in one recent study, the HPV negative cervical lesions appear to be associated with a poorer clinical prognosis in that they progress more rapidly and have higher metastatic potential than the HPV positive lesions (Riou *et al*, 1990).

ADDITIONAL FACTORS IN CERVICAL CARCINOGENESIS

Cervical carcinoma eventually develops in only a small percentage of women infected with "high risk" HPVs. This suggests that the infection with a "high risk" HPV constitutes only one step in cervical carcinogenesis. In agreement with this notion is the observation that HPV E6/E7 transformed human keratinocyte cell lines are generally not anchorage independent nor tumorigenic in nude mice (Dürst *et al*, 1987a,b; Pirisi *et al*, 1987; Kaur and McDougall, 1988; Schlegel *et al*, 1988). Progression to a fully transformed tumorigenic phenotype in HPV immortalized keratinocytes was observed upon cotransfection with an activated *ras* oncogene or after continuous passaging of the cell lines for extended periods of time (DiPaolo *et al*, 1989; Dürst *et al*, 1989; Hurlin *et al*, 1991; Pecoraro *et al*, 1991). These observations imply that additional cellular events may also be necessary for the development of cervical carcinoma.

Cytogenetic studies have shown that nine out of nine carcinomas of the uterine cervix had a loss of heterozygosity on the short arm of chromosome 3 (Yokota *et al*, 1989), implicating a possible tumour suppressor gene in that region of the genome. Lesions in the same region of chromosome 3p (3p21) have also been noted in small cell lung carcinoma (Yokota *et al*, 1987; Mori *et al*, 1989).

Additional evidence for host cell mutations in cervical cancers is provided by studies with somatic cell hybrids (Stanbridge *et al*, 1982). The cervical carcinoma cell lines HeLa and SiHa when fused with normal human cells reverted to a non-tumorigenic phenotype. Further studies with tumorigenic revertants of such hybrid cell lines or by microcell fusion have genetically mapped this effect to human chromosome 11 (Saxon *et al*, 1986; Koi *et al*, 1989). The exact molecular events and biological consequences of these host chromosomal lesions are not yet clearly understood. It has been proposed that some of these factors may control some aspects of HPV transcription (Rösl *et al*, 1988; Bosch *et al*, 1990; Smits *et al*, 1990; Miyasaka *et al*, 1991). Inactivation of such genes in cervical carcinoma cells would lead to deregulated expression of the HPV E6/E7 genes. In such models, infection with a "high risk" HPV would constitute an important initial event of carcinogenesis. A pool of highly replicative cells would be established, since some of the normal aspects of cell cycle, replication and differentiation control would be abolished by functional inactivation of key cellular regulatory proteins such as p53 and pRB. The expression of HPV E6 and E7 may contribute to chromosomal instability with the accumulation of chromosomal aberrations followed by clonal selection of malignant cells and tumorigenesis. Such models stress the importance of environmental mutagenic cofactors that may contribute to carcinogenic progression. Epidemiological studies have identified a small increase in the relative risk for the development of cervical cancers with cigarette smoking and long term use of oral contraceptives (Vessey, 1986).

SUMMARY

The HPVs associated with anogenital cancers encode two oncoproteins, E6 and E7. Both E6 and E7 can form specific complexes with tumour suppressor gene products. The E7 protein binds to the retinoblastoma tumour suppressor gene product pRB, with a preference for the underphosphorylated, "active" form of pRB. The E7 proteins derived from the "high risk" HPVs bind to pRB with a higher affinity than the E7 proteins from the "low risk" HPVs. The "high risk" HPV E6 proteins can associate with the p53 tumour suppressor protein. This interaction promotes the degradation of p53 in vitro, which presumably accounts for the very low levels of p53 in cervical carcinoma cell lines. The functional inactivation of pRB and p53 by the HPV oncoproteins E7 and E6, respectively, are likely to be important steps in cervical carcinogenesis, since mutations in the *RB* and *p53* genes were detected in HPV negative but not HPV positive cervical carcinoma cell lines. Cytogenetic studies strongly suggest, however, that additional chromosomal changes may be necessary for carcinogenic progression of HPV induced anogenital lesions.

References

Androphy EJ, Hubbert N, Schiller JT and Lowy DR (1987) Identification of the HPV-16 E6 protein from transformed mouse cells and human cervical carcinoma cell lines. *EMBO Journal* **6** 989–992

Bagchi S, Raychaudhuri P and Nevins JR (1990) Adenovirus E1A proteins can dissociate heteromeric complexes involving the E2F transcription factor: a novel mechanism for E1A trans-activation. *Cell* **62** 659–669

Baker CC (1990) Bovine papillomavirus type 1 transcription, In: Pfister H (ed). *Papillomaviruses and Human Cancer*, pp 91–112, CRC Press, Boca Raton, Florida

Baker CC, Phelps WC, Lindgren V, Braun MJ, Gonda MA and Howley PM (1987) Structural and translational analysis of human papillomavirus type 16 sequences in cervical carcinoma cell lines. *Journal of Virology* **61** 962–971

Banks L, Edmonds C and Vousden KH (1990) Ability of the HPV16 E7 protein to bind RB and induce DNA synthesis is not sufficient for efficient transformation in NIH3T3 cells. *Oncogene* **5** 1383–1389

Barbosa MS, Lowy DR and Schiller JT (1989) Papillomavirus polypeptides E6 and E7 are zinc-binding proteins. *Journal of Virology* **63** 1404–1407

Barbosa MS, Edmonds C, Fisher C, Schiller JT, Lowy DR and Vousden KH (1990) The region of the HPV E7 oncoprotein homologous to adenovirus E1a and SV40 large T antigen contains separate domains for Rb binding and casein kinase II. *EMBO Journal* **9** 153–160

Bedell MA, Jones KH, Grossman SR and Laimins LA (1989) Identification of human papillomavirus type 18 transforming genes in immortalized and primary cells. *Journal of Virology* **63** 1247–1255

Bernard BA, Bailly C, Lenoir M-C, Darmon M, Thierry F and Yaniv M (1989) The HPV18 E2 gene product is a repressor of the HPV18 regulatory region in human keratinocytes. *Journal of Virology* **63** 4317–4324

Bosch FX, Schwarz E, Boukamp P, Fusenig NE, Bartsch D and zur Hausen H (1990) Suppression in vivo of human papillomavirus type 18 E6-E7 gene expression in non-tumorigenic HeLa x fibroblast hybrid cells. *Journal of Virology* **64** 4743–4754

Boshart M, Gissmann L, Ikenberg H, Kleinheinz A, Scheurlen W and zur Hausen H (1984) A new type of papillomavirus DNA and its prevalence in genital cancer biopsies and in cell lines derived from cervical cancer. *EMBO Journal* **3** 1151–1157

Bubb V, McCance DJ and Schlegel R (1988) DNA sequence of the HPV-16 E5 ORF and structural conservation of its encoded protein. *Virology* **163** 243–246

Buchkovich K, Duffy LA and Harlow E (1989) The retinoblastoma protein is phosphorylated during specific phases of the cell cycle. *Cell* **58** 1097–1105

Cherington V, Brown M, Paucha E, St Louis J, Spiegelmann BM and Roberts TM (1988) Separation of simian virus 40 large-T antigen-transforming and origin binding functions from the ability to block differentiation. *Molecular and Cellular Biology* **8** 1380–1384

Coffey RJ, Bascom CC, Sipes NJ, Graves-Deal R, Weissman BE and Moses HL (1988) Selective inhibition of growth-related gene expression in murine keratinocytes by transforming growth factor beta. *Molecular and Cellular Biology* **8** 3088–3093

Cole ST and Danos O (1987) Nucleotide sequence and comparative analysis of the human papillomavirus type 18 genome: phylogeny of papillomaviruses and repeated structure of the E6 and E7 gene products. *Journal of Molecular Biology* **193** 599–608

Crook T, Fisher C and Vousden KH (1991a) Modulation of immortalizing properties of human papillomavirus type 16 E7 by p53 expression. *Journal of Virology* **65** 505–511

Crook T, Wrede D and Vousden KH (1991b) p53 point mutation in HPV negative human cervical carcinoma cell lines. *Oncogene* **6** 873–875

Cullen A, Reid R, Campion M and Lörincz A (1991) Analysis of the physical state of different human papillomavirus DNAs in intraepithelial and invasive cervical neoplasms. *Journal of Virology* **65** 606–612

DeCaprio JA, Ludlow JW, Figge J *et al* (1988) SV40 large tumor antigen forms a specific complex with the product of the retinoblastoma susceptibility gene. *Cell* **54** 275–283

DeCaprio JA, Ludlow JW, Lynch D *et al* (1989) The product of the retinoblastoma susceptibility gene has properties of a cell cycle regulatory element. *Cell* **58** 1085–1095

DeVilliers EM (1989) Heterogeneity of the human papillomavirus group. *Journal of Virology* **63**

4898–4903

DiMaio D and Neary K (1990) The genetics of bovine papillomavirus type 1 In: Pfister H (ed). *Papillomaviruses and Human Cancer*, pp 113–144, CRC Press, Boca Raton, Florida

DiPaolo JA, Woodworth CD, Popescu NC, Notario V and Doninger J (1989) Induction of human cervical squamous cell carcinoma by sequential transfection with human papillomavirus 16 DNA and viral Harvey ras. *Oncogene* **4** 395–399

Dürst M, Kleinheinz A, Hotz M and Gissmann L (1985) The physical state of human papillomavirus type 16 in benign and malignant genital tumors. *Journal of General Virology* **66** 1515–1522

Dürst M, Croce CM, Gissmann L, Schwarz E, and Huebner K (1987a) Papillomavirus sequences integrate near cellular oncogenes in some cervical carcinomas. *Proceedings of the National Academy of Sciences of the USA* **80** 3812–3815

Dürst M, Dzarlieva-Petrusevska RT, Boukamp P, Fusenig NE and Gissmann L (1987b) Molecular and cytogenetic analysis of immortalized human primary keratinocytes obtained after transfection with human papillomavirus type 16 DNA. *Oncogene* **1** 251–256

Dürst M, Gallahan D, Jay G and Rhim JS (1989) Glucocorticoid enhanced neoplastic transformation of human keratinocytes by human papillomavirus type 16 and an activated ras oncogene. *Virology* **173** 767–771

Dyson N, Howley PM, Münger K and Harlow E (1989a) The human papillomavirus-16 E7 oncoprotein is able to bind to the retinoblastoma gene product. *Science* **243** 934–937

Dyson N, Buchkovich K, Whyte P and Harlow E (1989b) The cellular 107K protein that binds to adenovirus E1A also associates with the large T antigens of SV40 and JC virus. *Cell* **58** 249–255

Edmonds C and Vousden KH (1989) A point mutational analysis of human papillomavirus type 16 E7 protein. *Journal of Virology* **63** 2650–2656

Ewen ME, Ludlow JW, DeCaprio JA et al (1989) An N-terminal transformation-governing sequence of SV40 large T antigen contributes to the binding of both p110^{Rb} and a second cellular protein, p120. *Cell* **58** 257–267

Firzlaff JM, Galloway DA, Eisenman RN and Lüscher B (1989) The E7 protein of human papillomavirus type 16 is phosphorylated by casein kinase II. *New Biologist* **1** 44–53

Firzlaff JM, Lüscher B and Eisenman RN (1991) Negative charge at the casein kinase II phosphorylation site is important for transformation but not for Rb protein binding by the E7 protein of the human papillomavirus type 16. *Proceedings of the National Academy of Sciences of the USA* **88** 5187–5191

Goldstein D and Schlegel R (1990) The E5 oncoprotein of bovine papillomavirus binds to a 16 kd cellular protein. *EMBO Journal* **9** 137–146

Green MR (1989) When the products of oncogenes and antioncogenes meet. *Cell* **56** 1–3

Grossman SR and Laimins L (1989) E6 protein of human papilllomavirus type 18 binds zinc. *Oncogene* **4** 1089–1093

Grossman SR, Mora R and Laimins L (1989) Intracellular localization and DNA-binding properties of human papillomavirus type 18 E6 protein expressed with a baculovirus vector. *Journal of Virology* **63** 366–374

Halbert CL and Galloway D (1988) Identification of the E5 open reading frame of human papillomavirus type 16. *Journal of Virology* **62** 1071–1075

Harlow E, Whyte P, Franza BR and Schley C (1986) Association of adenovirus early region 1A proteins with cellular polypeptides. *Molecular and Cellular Biology* **6** 1579–1589

Hawley-Nelson P, Vousden KH, Hubbert NL, Lowy DR and Schiller JT (1989) HPV16 E6 and E7 proteins cooperate to immortalize human foreskin keratinocytes. *EMBO Journal* **8** 3905–3910

Hurlin PJ, Kaur P, Smith PP, Perez-Reyes N, Blanton RA and McDougall JK (1991) Progression of human papillomavirus type 18-immortalized human keratinocytes to a malignant phenotype. *Proceedings of the National Academy of Sciences of the USA* **88** 571–574

Imai Y, Tsunokawa Y, Sugimura T and Terada M (1989) Purification and DNA-binding properties of human papillomavirus type 16 E6 protein expressed in Escherichia coli. *Biochemical and Biophysical Research Communications* **164** 1402–1410

Jones RE, Wegrzyn RJ, Patrick DR *et al* (1990) Identification of HPV-16 E7 peptides that are potent antagonists of E7 binding to the retinoblastoma suppressor protein. *Journal of Biological Chemistry* **265** 12782–12785

Kalderon D and Smith AE (1984) In vitro mutagenesis of a putative DNA binding domain of SV40 large-T. *Virology* **139** 109–137

Kanda T, Watanabe S and Yoshiike K (1988) Immortalization of primary rat cells by human papillomavirus type 16 subgenomic fragments controlled by the SV40 promoter. *Virology* **165** 321–325

Kaur P and McDougall JK (1988) Characterisation of primary human keratinocytes transformed by human papillomavirus type 18. *Journal of Virology* **62** 1917–1924

Koi M, Morita H, Yamada H, Satoh H, Barrett JC and Oshimura H (1989) Normal human chromosome 11 suppresses tumorigenicity of human cervical tumor cell line SiHa. *Molecular Carcinogenesis* **2** 12–21

Lambert PF (1991) Papillomavirus DNA replication. *Journal of Virology* **65** 3417–3420

Lamberti C, Morrissey LC, Grossman SR and Androphy EJ (1990) Transcriptional transactivation by the human papillomavirus E6 zinc finger oncoprotein. *EMBO Journal* **9** 1907–1913

Lane DP and Crawford LV (1979) T antigen is bound to a host protein in SV40-transformed cells. *Nature* **278** 261–263

Larose A, Dyson N, Sullivan M, Harlow E and Bastin M (1991) Polyomavirus large T mutants affected in retinoblastoma protein binding are defective in immortalization. *Journal of Virology* **65** 2308–2313

Lillie JW, Lowenstein PM, Green MR and Green M (1987) Functional domains of adenovirus type 5 E1A proteins. *Cell* **50** 1091–1100

Linzer DIH and Levine AJ (1979) Characterization of a 54K dalton cellular SV40 tumor antigen present in SV40-transformed cells and uninfected embryonal carcinoma cells. *Cell* **17** 43–52

Ludlow JW, DeCaprio JA, Huang C-M, Lee W-H, Paucha E and Livingston DM (1989) SV40 large T antigen binds preferentially to an underphosphorylated member of the retinoblastoma gene product family. *Cell* **56** 57–65

Mallon RG, Wojciechowicz D and Defendi V (1987) DNA-binding activity of papillomavirus proteins. *Journal of Virology* **61** 1655–1660

Martin P, Vass WC, Schiller JT, Lowy DR and Velu TJ (1989) The bovine papillomavirus E5 transforming protein can stimulate the transforming activity of EGF and CSF-1 receptors. *Cell* **59** 21–32

Matlashewski G, Banks L, Pim D and Crawford L (1986) Analysis of human p53 proteins and mRNA levels in normal and transformed cells. *European Journal of Biochemistry* **154** 665–672

Matlashewski G, Schneider J, Banks L, Jones N, Murray A and Crawford L (1987) Human papillomavirus type 16 cooperates with activated ras in transforming primary cells. *EMBO Journal* **6** 1741–1746

Matsukura T, Kanda T, Furuno A, Yoshikawa H, Kawana T and Yoshiike K (1986) Cloning of monomeric human papillomavirus type 16 integrated within cell DNA from a cervical carcinoma. *Journal of Virology* **58** 979–982

Matsukura T, Koi S and Sugase M (1989) Both episomal and integrated forms of human papillomavirus type 16 are involved in invasive cervical cancers. *Virology* **172** 63–72

McBride AA, Spalholz BA, Lambert PF and Howley PM (1989) Functional domains of the papillomavirus E2 proteins, In: Villareal LP (ed). *Common Mechanisms of Transformation by Small DNA Tumor Viruses*, pp 115–126, ASM Publications, Washington DC

Mihara K, Cao X-R, Yen A *et al* (1989) Cell-cycle dependent regulation of phosphorylation of the human retinoblastoma gene product. *Science* **246** 1300–1303

Miyaska M, Takami Y, Inoue H and Hakura A (1991) Rat embryo fibroblast cells suppress transformation by the E6 and E7 genes of human papillomavirus type 16 in somatic hybrid cells. *Journal of Virology* **65** 479–482

Moran E and Mathews MB (1987) Multiple domains in the adenovirus E1A gene. *Cell* **48** 177–178

Moran E and Zerler B (1988) Interactions between cell growth-regulating domains in the products of the adenovirus E1A oncogene. *Molecular and Cellular Biology* **8** 1756–1764

Mori N, Yokota J, Oshimura M *et al* (1989) Concordant deletions of chromosome 3p and loss of heterozygosity for chromosome 13 and 17 in small cell lung carcinoma. *Cancer Research* **49** 5130–5135

Moses HL, Yang EY and Pietenpol JA (1990) TGF-β stimulation and inhibition of cell proliferation: new mechanistic insights. *Cell* **63** 245–247

Mueller C, Graessmann A and Graessmann M (1978) Mapping of early SV40-specific functions by microinjection of different early viral DNA fragments. *Cell* **15** 579–585

Münger K, Werness BA, Dyson N, Phelps WC, Harlow E and Howley PM (1989a) Complex formation of human papillomavirus E7 proteins with the retinoblastoma tumor suppressor gene product. *EMBO Journal* **8** 4099–4105

Münger K, Phelps WC, Bubb V, Howley PM and Schlegel R (1989b) The E6 and E7 genes of the human papillomavirus type 16 together are necessary and sufficient for transformation of primary human keratinocytes. *Journal of Virology* **63** 4417–4421

Münger K, Yee CL, Phelps WC, Pietenpol JA, Moses HL and Howley PM (1991) Biochemical and biological differences between E7 oncoproteins of the high and low risk HPV types are determined by aminoterminal sequences. *Journal of Virology* **65** 3943–3948

Nevins JR (1989) Mechanisms of viral-mediated trans-activation of transcription. *Advances in Virus Research* **37** 35–87

Oren M, Maltzman W and Levine AJ (1981) Post-translational regulation of the 54 K cellular tumor antigen in normal and transformed cells. *Molecular and Cellular Biology* **1** 101–110

Pecoraro G, Lee M, Morgan D and Defendi V (1991) Evolution of in vitro transformation and tumorigenesis of HPV 16 and HPV 18 immortalized primary cervical epithelial cells. *American Journal of Pathology* **173** 1–8

Petti L, Nilson LA and DiMaio D (1991) Activation of the platelet-derived growth factor receptor by the bovine papillomavirus E5 transforming protein. *EMBO Journal* **10** 845–855

Phelps WC and Howley PM (1987) Transcriptional trans-activation by the human papillomavirus type 16 E2 gene product. *Journal of Virology* **61** 1630–1638

Phelps WC, Yee CL, Münger K and Howley PM (1988a) The human papillomavirus type 16 E7 gene encodes transactivation and transformation functions similar to adenovirus E1a. *Cell* **53** 539–547

Phelps WC, Yee CL, Münger K and Howley PM (1988b) Functional and sequence similarities between HPV16 E7 and adenovirus E1A. *Current Topics in Microbiology and Immunology* **144** 153–166

Phelps WC, Münger K, Yee CL and Howley, PM (1990) Site directed mutagenesis of the HPV16 E7 gene, In: Howley PM and Broker T (eds). *UCLA Symposia on Molecular and Cellular Biology*, new series vol 124: *Papillomaviruses*, pp 305–311, AR Liss Inc, New York

Phelps WC, Bagchi S, Barnes JA *et al* (1991) Analysis of *trans*-activation by HPV16 E7 and adenovirus 12S E1A suggests a common mechanism. *Journal of Virology* **65** 6922–6930

Pietenpol JA, Holt JT, Stein RW and Moses HL (1990a) Transforming growth factor β1 suppression of c-*myc* gene transcription: role in inhibition of keratinocyte proliferation. *Proceedings of the National Academy of Sciences of the USA* **87** 3758–3762

Pietenpol JA, Stein RW, Moran E *et al* (1990b) TGF-β1 inhibition of transcription and growth in keratinocytes is abrogated by viral transforming proteins with pRB binding domains. *Cell* **61** 777–785

Pirisi L, Yasumoto S, Fellerey M, Doninger JK and DiPaolo JA (1987) Transformation of human fibroblasts and keratinocytes with human papillomavirus type 16 DNA. *Journal of Virology* **61** 1061–1066

Reich NC, Oren M and Levine AJ (1983) Two distinct mechanisms regulate the levels of a cellular tumor antigen. *Molecular and Cellular Biology* **3** 2134–2150

Riou G, Favre M, Jeannel DJ, Bourhis J, Le Doussal V and Orth G (1990) Association between poor prognosis in early-stage invasive cervical carcinomas and non-detection of HPV DNA. *Lancet* **335** 1171–1174

Romanczuk H, Thierry F and Howley PM (1990) Mutational analysis of cis elements involved in E2 modulation of human papillomavirus type 16 P_{97} and type 18 P_{105} promoters. *Journal of Virology* **64** 2849–2859

Rösl F, Dürst M and zur Hausen H (1988) Selective suppression of human papillomavirus transcription in non-tumorigenic cells by 5-azacytidine. *EMBO Journal* **7** 1321–1327

Sarnow P, Ho YS, Williams J and Levine AJ (1982) Adenovirus E1b-58kd tumor antigen and SV40 large tumor antigen are physically associated with the same 54kd cellular protein in transformed cells. *Cell* **28** 387–394

Sato H, Watanabe S, Furuno A and Yoshiike K (1989a) Human papillomavirus type 16 E7 protein expressed in Escherichia coli and monkey COS-1 cells: immunofluorescence detection of the nuclear E7 protein. *Virology* **170** 311–315

Sato H, Furuno A and Yoshiike K (1989b) Expression of human papillomavirus type 16 E7 gene induces DNA synthesis in rat 3Y1 cell. *Virology* **168** 195–199

Saxon PJ, Srivatsan ES and Stanbridge EJ (1986) Introduction of chromosome 11 via microcell transfer control tumorigenic expression of HeLa cells. *EMBO Journal* **5** 3461–3466

Scheffner M, Werness BA, Huibregtse JM, Levine AJ and Howley PM (1990) The E6 oncoprotein encoded by the human papillomavirus types 16 and 18 promotes the degradation of p53. *Cell* **63** 1129–1136

Scheffner M, Münger K, Byrne JC and Howley PM (1991) The state of the p53 and retinoblastoma genes in human cervical carcinoma cell lines. *Proceedings of the National Academy of Sciences of the USA* **88** 5523–5527

Schlegel R, Phelps WC, Zhang Y-L and Barbosa M (1988) Quantitative keratinocyte assay detects two biological activities of human papillomavirus DNA and identifies viral types associated with cervical carcinoma. *EMBO Journal* **7** 3181–3187

Schwarz E, Freese UK, Gissmann L *et al* (1985) Structure and transcription of human papillomavirus sequences in cervical carcinoma cells. *Nature* **314** 111–114

Smits PHM, Smits HL, Jebbink MF and ter Schegget J (1990) The short arm of chromosome 11 likely is involved in the regulation of the human papillomavirus type 16 early enhancer-promoter and in the suppression of the transforming activity of the viral DNA. *Virology* **176** 158–165

Smotkin D and Wettstein FO (1986) Transcription of human papillomavirus type 16 early genes in cervical cancer and a cervical cancer derived cell line and identification of the E7 protein. *Proceedings of the National Academy of Sciences of the USA* **83** 4680–4684

Smotkin D, Prokoph H and Wettstein FO (1989) Oncogenic and nononcogenic human genital papillomaviruses generate the E7 mRNA by different mechanisms. *Journal of Virology* **63** 1441–1447

Stanbridge E, Dez CJ, Dorsen C-J *et al* (1982) Human cell hybrids: analysis of transformation and tumorigenicity. *Science* **215** 252

Storey A, Pim D, Murray A, Osborn K, Banks L and Crawford L (1988) Comparison of the in vitro transforming activities of human papillomavirus types. *EMBO Journal* **7** 1815–1820

Storey A, Osborn K and Crawford L (1990) Co-transformation by human papillomavirus types 6 and 11. *Journal of General Virology* **71** 165–171

Tanaka A, Noda T, Yajima H, Hatanaka M and Ito Y (1989) Identification of a transforming gene of human papillomavirus type 16. *Journal of Virology* **63** 1465–1469

Thierry F and Yaniv M (1987) The BPV-1 E2 trans-acting protein can be either an activator or repressor of the HPV-18 regulatory region. *EMBO Journal* **6** 3391–3397

Thierry F and Howley PM (1991) Functional analysis of E2-mediated repression of the HPV18 P_{105} promoter. *New Biologist* **3** 90–100

Vessey MP (1986) Epidemiology of cervical cancer: role of hormonal factors, cigarette smoking and occupation. *Banbury Report* **21** 29–43

Vousden KH, Doninger J, DiPaolo JA and Lowy DR (1988) The E7 open reading frame of human papillomavirus type 16 encodes a transforming gene. *Oncogene Research* **3** 167–175

Watanabe S and Yoshiike K (1988) Transformation of rat 3Y1 cells by human papillomavirus type 18 DNA. *International Journal of Cancer* **41** 896–900

Watanabe S, Kanda T and Yoshiike K (1989) Human papillomavirus type 16 transformation of primary human embryonic fibroblasts requires expression of open reading frames E6 and E7. *Journal of Virology* **63** 965–969

Watanabe S, Kanda T, Sato H, Furuno A and Yoshiike K (1990) Mutational analysis of human papillomavirus type 16 E7 functions. *Journal of Virology* **64** 207–214

Werness BA, Levine AJ and Howley PM (1990) Association of human papillomavirus types 16 and 18 E6 proteins with p53. *Science* **248** 76–79

Whyte P, Ruley HE and Harlow E (1988a) Two regions of the adenovirus early region 1A proteins are required for transformation. *Journal of Virology* **62** 257–265

Whyte P, Buchkovich KJ, Horowitz JM *et al* (1988b) Association between an oncogene and an antioncogene: the adenovirus E1a proteins bind to the retinoblastoma gene product. *Nature* **334** 124–129

Whyte P, Williamson NM and Harlow E (1989) Cellular targets for transformation by the adenovirus E1A proteins. *Cell* **56** 67–75

Yee S and Branton PE (1985) Detection of cellular proteins associated with human adenovirus type 5 early region E1A polypeptides. *Virology* **147** 142–153

Yokota J, Wada M, Shimosato Y, Terada M and Sugimura T (1987) Loss of heterozygosity on chromosomes 3, 13, and 17 in small-cell carcinoma and on chromosome 3 in adenocarcinoma of the lung. *Proceedings of the National Academy of Sciences of the USA* **84** 9252–9256

Yokota J, Tsukada Y, Nakajima T *et al* (1989) Loss of heterozygosity on the short arm of chromosome 3 in carcinoma of the uterine cervix. *Cancer Research* **49** 3598–3601

zur Hausen H and Schneider A (1987) The role of papillomaviruses in human anogenital cancers, In: Salzman N and Howley PM (eds). *The Papovaviridae* vol 2 pp 245–263, Plenum Press, New York

The authors are responsible for the accuracy of the references.

Biographical Notes

Sam Benchimol graduated from the Department of Medical Biophysics, University of Toronto, in 1981. He worked on bacteriophage λ assembly with Andy Becker and began his studies on p53 as a postdoctoral fellow with Lionel Crawford at the Imperial Cancer Research Fund. He has been at the Ontario Cancer Institute since 1983, where he is currently a Senior Staff Scientist and Associate Professor in the Department of Medical Biophysics, University of Toronto.

Sela Cheifetz is an assistant laboratory member in the cell biology and genetics programme at Memorial Sloan-Kettering Cancer Center. Her PhD degree in biochemistry was awarded in 1985 by the University of Toronto for work, with M A Moscarello, on protein-lipid interactions in model membrane systems. She was a postdoctoral fellow with Joan Massagué at the University of Massachusetts Medical School and took her present position in 1989. Her main contributions are in the area of TGF-βs and their receptors.

Nicholas Dyson is an Assistant Member of the Massachusetts General Hospital Cancer Center and an Assistant Professor at Harvard University Medical School.

Eric R Fearon is currently a postdoctoral fellow in the Oncology Center and the Department of Medicine at the Johns Hopkins University School of Medicine in Baltimore. He is a graduate of the Johns Hopkins University and received his MD and PhD degrees from Johns Hopkins in 1990. His research interests include tumour suppressor gene function and genetic alterations in human cancer.

Daniel A Haber was born in 1957 in Paris, France. He received both his MD and PhD degrees from Stanford University in 1983 and went on to train in internal medicine and medical oncology at Massachusetts General Hospital and the Dana-Farber Cancer Institute. He has completed his postdoctoral research with Dr Housman at the Massachusetts Institute of Technology and is now Assistant Professor at Harvard Medical School and member of the Massachusetts General Hospital Cancer Center. His research interests are in molecular oncology, in particular the characterization of the Wilms' tumour gene *WT1*.

Ed Harlow is a Professor in Genetics at Harvard University Medical School and Director of the Laboratory of Molecular Oncology at the Massachusetts General Hospital Cancer Center.

David E Housman was born in 1946 in New York City. He received his PhD in biology from Brandeis University in 1971 and then went on to a postdoctoral fellowship at the Massachusetts Institute of Technology (MIT). Following an initial appointment at the University of Toronto, he returned to the Center for Cancer Research at MIT, where he is now Professor of Biology. His research interests are focused on the field of human genetics, with special emphasis on neurogenetics and the genetics of cancer.

Peter M Howley, MD, has received degrees from Princeton University, Rutgers Medical School and Harvard Medical School. He trained as an anatomic pathologist at Massachusetts General Hospital and at the National Cancer Institute. In 1973, he went to the National Institute of Allergy and Infectious Diseases to do a fellowship with Malcolm Martin in molecular virology. In 1977, he joined the staff of the Laboratory of Pathology at the National Cancer Institute, and in 1984, he became Chief of the Laboratory of Tumor Virus Biology at the National Cancer Institute. His research interests include the molecular biology of the papillomaviruses and their role in carcinogenesis.

Jon M Huibregtse, PhD, received his BS and PhD degrees in biological chemistry from the University of Michigan. He joined the Laboratory of Tumor Virus Biology at the National Cancer Institute in 1989 and is working on problems related to human papillomavirus E6 functions and p53.

Penny Johnson completed her MS at the University of Ottawa in 1987. Currently, she is completing a doctorate in the Department of Medical Biophysics, University of Toronto.

Marikki Laiho has been Assistant Professor in the School of Medicine at University of Helsinki, Finland, since 1990. She obtained her MD degree in 1987 and her PhD degree in 1988 from the University of Helsinki and was a postdoctoral fellow at the University of Massachusetts Medical School and at Memorial Sloan-Kettering Cancer Center with Joan Massagué. Since her graduate work with Jorma Keski-Oja, her main reseach interest has been on TGF-β as a regulator of the extracellular matrix and as a growth inhibitor.

Arnold J Levine, currently Harry C Weiss Professor in Life Sciences and Chairman of the Department of Molecular Biology at Princeton University, is a graduate of Harpur College (SUNY, Binghamton) and the University of Pennsylvania. He did postdoctoral research at the California Institute of Technology and then went to Princeton as an Assistant Professor in 1968. He became full professor before leaving Princeton in 1979 to chair the Department of Microbiology at the State University of New York, Stony Brook. His interests span a wide spectrum of the life sciences, and one of his principal responsibilities at Princeton has been to help coordinate work in molecular biology with research and teaching already under way in biology, chemistry and related fields. He is a member of the National Academy of Sciences.

David M Livingston, MD, is Director and Physician-in-Chief of the Dana Farber Cancer Institute (DFCI) and Chief of the Division of Neoplastic Disease Mechanisms and Professor of Medicine at Harvard Medical School. He graduated cum laude from Harvard University and received his MD magna cum laude from Tufts University School of Medicine, Boston. He received his clinical training at the Peter Bent Brigham Hospital in Boston. He has been associated with Brigham & Women's Hospital as a physician and with the National Cancer Institute as a senior investigator. He was a member (1979–1983), then Chairman (1986–1988), of the National Institutes of Health Virology Study Section. His research interests are oncogenes and tumour suppressor genes, and he is the author of more than 90 publications.

Joan Massagué is a Howard Hughes Medical Institute Investigator and member of the cell biology and genetics programme at Memorial Sloan-Kettering Cancer Center in New York. His research interests lie in aspects of intercellular signalling via peptide growth factors and their receptors. He received his PhD degree in biochemistry from the University of Barcelona, Spain, in 1978. He was a postdoctoral fellow at Brown University working on the identification of insulin like growth factor receptors with Michael P Czech. He initiated his research programme on transforming growth factors as an Assistant and Associate Professor of Biochemistry at the University of Massachusetts Medical School and continued working on this subject after moving to his present position in 1989.

Frank McCormick took his BSc at the University of Birmingham and his PhD at the University of Cambridge. He did postdoctoral research at the State University of New York, Stony Brook, with Dr Seymour S Cohen, working on polyamine metabolism in mammalian cells, and at the Imperial Cancer Research Fund, London, with Dr Alan Smith, working on the association between p53 and SV40 large T antigen. He joined Cetus in 1981, set up the organization's oncogene project in 1984 and is now Vice President of Research.

Karl Münger, Dr phil II, received his degree in biochemistry from the University of Zürich, Switzerland. He joined the Laboratory of Tumor Virus Biology at the National Cancer Institute in 1986. His research interests include the molecular mechanisms of cellular transformation by DNA tumour viruses, in particular the E7 protein of the human papillomaviruses.

Paul Polakis received his PhD from the biochemistry department at Michigan State University in 1984. In 1985, he became Assistant Professor in the chemistry department at Oberlin College, Ohio. He followed this appointment with postdoctoral research in the immunology department of Howard Hughes Institute at Duke University (1987) and at Genentech Inc (1989). He is currently Senior Scientist at Cetus.

David Ralph obtained his PhD in molecular biology and genetics in 1986 from Ohio State University. His graduate work was on the evolution of cytoplasmic genomes. He has been a postdoctoral fellow at Columbia University studying RNA processing in trypanosomes with Lex Van der Ploeg and at the University of Massachusetts Medical School and Memorial Sloan-Kettering Cancer Center with Joan Massagué. His current interests are on mechanisms of growth suppression.

Martin Scheffner, Dr rer nat, graduated from the University of Konstanz, Germany. In 1990, he joined the Laboratory of Tumor Virus Biology at the National Cancer Institute and is studying the effect of human papillomavirus E6 proteins on p53 stability.

Eric J Stanbridge received his PhD at Stanford University and is currently Professor of Microbiology and Molecular Genetics at the University of California, Irvine, College of Medicine.

Robert A Weinberg, Professor of Biology at the Massachusetts Institute of Technology (MIT), Cambridge, Massachusetts and a member of the Whitehead Institute for Biomedical Research, Cambridge, gained a BS in biology at MIT in 1964 and a PhD, also at MIT. in 1969. He did postdoctoral research at the Weizmann Institute, Rehovoth, Israel, and at the Salk Institute. He joined MIT in 1972 as a research associate of Dr David Baltimore, progressed to become Assistant Professor and then Associate Professor in the department of biology and was appointed to his present position in 1982. His research interests are in the mechanisms of action of oncogenes and tumour suppressor genes.

Frances Weis is a graduate student in the Cornell–Sloan-Kettering Graduate School of Medical Sciences and her research is on growth inhibitor signal transduction. She has conducted research on epidermal growth factor receptors under Roger Davis at the University of Massachusetts Medical School.

Alejandro Zentella is a Howard Hughes Medical Institute postdoctoral fellow at Memorial Sloan-Kettering Cancer Center. He obtained his PhD degree in 1990 from the Rockefeller University for studies with Anthony Cerami on the mechanism of action of tumour necrosis factor. He is currently working on negative regulation of the cell cycle.

Index

LIST OF PREVIOUS ISSUES

VOLUME 1 1982

No. 1: Inheritance of Susceptibility to Cancer in Man
Guest Editor: W F Bodmer

No. 2: Maturation and Differentiation in Leukaemias
Guest Editor: M F Greaves

No. 3: Experimental Approaches to Drug Targeting
Guest Editors: A J S Davies and M J Crumpton

No. 4: Cancers Induced by Therapy
Guest Editor: I Penn

VOLUME 2 1983

No. 1: Embryonic & Germ Cell Tumours in Man and Animals
Guest Editor: R L Gardner

No. 2: Retinoids and Cancer
Guest Editor: M B Sporn

No. 3: Precancer
Guest Editor: J J DeCosse

No. 4: Tumour Promotion and Human Cancer
Guest Editors: T J Slaga and R Montesano

VOLUME 3 1984

No. 1: Viruses in Human and Animal Cancers
Guest Editors: J Wyke and R Weiss

No. 2: Gene Regulation in the Expression of Malignancy
Guest Editor: L Sachs

No. 3: Consistent Chromosomal Aberrations and Oncogenes in Human Tumours
Guest Editor: J D Rowley

No. 4: Clinical Management of Solid Tumours in Childhood
Guest Editor: T J McElwain

VOLUME 4 1985

No. 1: Tumour Antigens in Experimental and Human Systems
Guest Editor: L W Law

No. 2: Recent Advances in the Treatment and Research in Lymphoma and Hodgkin's Disease
Guest Editor: R Hoppe

No. 3: Carcinogenesis and DNA Repair
Guest Editor: T Lindahl

No. 4: Growth Factors and Malignancy
Guest Editors: A B Roberts and M B Sporn

VOLUME 5 1986

No. 1: Drug Resistance
Guest Editors: G Stark and H Calvert

No. 2: Biochemical Mechanisms of Oncogene Activity: Proteins Encoded by Oncogenes
Guest Editors: H E Varmus and J M Bishop

No. 3: Hormones and Cancer: 90 Years after Beatson
Guest Editor: R D Bulbrook

No. 4: Experimental, Epidemiological and Clinical Aspects of Liver Carcinogenesis
Guest Editor: E Farber

VOLUME 6 1987

No. 1: Naturally Occurring Tumours in Animals as a Model for Human Disease
Guest Editors: D Onions and W Jarrett

No. 2: New Approaches to Tumour Localization
Guest Editor: K Britton

No. 3: Psychological Aspects of Cancer
Guest Editor: S Greer

No. 4: Diet and Cancer
Guest Editors: C Campbell and L Kinlen

VOLUME 7 1988

No. 1: Pain and Cancer
Guest Editor: G W Hanks

ERRATA

Cancer Surveys Volume 10: Cancer, HIV and AIDS

1. Owing to a computer error, Table 1 (p 112) in the chapter by Luxton, Thomas and Crawford was printed incorrectly. See corrected version below.

TABLE 1. Characteristics of non-Hodgkin lymphoma in AIDS

Tumour group	Chromosomal translocation	EBV genome	Tumour type/ no. of cases	References[a]
BL like tumours	+ (endemic)	+	1 SNCC	1
	+ (sporadic)	+	2 SNCC, 1 LNCC 1 LC-IBP	2
	+	+	2 BL type 1 SNCC 1 diffuse LC	3, 4, 5
	+ (endemic)	–	3 SNCC	2
	+	–	1 LNCC	
Non-BL tumours	–	+	3 of uncertain type 2 LC-IBP	6, 2, 7
	–	–	5 SNCC 2 LNCC 1 LC-IBP	7, 2

The table summarizes the information available from reports of AIDS NHL, where the presence of chromosomal translocation and EBV genomes have been examined. Endemic, chromosomal translocations characteristic of endemic BL (see text). Sporadic, chromosomal translocations characteristic of sporadic BL, otherwise data not available. SNCC, small non-cleaved cell lymphoma. LC-IBP, large cell immunoblastic plasmacytoid. BL, Burkitt's lymphoma type (all high grade lymphomas). LNCC, large non-cleaved cell (intermediate grade lymphoma).

[a] 1 Haluska *et al*, 1989
 2 Subar *et al*, 1988
 3 Whang-Peng *et al*, 1984
 4 Petersen *et al*, 1985
 5 Groopman *et al*, 1986
 6 Knowles *et al*, 1988
 7 Boiocchi *et al*, 1990

2. Figures 1 and 2 (p 10 and 13) in the chapter by Beral were transposed.